ADVANCES IN RESEARCH ON CHOLERA AND RELATED DIARRHEAS

NEW PERSPECTIVES IN CLINICAL MICROBIOLOGY

Other volumes in this series:

Brumfitt W, ed Hamilton-Miller JMT, assist. ed: New perspectives in clinical microbiology. 1978. ISBN 90-247-2074-5
Tyrrell DAJ, ed: Aspects of slow and persistent virus infections. 1979. ISBN 90-247-2281-0
Brumfitt W, Curcio L, Silvestri L, eds: Combined antimicrobial therapy. 1979. ISBN 90-247-2280-2
van Furth R, ed: Developments in antibiotic treatment of respiratory infections. 1981. ISBN 90-247-2493-7
van Furth R, ed: Evaluation and management of hospital infections. 1982. ISBN 90-247-2754-5

ADVANCES IN RESEARCH ON CHOLERA AND RELATED DIARRHEAS

edited by

S. KUWAHARA

Department of Microbiology
Toho University
Tokyo, Japan

N. F. PIERCE

Baltimore Hospitals and Johns Hopkins University School of Medicine
Baltimore, Maryland, U. S. A.

1983 **MARTINUS NIJHOFF PUBLISHERS**
a member of the KLUWER ACADEMIC PUBLISHERS GROUP
BOSTON / THE HAGUE / DORDRECHT / LANCASTER

Distributors

for the United States and Canada: Kluwer Boston, Inc., 190 Old Derby Street, Hingham, MA 02043, USA
for Japan: KTK Scientific Publishers, 307 Shibuyadai-haim, 4-17 Sakuragaoka-cho, Shibuya-ku, Tokyo 150, Japan
for all other countries: Kluwer Academic Publishers Group, Distribution Center, P.O. Box 322, 3300 AH Dordrecht, The Netherlands

Library of Congress Cataloging in Publication Data

Main entry under title: CIP

Advances in research on cholera and related diarrheas.

(New perspectives in clinical microbiology ; v. 6)
Bibliography: p.
Includes index.
1. Cholera, Asiatic--Immunological aspects--Addresses, essays, lectures. 2. Cholera, Asiatic--Preventive inoculation--Addresses, essays, lectures. 3. Diarrhea--Immunological aspects--Addresses, essays, lectures. I. Kuwahara, S. (Shōgo), 1921- . II. Pierce, N. F. III. Series. [DNLM: 1. Cholera. 2. Diarrhea. W1 NE484C v. 6 / WI 407 A244]
RC126.A2 1983 616.9'32 83-13220
ISBN-13:978-94-009-6737-3 e-ISBN-13:978-94-009-6735-9
DOI: 10.1007/978-94-009-6735-9

Book Information

Joint edition published by: KTK Scientific Publishers, Tokyo, Japan and Martinus Nijhoff Publishers, Boston, USA

PREFACE

The United States–Japan Cooperative Medical Science Program was initiated in 1965 by joint agreement between the President of the United States and the Prime Minister of Japan. The purpose of the Program was to promote cooperative biomedical research between the two countries, especially on health problems of recognized importance in Asia. Cholera was designated as one topic of mutual interest. Panels of scientists from each country were formed, and these met to select priority areas for research. The Cholera Panels initially defined two major goals: 1) improved and simplified therapy for cholera, and 2) better methods for immunization. Progress in the pursuit of these goals led to the recognition that bacteria other than *Vibrio cholerae* are also important causes of acute dehydrating diarrhea which resembles cholera in its manifestations and pathogenesis; most notable among these are enterotoxinogenic strains of *Escherichia coli.* Accordingly, panel guidelines were expanded to include all diarrheal diseases that involve fluid loss caused by an enterotoxin. More recently, studies have shown that vibrios, including *V. cholerae*, have a distinct environmental life cycle that is probably an important factor in the epidemiology of vibrio infections. For this reason, the panel guidelines were again expanded to include studies on the environmental ecology of vibrios.

A major project of the Joint Cholera Panels has been the organization and sponsorship of an annual conference on cholera and related diarrheal diseases. These meetings, held alternatively in Japan and the United States, have provided an unique forum for the presentation of new research on topics falling within the guidelines of the Panels. The very rapid increase in both basic and practical knowledge concerning these diseases, and the fact that this is the only regularly held international meeting on this subject, have added considerably to the value and importance of these conferences.

This volume, the first in a planned series entitled "Advances in Research on Cholera and Related Diarrheas", contains papers presented at the Seventeenth Joint Conference on Cholera, held in Baltimore, Maryland, October 26-28, 1981. The proceedings of the previous 16 conferences, beginning with the first, held in Hawaii in 1965, have also been published by either the United States or Japanese Cholera Panels. It is sincerely hoped that publication in this new format will make these proceedings available to a larger number of researchers, public health officials, and clinicians who are concerned with cholera and related acute diarrheal diseases.

Shogo Kuwahara, M. D.
Chairman, Japanese Cholera Panel

Nathaniel F. Pierce, M. D.
Chairman, United States Cholera Panel

Contents

GENETICS

ENTEROTOXINS

IMMUNOLOGY AND VACCINE DEVELOPMENT

Advances in Research on Cholera and Related Diarrheas, eds., S. Kuwahara, N. F. Pierce, 3–5.

ROLE OF COLONIZATION FACTOR ANTIGEN IN IMMUNOPROTECTION AGAINST ENTEROTOXIGENIC *ESCHERICHIA COLI* DIARRHEA

Dolores G. Evans, Francisco F. J. de la Cabada, and Doyle J. Evans, Jr.

Department Medicine, Baylor Collage of Medicine, VA Medical Center
Houston, Texas 77030, U. S. A.

Colonization factor antigens CFA/I and CFA/II of human-associated enterotoxigenic *E. coli* (ETEC) are good candidates as immunoprotective antigens because of their primary role as ETEC virulence factors which involves specific interaction with the intestinal epithelium. We used the temporary intestinal ligation technique with adult rabbits to investigate the local and systemic immune responses to purified CFA/I and to CFA/I^+ ETEC (strain H-10407; 078:Hll:CFA/I; ST^+ LT^+). Local immune responses were determined by quantitating the number of IgG–, IgM–, –IgA and anti-CFA/I–producing cells in the lamina propria of the test animals; immunoprotection was determined by challenging the antigen-primed animals or rechallenging rabbits which were allowed to survive an initial challenge with the same dose of strain H-10407 (1×10^8 CFU per animal) given 5 to 6 weeks previously (1).

Rabbits (seven; Group II) re-challenged with strain H-10407 showed some protection (4 of 7, or 57%) from diarrhea with significantly ($P<0.0001$) less fluid response than a control group of ten rabbits (Group I) but no protection against colonization of the intestine (1); Table 1. However, rabbits previously exposed to two oral doses of purified CFA/I (1.0 mg antigen per dose for one group of nine animals (Group III) and 5.0 mg antigen per dose for another group of seven animals, Group IV) showed protection against both diarrhea (77% and 100%, respectively) and colonization of the intestine. None of the animals immunized with 5.0 mg doses of CFA/I showed a diarrhea response (Group IV) although a group of five animals similarly immunized with CFA/I (Group V) showed no protection against a challenge dose of a CAF/II-positive ETEC strain (06:H1-6:CFA/II; ST^+ LT^+), as seen in Table 1.

Comparison of the local and systemic immune response to the purified antigen and to the CFA/I-positive bacteria clearly indicate that the cell-free antigen favored the local response whereas the bacteria favored a systemic response; for example, only the bacteria stimulated significant anti-CFA/I serum titers (data not shown). Protection did not correlate with serum titers (either anti-LT, anti-078 or anti-CFA/I) but did correlate with the local immune response. The oral doses of CFA/I produced a relatively poor response in terms of IgG and IgM-producing cells but did produce a vigorous response in terms of IgA- and anti-CFA/I-producing cells in the lamina propria of the animals (Tables 2 and 3).

Table 1. Diarrhea response of rabbits in five different experimental groups.

Rabbit Group*	Number tested	Fluid accumulation in ml (mean ± standard error)
I	10	65.10 ± 12.05
II	7	16.42 ± 7.22
III	9	13.66 ± 5.24
IV	7	1.85 ± 1.85
V	5	51.60 ± 16.79

*Rabbit groups described in text.

Table 2. Mucosal antibody responses of rabbits immunized perorally with CFA/I or by exposure to CFA/I-positive bacteria.

Rabbit group	Number tested	Number of antibody-producing cells per $mm^3 \times 10^3$		
		IgA	IgM	IgG
I	5	2.472 ± 0.248	1.232 ± 0.160	1.679 ± 0.122
II	7	3.832 ± 0.160	2.146 ± 0.601	4.126 ± 1.348
III	9	7.251 ± 1.240	3.808 ± 0.541	4.098 ± 0.761
IV	7	10.844 ± 2.025	3.924 ± 0.925	4.309 ± 0.828
V	5	11.661 ± 2.523	3.886 ± 0.257	4.987 ± 1.193

Table 3. Mucosal anti-CFA/I response of rabbits immunized perorally with CFA/I or by exposure to CFA/I-positive bacteria.

Rabbit group	Number tested	Number of anti-CFA/I-producing cells per $mm^3 \times 10^3$ (Mean ± standard deviation)
I	10	0.0
II	7	4.685 ± 4.669
III	9	8.403 ± 3.724
IV	5	8.563 ± 2.332
V	5	12.783 ± 5.652

There was a highly significant inverse relationship between the numbers of IgA- and anti-CFA/I-producing cells in the lamina propria of the animals and the diarrhea response to strain H-10407; with correlation coefficients of -0.616 and -0.678, respectively. These results support the hypothesis that oral immunization with purified CFA/I should be immunoprotective in humans.

This work was supported in part by Public Health Service grants AI-13385 (DGE) and AI-15379 (DJEJr) from the National Institute of Allergy and Infectious Diseases, NIH.

REFERENCE

1. Cabada, F. J. de la, D. G. Evans, and D. J. Evans, Jr. 1981. Immunoprotection against enterotoxigenic *Escherichia coli* diarrhea in rabbits by peroral administration of purified colonization factor antigen I (CFA/I). *FEMS. Microbiol. Lett.* **11**:303-307.

Advances in Research on Cholera and Related Diarrheas, eds., S. Kuwahara, N. F. Pierce, 7–11.

THE ILEAL LOOP TEST ON MICE WHICH WERE ORALLY IMMUNIZED WITH IF30

T. Ishihara[1] and A. Ghoda[1,2]

1) Department of Microbiology, School of Hygienic Sciences, Kitasato University, Sagamihara-shi, Kanagawa-ken 228, Japan
2) The Kitasato Institute, Minato-ku, Tokyo 108, Japan

We have reported that the oral administration of fraction IF30 of *Vibrio cholerae eltor* Inaba V86 strain protects mice from the intraperitoneal challenge with V86 strain (1, 2, 3). This time we will report the result of the loop test on orally immunized mice and rabbits.

MATERIALS AND METHODS

1. Materials
   a. Animals: Six-week-old closed colony, ddY and ICR strains, of female mice and 2-month-old New Zealand white male rabbits were used.
   b. Antigen: IF30 was used as the antigen. IF30 was made as follows (4, 5, 6): *Vibrio cholerae eltor* Inaba V86 strain was grown on heart infusion agar (Difco), pH 8.0, at 37 C for 18 to 20 hours, harvested in sterile PBS of 1/75 M, pH 7.2, and the same volume of 5 M urea solution was added. The material was sonicated at 20 KC for 20 minutes, and centrifuged to obtain the supernatant. The supernatant was dialyzed against distilled water and centrifuged. Ammonium sulfate was added to the supernatant and the precipitate formed at 30% saturation was obtained. The precipitate was resuspended in PBS of 1/75 M, dialyzed against PB of 0.005 M, pH 7.6, and lyophilized.
   c. Challenging organisms: *V. cholerae eltor* V86 strain was grown on heart infusion agar (pH 8.0) at 37 C for 18 to 20 hours, harvested in sterile saline and suspended in heart infusion broth at desired concentrations.

2. Methods
   a. Oral administration: In case of mice, 1 mg to 10 mg of IF30 was dissolved in 1 ml of sterile distilled water and administered by gastric tubes once a day for three successive days. In case of rabbits, 100 mg or 300 mg of IF30 was dissolved in 50 ml of sterile distilled water and administered by silicon tubes once a day for three successive days.
   b. Immunization by means of drinking water: IF30 was dissolved in sterile distilled water at concentrations of 1 mg, 5 mg and 10 mg/100 ml and was given freely through drinking bottles for one or three weeks.

c. Loop test: In case of mice, 7 to 10 days after the last administration of the antigen, one loop per mouse was made and 0.2 ml of a suspension of V86 which contained 10 to 10^4 organisms was inoculated. Seventeen to 20 hours later mice were sacrificed and swelling was macroscopically observed and then the loops were cut out to measure the length and volume and to calculate the ratio of the volume to length. In case of rabbits, five loops per rabbit were made after 15 days of the last administration of the antigen and 0.5 ml each of V86 suspension which contained 10^2, 10^4 and 10^6 organisms was inoculated in 3 loops, one loop was inoculated with heart infusion broth, and the last one was left as the uninoculated control. Twenty hours later the rabbits were sacrificed and swelling of the loops were observed, for measurement of the volume of fluid in the loops and the length of the loops as well as the ratios of the volume to length.

RESULTS

1. Loop tests in orally immunized ddY strain of mice: As is shown in Table 1, in groups immunized with 10 mg of antigen for 3 successive days and challenged with 1.2×10^2 to 4×10^2 organisms 44.4% became positive while in those similarly immunized and challenged with 8 to 56 organisms 30% became positive, and these rates were much lower than in the control groups whose rates were 63.6% and 65%, respectively.

2. Loop tests in orally immunized ICR strain of mice: As is shown in Table 2, when challenged with 10^3 organisms no difference was observed between any of the immunized groups and the control group, but the positive rates were much lower than control in groups immunized with 5 mg and 10 mg and challenged with 25 to 100 organisms. The difference was significant with the X^2 test at the 5% level in the 10 mg immunization group.

In the above two experiments, it was shown that when mice were immunized orally with 10 mg of antigen for 3 successive days and challenged with a small number of the organisms the loops were protected from swelling regardless of the mouse strain.

Table 1. Loop tests in orally immunized ddY strain of mice.

Dose per day (Total dose) mg. D.W.	Challenge dose (1.2 ~ 4.2) x 10^2			8 ~ 56		
	No. of loops examined	positive	(Positive rate,%)	No. of loops examined	positive	(Positive rate,%)
10 (30)	9	4	(44.4)	10	3	(30.0)
5 (15)	6	6	(100)	10	7	(70.0)
2 (6)				10	5	(50.0)
1 (3)	8	6	(75.0)	10	3	(30.0)
Control	11	7	(63.6)	20	13	(65.0)

Table 2. Loop tests in orally immunized ICR strain of mice.

Dose per day (Total dose) mg. D.W.	Challenge dose (1.5 ~ 1.7) x 10^3			Challenge dose 25 ~ 100		
	No. of loops examined	No. of loops positive	(Positive rate,%)	No. of loops examined	No. of loops positive	(Positive rate,%)
10 (30)	7	6	(85.7)	10	3	(30.0)※
5 (15)	6	3	(50.0)	5	2	(40.0)
2 (6)				5	5	(100)
1 (3)	6	5	(83.3)	5	3	(60.0)
Control	9	7	(77.8)	23	16	(69.6)※

※ : The difference was significant with the X^2 test at the 5% level.

3. Loop tests in orally immunized rabbits: As is seen in Table 3, when rabbits were orally immunized with one dose of 300 mg, the rates of positive loops were 83.3%, 66.7% and 33.3% after challenge with 10^6, 10^4 and 10^2 organisms, respectively. This result indicates that the rate of positive loops decreased with the decrease of the challenging dose. The v/1 rate was also decreased even at the positive loop in the immunized groups. When the immunizing dose was lowered the rate of protection was decreased.

4. Loop tests in ddY strain of mice which were orally immunized by means of drinking water: As is seen in Table 4, in the group immunized with 5 mg/100 ml of the antigen for 3 weeks and challenged with 10^3 to 10^4 organisms or 6 to 20 organisms the rates of positive loops were 25% and 44.4%, respectively, which were lower than in the control groups, but the number of mice used was small, therefore, it will be necessary to add more data before drawing conclusion.

Table 3. Loop tests in orally immunized rabbits.

Dose per day (Total dose) mg. D.W.	Challenge dose (0.8 ~ 1) x 10^6			Challenge dose (0.8 ~ 1) x 10^4			Challenge dose (0.9 ~ 1) x 10^2		
	No.of loops ※1	No.of loops ※2	(Positive rate,%)	No.of loops ※1	No.of loops ※2	(Positive rate,%)	No.of loops ※1	No.of loops ※2	(Positive rate,%)
300 (900)	6	5 [1.52] ※3	(83.3)	6	4 [0.90]	(66.7)	6	2 [0.74]	(33.3)
100 (300)	6	6 [1.74]	(100)	6	6 [1.54]	(100)	6	6 [1.15]	(100)
Control	7	7 [1.73]	(100)	7	7 [1.25]	(100)	7	6 [1.13]	(85.7)

※1 : No. of loops examined ; ※2 : No. of positive loops.

※3 : Numbers in [ ] are average ratio of volume per length of the loop examined.

Table 4. Loop tests in ddY strain of mice which were orally immunized by means of drinking water.

Administration Dose*- Period (Range of IF30 intake per mouse)	Challenge dose 10^3 ~ 10^4 No. of loops examined	positive	(Positive rate,%)	6 ~ 20 No. of loops examined	positive	(Positive rate,%)
$10^{mg.}$ - $1^{w.}$ (4.5~5.5)$^{mg.}$	6	5	(83.3)	6	4	(66.7)
5 - 3 (5.4~7.1)	4	1	(25.0)	9	4	(44.4)
1 - 3 (1.4~1.8)	4	2	(50.0)	8	6	(75.0)
Control	10	8	(80.0)	19	12	(63.2)

*: IF30 content in 100 ml. of drinking water.

Table 5. Loop tests in ICR strain of mice which were orally immunized by means of drinking water.

Administration Dose* - Period (Range of IF30 intake per mouse)	Challenge dose 10^3 ~ 10^4 No. of loops examined	positive	(Positive rate,%)	4 ~ 26 No. of loops examined	positive	(Positive rate,%)
$10^{mg.}$ - $1^{w.}$ (4.0 - 6.0)$^{mg.}$	8	5	(62.5)	6	2	(33.3)
5 - 3 (5.5 - 6.5)	8	6	(75.0)	4	3	(75.0)
1 - 3 (1.1 - 1.5)	9	4	(44.4)	4	2	(50.0)
Control	23	16	(69.6)	16	10	(62.5)

*: IF30 content in 100 ml of drinking water.

5. Loop tests in ICR strain of mice which were orally immunized by means of drinking water: As is seen in Table 5, in the group immunized with 10 mg of the antigen and challenged with 4 to 26 organisms the rate of positive loops was 33.3% and in the group immunized with 1 mg of the antigen and challenged with 10^3 to 10^4 organisms the rate was 44.4%, both being lower than that of the control groups.

CONCLUSION

When mice were immunized orally for three successive days with 30 mg of the antigen and challenged with a small number of organisms, the mice were protected regardless of the mouse strain, and in rabbits the rate of positive loops decreased with the decrease of the challenge dose. When mice were immunized by means of drinking water giving 5 mg or 10 mg per 100 ml of IF30, the loops were protected from the challenge but the results were inconsistent.

REFERENCES

1. Ghoda, A., Takeuchi, S. and Ishihara, T. 1977. Protection of experimental cholera by oral administration of the cellular fraction of *Vibrio cholerae eltor.* Proc. 13th Joint. conf. on Cholera.
2. Ishihara, T., Komagata, Y., Takeuchi, S. and Ghoda, A. 1978. Protection of experimental cholera by oral administration of the cellular fraction of *Vibrio cholerae eltor.* 2) Protection in ddN strain of mice. Proc. 14th Joint Conf. on Cholera.
3. Ishihara, T., Komagata, Y. and Ghoda, A. 1980. Protection of experimental cholera by oral administration of the cellular fraction of *Vibrio cholerae eltor.* 4) Protection against different strains. Proc. 16th Joint Conf. on Cholera (in press)
4. Yoshioka, M., Ghoda, A., Kazuno, Y., Takahashi, K., Hirano, T., Suzuki, T., Ando, Y. and Akiba, Y. 1968. Analytical studies on infection and immunity of cholera. Proc. 4th Joint Conf. on Cholera.
5. Yoshioka, M., Takahashi, K., Hirano, T., Kazuno, Y., Takeuchi, S., Akiba, Y., Ghoda, A., Suzuki, T. and Suzuki, Y. 1970. Separation of protective bacterial substances against experimental vibrio infection. Jour. Infect. Diseases. **121**, Suppl.
6. Ghoda, A., Takeuchi, S. and Ishihara, T. 1976. Oral immunization of experimental animals with IF30. Proc. Joint Conf. on Cholera.

Advances in Research on Cholera and Related Diarrheas, eds., S. Kuwahara, N. F. Pierce, 13–18.

LOCAL IgA ANAMNESTIC RESPONSE FOLLOWING PERORAL IMMUNIZATION WITH *SHIGELLA FLEXNERI* ANTIGENS

David F. Keren

Department of Pathology, The University of Michigan Medical Center
Ann Arbor, MI 48109

It is clear that secretory IgA is the main immunoglobulin class secreted from the mucosal surface of the gastrointestinal tract (1). The mechanism involved in optimally stimulating a mucosal IgA response to enteric pathogens is unclear. Further, it is unclear whether a mucosal memory response similar to the systemic anamnestic response can be found in intestinal secretions after oral or parenteral immunization. In this presentation, we outline a method to probe the IgA memory response in intestinal secretions after oral immunization with the enteric pathogen *Shigella flexneri.*

In previous studies, we have shown that chronically isolated intestinal loops can be created in rabbits (2), and that by directly immunizing such isolated ileal loops one can demonstrate the kinetics of the primary secretory IgA response to *Shigella flexneri* antigens in the daily secretions collected from these loops (3-5).

Our previous studies have shown that intestinal secretions from isolated loops stimulated directly with various Shigella preparations will contain considerable secretory IgA activity, but no or minimal IgG directed against the *Shigella flexneri* antigens (3-5). No or trivial IgG or IgA directed against these *Shigella flexneri* antigens are found in the sera of these rabbits. The antigen form used to directly immunize these loops is of significance (5). As shown in figure 1, the best response was achieved with live bacteria, however, acetone killed *Shigella flexneri* could also achieve an effective mucosal IgA response. Purified Westphal preparation lipolysaccharide when given directly into the isolated loop was not able to achieve an effective mucosal immune response (figure 1).

It has been difficult to study the mucosal memory response with this model for local immunity. In the first place, it is technically difficult to maintain the chronically isolated ileal loops for long periods of time in these animals. The animals that do survive (we have kept some for over 200 days), will usually require several surgical procedures to relieve abdominal problems and drain abscesses. Obviously, these are undesirable events in an experimental model against an infectious disease. In the second place, by directly immunizing the chronically isolated ileal loops we have created an extremely artificial situation. In the natural course of events an enteric vaccine or an enteric pathogen would pass through gastric acid, bile, pancreatic digestive enzymes, normal intestinal flora, and food products. Any or all of these might be able to alter the ability of the orally admin-

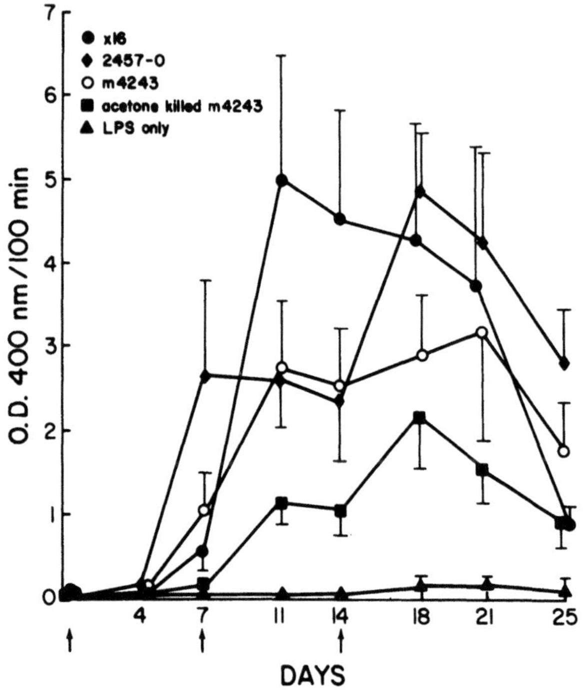

Figure 1. Mean IgA anti-*Shigella flexneri* response in secretions from isolated ileal loops immunized directly with the indicated preparations. IgA activity expressed as O.D. 400 nm/100 min. Arrows indicate days when antigen was administered intraloop. Standard errors of means indicated.

istered *Shigella flexneri* to stimulate the mucosal immune response. Therefore, although the findings by directly immunizing these isolated ileal loops have been useful in studying the development of the local immune response under controlled conditions, the artificial method of stimulation may limit the relevance of the study of natural local immune defenses.

In the present studies, rather than directly stimulating the isolated ileal loops, we choose to immunize the animals orally. The mucosal IgA immune response was followed by studying the secretions from isolated ileal loops for their specific IgA activity at various times after the oral immunization. It should be noted that the isolated ileal loops never receive the *Shigella flexneri* antigens directly.

The feasibility of this approach evolves from studies of antigen stimulation of mucosal immunity and leukocyte trafficking in the bowel. In the bowel, Owen has demonstrated that macromolecules are taken up by specialized epithelial cells called M cells that overlie Peyer's patches (6). Work from several laboratories has shown that precursor B lymphocytes and regulatory T lymphocytes in Peyer's patches and other gut associated lymphoid tissue migrate to mesenteric lymph nodes, the thoracic duct, the systemic circulation, and lastly to several mucosal surfaces including other areas of the gut where antigen was not directly applied and even other mucosal surfaces such as the bronchus, mammary glands, and salivary glands (7).

If such a common mucosal immune system as described above does in fact exist, it should be possible to create an isolated ileal loop in a animal, give an oral dose of antigen to that animal and follow the intestinal IgA response achieved in that animal in the chronically isolated ileal loop. Such was the basis for the present study.

Chronically isolated ileal (Thiry-Vella) loops were created in rabbits using previously described techniques (2). The rabbits were immunized orally with live *Shigella* X16 (a hybrid of *Shigella flexneri* and *Escherichia coli*) according to the schedule listed in Table 1. Secretions were collected daily from the chronically isolated loops and serum samples were taken weekly. Secretions and sera were assayed for their specific IgA and IgG activities against *Shigella flexneri* antigens using a previously described enzyme-linked immunosorbent assay (ELISA) (8).

The mean IgA response against *Shigella flexneri* antigens in secretions from 19 rabbits in group 1 are shown in figure 2. The kinetics of this local IgA response are the same as those shown in figure 2 when the isolated ileal loops were directly exposed to the *Shigella flexneri* antigens. It is noted, however, that the overall magnitude of this response is low.

Since previous studies have shown that multiple intraloop immunizations result in a stronger local immune response to *Shigella flexneri* antigens than a single stimulation (5), we administered live *Shigella* X16 orally to 8 rabbits on day 0, 7 and 14 (first dose given the day after surgical creation of the isolated ileal loops). The response obtained from these animals was not significantly greater than that from the animals given only a single dose of *Shigella flexneri* antigen (figure 2).

Table 1. Immunization schedule.

Group	Antigen	Dose	Route	Day(s)[(1)] Given
I	Live Shigella X16	10^{10}	Oral[(2)]	0
II	Live Shigella X16	10^{10}	Oral	0,7,14
III	Killed Shigella X16	10^{10}	Oral	–75,–68,–61,0
IV	Killed Shigella X16	10^{10}	Oral	0
V	Live Shigella X16	10^{10}	Oral	0,7,14
VI	Killed Shigella X16	10^{10}	Oral	–75,–68,–61,0

(1) Day of surgical creation of isolated loops = day -1 for all groups.

(2) Shigella placed in stomach via orogastric feeding tube. Isolated loop *not* directly exposed to shigella.

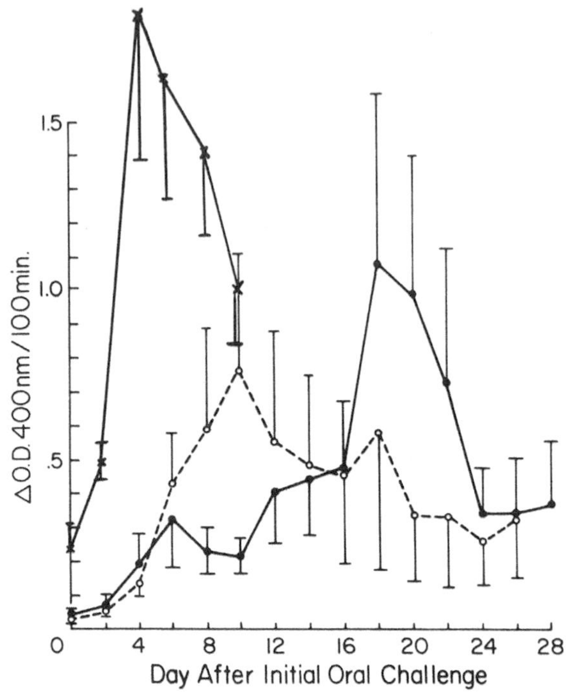

Figure 2. Mean IgA anti-*S. flexneri* response in secretions from animals (not primed) given a single *oral* challenge with live *Shigella* X16 (Group I - ●); animals (not primed) given 3 *oral* doses of live *Shigella* X16 on days 0,7 and 14 (Group II - o); and animals primed with 3 oral doses of live *Shigella* X16 on days -75, -68, -61 and then given a single oral challenge on day 0 (Group III - X).

As we have previously shown that local immunization with killed *Shigella* X16 can result in a significant secretory IgA response, a single dose of heat-killed *Shigella* X16 was given orally to each of 12 rabbits on day 0 (the day after surgical creation of the isolated ileal loops). A second group was given three oral doses of this same heat-killed *Shigella* X16 antigen. The results of this study, shown in fugure 3, demonstrate that a primary IgA response was obtained in both groups with no significant enhancement noted by the three dose regimen. The kinetics of this response, however, were the same as when the *Shigella* were instilled directly into the isolated loops.

No, or minimal IgG was found in the serum or loop secretions of any of these animals. No IgA against *Shigella* was found in sera of any animals tested.

To study the mucosal memory response a group of 10 rabbits that did not have chronically isolated ileal loops was primed by giving three oral doses of live *Shigella* X16. After the third dose, the animals were allowed to rest for two months; at this time, a chronically isolated ileal loop was created and a single oral challenge of the same live *Shigella* X16 antigen was given. The striking IgA anti *Shigella flexneri* response that resulted in the intestinal secretions is shown in figure 2.

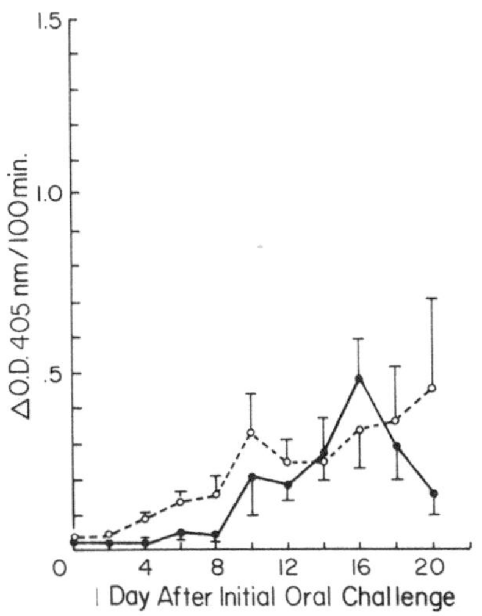

Figure 3. Mean IgA anti-*Shigella* response in intestinal secretions from rabbits given one (Group IV-o) or three doses of killed (Group V - ●) oral *Shigella* X16.

It is clear from the data in figure 2 that when primed with three oral doses of live *Shigella* X16, a rabbit maintains a low level of secretory IgA against the *Shigella flexneri* antigens. Following a single oral challenge, these primed animals exhibit a striking, rapid IgA anamnestic response to this antigen.

Another group of rabbits was primed by three oral doses with killed *Shigella* X16 60 days prior to creation of isolated ileal loops. When these animals were challenged by a single oral dose of the same heat-killed antigen that they were primed with, no enhancement of their local secretory IgA response was seen. (Data not shown).

The fact that the kinetics of the IgA anti-*Shigella flexneri* response seen in the isolated loops after a single oral immunization followed the same kinetics as our previously described systems wherein the isolated loops were directly stimulated with *Shigella flexneri* antigens is further evidence that there is a common mucosal immune system and that our chronically isolated ileal loop model can be a useful probe to study the secretory IgA responses in the actual secretions. The present study has taken advantage of this model system to achieve the direct demonstration of a secretory IgA memory response to *Shigella flexneri* antigens.

In the present study a mucosal IgA memory response to *Shigella flexneri* antigens was only achieved after oral immunization with three doses of live locally invasive *Shigella* X16. Such a memory response was not found in those animals that were given three oral doses of heat-killed *Shigella flexneri* antigens. Obviously, the memory response of the animals given three doses of live *Shigella* X16 may relate to a difference in actual antigen load. The live *Shigella* X16 can multiply in the gastrointestinal tract and consequently the actual antigen load given to these animals cannot be calculated. Secondly, the

Shigella X16 strain is capable of local invasion. It does not persist after local invasion (which is what originally made it attractive as a potential vaccine strain). This local invasion may allow more efficient presentation of the antigen to prime for the mucosal memory response. Clearly, the animals given heat-killed *Shigella* would have had a lower antigen load and would not have had antigen directly entering the intestinal epithelial cells. Lastly, perhaps the animals given killed *Shigella* were primed for a mucosal memory response, but to express that response, they may need to be challenged by live and/or locally invasive *Shigella*. Work is currently underway in our laboratory to distinguish between these various possibilities.

In this study, we present a direct demonstration in intestinal secretions of an IgA amnestic response to *Shigella flexneri* antigens. This was achieved by oral immunization with 3 doses of live *Shigella* X16. Heat-killed *Shigella* X16 was ineffective in eliciting a mucosal memory response in the dosages used in this study when the challenge was given with the same heat-killed antigen. Continued use of chronically isolated ileal loops as a probe to monitor the mucosal memory response should help to elucidate the optimal schedule to stimulate the mucosal memory response.

The author would like to thank Ms. MaryAnn Byrnes for her excellent assistance in preparing this manuscript.

This work was supported in part by U.S. Army Medical Research and Development Command Contract #DAMD 17-80-C-0113.

REFERENCES

1. Crabbe, P. A., A. O. Carbonara, and J. F. Heremans. 1965. The normal human intestinal mucosa as a major source of plasma cells containing A immunoglobulin. *Lab. Invest.* **14**:135.
2. Keren, D. F., H. L. Elliott, G. D. Brown, and J. H. Yardley. 1975. Atrophy of villi with hyper–trophy and hyperplasia of Paneth cells in isolated (Thiry-Vella) ileal loops in rabbits. *Gastroenterol.* **68**:83.
3. Keren, D. F., P. S. Holt, H. H. Collins, P. Gemski, and S. B. Formal. 1978. The role of Peyer's patches in the local immune response of rabbit ileum to live bacteria. *J. Immunol.* **120**:1892.
4. Keren, D. F., P. S. Holt, H. H. Collins, P. Gemski, and S. B. Formal. 1980. Variables affecting local immune response in ileal loops. I. Role of immunization schedule, bacterial flora and postsurgical inflammation. *Infect. Immun.* **28**:950.
5. Keren, D. F., H. H. Collins, P. Gemski, P. S. Holt, and S. B. Formal. 1981. Role of antigen form in development of mucosal immunoglobulin A response to *Shigella flexneri* antigens. *Infect. Immun.* **31**:1193.
6. Owen, R. L. 1977. Sequential uptake of horseradish peroxidase by lymphoid follicle epithelium of Peyer's patches in the normal unobstructed mouse intestine: an ultrastructural study. *Gastroenterol.* **72**:440.
7. Cebra, J. J., R. Kamat, P. Gearhart, S. Robertson, and J. Tseng. 1977. The secretory IgA system of the gut. In *Immunology of the Gut.* Ciba Foundation Symposium. R. Porter and E. Knight editors. Elsevier North-Holland, Inc. **46**:5.

Advances in Research on Cholera and Related Diarrheas, eds., S. Kuwahara, N. F. Pierce, 19–27.

EFFECTS OF THE ORAL IMMUNIZATION WITH LIVE V. CHOLERAE ON THE ANTIBODY FORMATION

Y. Komagata[1] and A. Ghoda[1,2]

1) The Kitasato Institute, Minato-ku, Tokyo 108, Japan
2) Department of Microbiology, School of Hygienic Sciences, Kitasato University, Sagamihara-shi, Kanagawa-ken 228, Japan

We have shown that the cell and a fraction, IF52, of *Vibrio cholerae eltor* V86 enhanced the induction of IgE antibody and also have shown that another fraction IF30 depressed the induction of IgE antibody production and enhanced the induction of vibriocidal antibody (1). This time we examined the influence of the oral administration of live cholera vibrio on the induction of antibodies.

MATERIALS AND METHODS

1. Animals used were 6 weeks old male and female SPF BALB/c mice.
2. Bacterial strains used was *Vibrio cholerae eltor* V86 strain.
3. Method of pretreatment: Antigens were given orally or intraperitoneally once or more frequently depending on each experiment.
4. Oral administration: A given amount of the antigen was suspended or dissolved in 0.2 ml of saline and given intragastrically with a gastric tube.
5. Method of immunization: 10^{10} cells/mouse of DNP conjugated heat killed V86 were inoculated intraperitoneally with alum adjuvant.
6. Measurement of the anti-haptenic IgE antibody: PCA was performed in Sprague Dawley rats using DNP conjugated human albumin as the antigen and titers are shown by the dilution factor of the serum (2).
7. Vibriocidal antibody titer: Microtiter method was used and titers are shown by the dilution factor (3).
8. Carbon clearance: According to Benacerraf's method carbon was injected through the tail vein of mice and the carbon density in blood was measured during a scheduled time course.

RESULTS

The following experiment was carried out to examine how long the organisms persist and how the organisms proliferate in organs when vibrio was given orally. 10^7 cells/mouse of vibrio were given orally and mice were sacrificed during the time course and several parts of the intestines were cut out aseptically, homogenized, diluted with saline, spread on

Table 1. Distribution of live vibrios in the intestines after oral administration.

Hours after challenge	Small intestine upper	middle	under	Large intestine
2 hrs	0	1	6	6.0×10^4
4	0	0	0	2.6×10^1
6	0	0	1.6×10^1	3
8	0	2.3×10^3	0	2
10	2.2×10^1	1.1×10^1	0	0
18	0	0	0	0
24	0	0	0	0
30	0	0	0	0
48	0	0	0	0

Number of Oral Administration 2.4×10^7/mouse
Medium : TCBS

TCBS plates and the number of colonies counted. As is shown in Table 1, until 10 hours organisms were found in some parts of the intestines but completely disappeared at 18 hours. Also, it seems likely that the organisms first proliferated in the colon and ascended to the small intestines.

We examined the oral pretreatment with live, killed organisms or IF30 on the production of antibodies. 10^7 cells/mouse of live vibrio, 10^{10} cells/mouse of killed organisms or 2.5 mg/mouse of IF30 was orally given to mice and 3 days later the animals were immunized with DNP heat killed vibrio. The anti-DNP IgE antibody and vibriocidal antibody titers were measured during the time course. As is shown in Fig. 1, IgE antibody production was depressed by the pretreatment with IF30, and the pretreatment with live or killed organisms had no effect. Vibriocidal antibody production was enhanced by the treatment with IF30 but rather depressed by the pretreatment with live or killed vibrio.

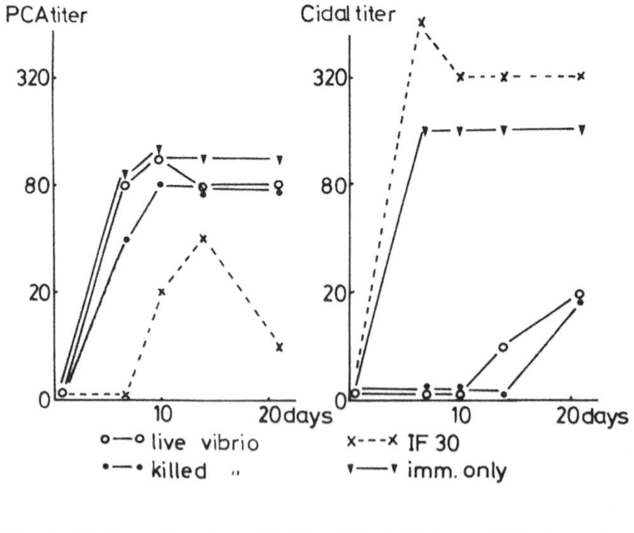

Fig. 1. Oral sensitization with live, killed vibrios or IF30 (one time).

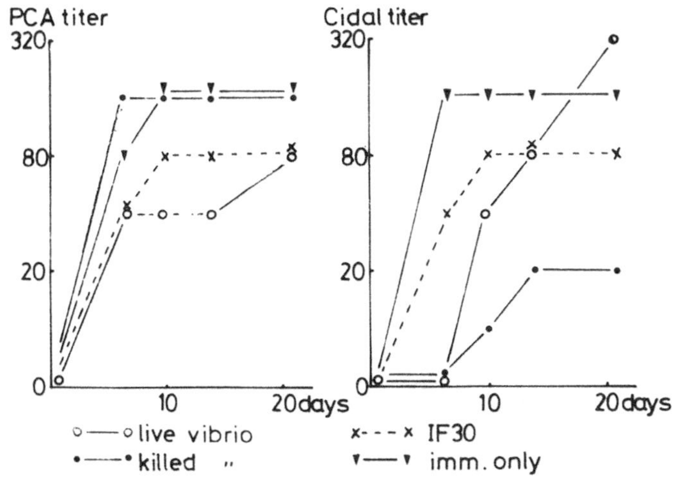

Fig. 2. Oral sensitization with live, killed vibrios or IF30 (3 successive days).

We examined the effect of repeated pretreatment with live or killed vibrio or IF30 on the production of antibodies. The same dose as was used in the previous experiment was given three successive days and 3 days later the animals were immunized with DNP heat killed vibrio, and IgE and vibriocidal antibodies were measured. As is shown in Fig. 2, IgE antibody production was depressed a little by the pretreatment with live vibrio but the degree was weaker than after pretreated once with IF30, as is shown in Fig. 1. The vibriocidal antibody titer was also enhanced by live vibrio at the later stage of immunization.

In this experiment the interval of the pretreatment was changed. Pretreatments were given 3 times with intervals of 3 days and 3 days later the animals were immunized with DNP-heat killed vibrio. As is shown in Fig. 3, IgE production was depressed a little by the pretreatment with live vibrio at an early stage of immunization but the other pretreatments showed no effect. As for vibriocidal antibody, repeated pretreatments with live vibrio enhanced the production but to no higher level than in the non-treated control groups.

In the preceding three experiments, it was shown that IgE production was best suppressed and vibriocidal antibody was best enhanced when IF30 given once as the pretreatment but the effect was diminished when IF30 was given repeatedly. By repeated pretreatments with live vibrio, IgE production was depressed, and the vibriocidal antibody titer rose by the same treatment. Heat killed vibrio showed no effect at all.

We examined the effect of repeated pretreatments with live vibrio on the production of antibodies. 10^7 cells/mouse of live vibrio were given once, twice, three times or four times successively and the animals were immunized at the last day of the pretreatment and the antibody production was compared. As is shown in Fig. 4, IgE production was best depressed by the two times repeated pretreatments but the effect was increasingly

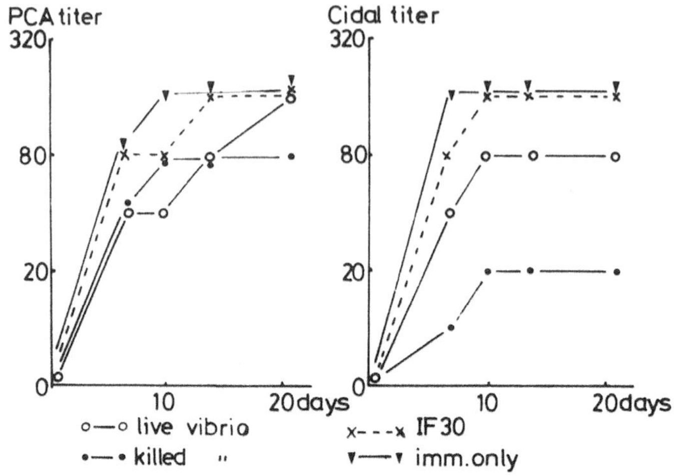

Fig. 3. Oral sensitization with live, killed vibrios or IF30 (3 times with 3 days interval).

less marked by three times and four times repeated pretreatments, and one pretreatment has no depressive effect on the IgE production. The vibriocidal antibody production was also depressed by the two times pretreatment, but four times and three times pretreatment enhanced the production.

We have previously shown that when IF30 was given intraperitoneally as the pretreatment, IgE production was depressed and the vibriocidal antibody production was enhanced (1). Also, we have shown that killed vibrio enhanced the IgE production and vibriocidal antibody production (4). We, therefore, examined the combination of pretreatments with live vibrio and killed vibrio or with IF30. Mice were first pretreated

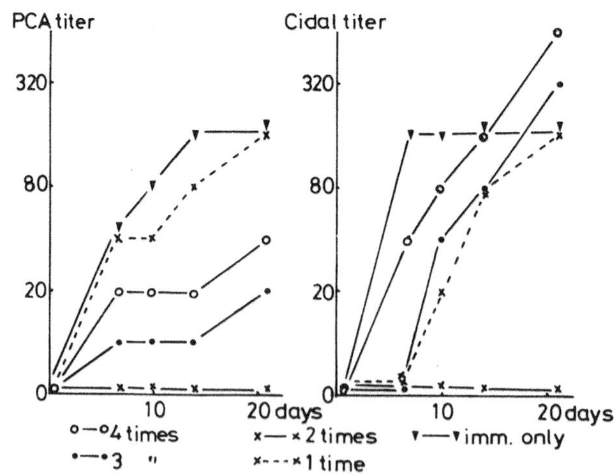

Fig. 4. Effect of repeated oral sensitizations with live vibrios on antibody production.

orally with live vibrio and 0, 1, 2 and 3 days later intraperitoneally injected with killed vibrio or IF30 as the second sensitization. Then 7 or 14 days later they were immunized with DNP heat killed vibrio and the effect of the pretreatment to antibody production was examined.

As is shown in Table 2, regardless of the interval between the first and second sensitizations, the combination of live and killed vibrios depressed IgE production a little while vibriocidal antibody production was enhanced. The combination of live vibrio and IF30 depressed IgE production strongly especially when the interval between the first and second sensitizations was one day and immunization was given 14 days later, whereby IgE was not detected. Vibriocidal antibody production was strongly enhanced by the combination of live vibrio and IF30.

These results suggest that IF30 depresses the production of IgE which is enhanced by live vibrio, but killed vibrio has lesser effect.
Also, the oral administration of live vibrio depresses vibriocidal antibody production but combination with either killed vibrio or IF30 diminishes the effect and enhances the production.
In this experiment, the effect of combination of the oral pretreatment with live or killed vibrio or IF30 and intrapritoneal pretreatment with killed vibrio or IF30 with adjuvant

Table 2. Combination of oral administration with intraperitoneal injection.

Sensitization			Interval	Immunization	PCA titer			Cidal titer		
First oral	Interval	Second I.P			7	14 days	21	7	14 days	21
live	1 day	killed	7 days	DNP-W.C.	40	80	80	160	640	320
″	2	″	″	″	40	80	80	320	640	160
″	3	″	″	″	40	40	40	640	640	640
″	0	″	″	″	40	80	80	320	640	640
live	1	″	14 days	″	40	40	40	1280	640	640
″	2	″	″	″	80	80	80	1280	640	640
″	3	″	″	″	80	80	80	1280	1280	640
″	0	″	″	″	20	80	80	1280	1280	1280
live	1	IF30	7 days	″	<10	20	20	640	1280	1280
″	2	″	″	″	<10	20	20	640	2560	1280
″	3	″	″	″	<10	20	20	640	640	320
″	0	″	″	″	10	10	<10	640	640	640
live	1	″	14 days	″	<10	<10	<10	640	1280	1280
″	2	″	″	″	<10	20	20	1280	2560	2560
″	3	″	″	″	10	10	10	640	640	640
″	0	″	″	″	<10	10	<10	2560	2560	2560
(–)		(–)			80	160	160	160	160	160

I.P. : intraperitoneal
DNP-W.C. : DNP whole cells

on the production of antibodies was examined. As the first treatment, live or killed vibrio or IF30 was given orally and 3 days later the second treatment with killed vibrio or IF30 was given intraperitoneally with adjuvant. Then, 14 days later the animals were immunized with DNP heat killed vibrio and production of antibodies was examined. As is shown in Fig. 5, IgE production was best depressed by the combined treatment with IF30 followed by the combination of the second treatment with IF30 with any first treatment. Vibriocidal antibody production was enhanced in all combinations.

In this experiment, activation of macrophages after the oral administration or the intraperitoneal inoculation of live or killed vibrio or IF30 was examined. Live or killed vibrio or IF30 was given orally or intraperitoneally and 3 days later carbon clearance was examined. As is shown in Fig. 6, activation of macrophages was observed with the intraperitoneal injection of killed vibrio or IF30, and also a slight activation was seen with the oral administration of live or killed vibrio, but the oral administration of IF30 showed no effect.

As the live vibrio activated macrophages, we examined when the activation began. Mice were orally treated with live vibrio and carbon clearance was examined at 0, 1, 2 and 3 days after the oral treatment. As is shown in Fig. 7, the activation of macrophages appeared at 1 day after the treatment and persisted at least for three days.

In this experiment, the effect of the oral or peritoneal treatment of mice with live or killed vibrio or IF30 on the number of viable cells in the liver and spleen after an intravenous challenge with the vibrio was examined. Three days after the treatment the mice

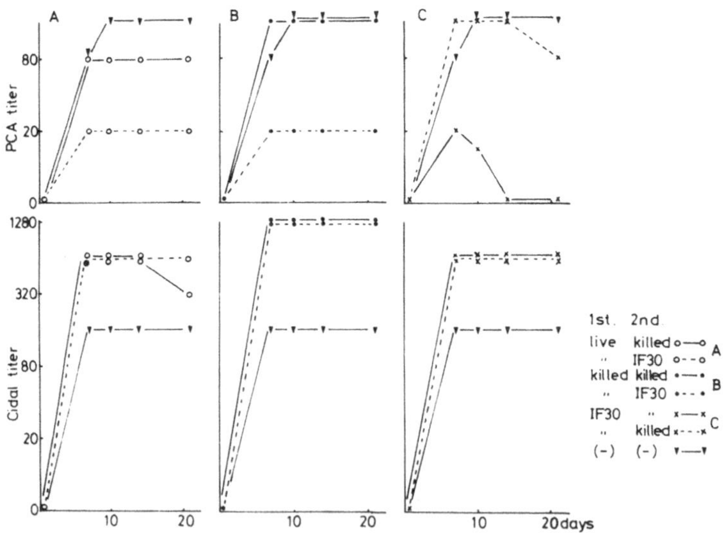

Fig. 5. Sensitization with the combination of live and killed vibrios or IF30 (1st sensitization = oral, 2nd sensitization = intraperitoneal).

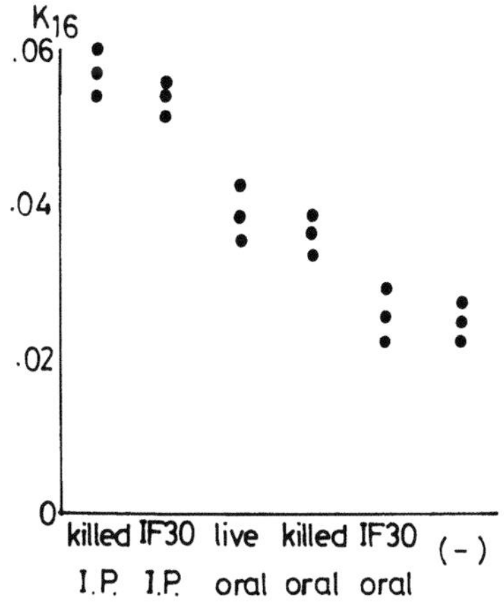

Fig. 6. Carbon clearance after oral administration or intraperitoneal injection.

were intravenously inoculated with $2x10^5$ vibrios and 4 hours later the number of viable cells in the liver and spleen was counted.

As is shown in Fig. 8, the numbers of viable cells in both the liver and spleen decreased as compared to the control in the group intraperitoneally treated with killed vibrio or IF30. In the group orally treated with killed vibrio or IF30, too, the number of viable cells in the liver was decreased, but in the group treated orally with live vibrio, the number of viable cells in the liver was higher than in the control.

DISCUSSION

In a series of studies we have shown that a fraction, IF52, and heat killed whole cells of *Vibrio cholerae eltor* enhanced IgE antibody production and depressed induction of IgG, whereas another fraction, IF30, enhanced production of vibriocidal antibody and depressed IgE induction. We, therefore, examined whether or not live whole cells of *V. cholerae* had any effect on the induction of IgE when the organisms were given orally (4).

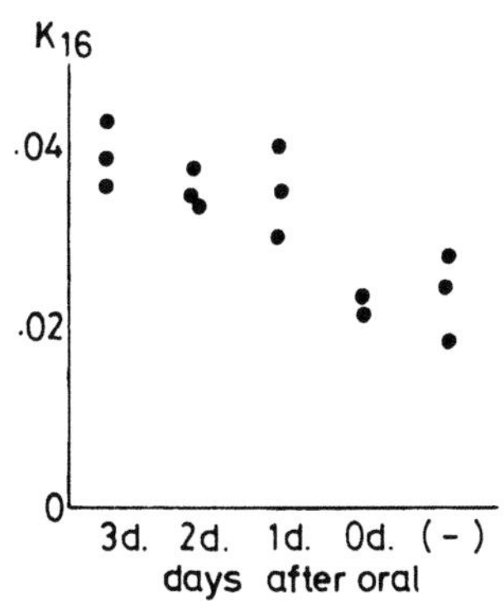

Fig. 7. Carbon clearance after live vibrio oral administration in the time course.

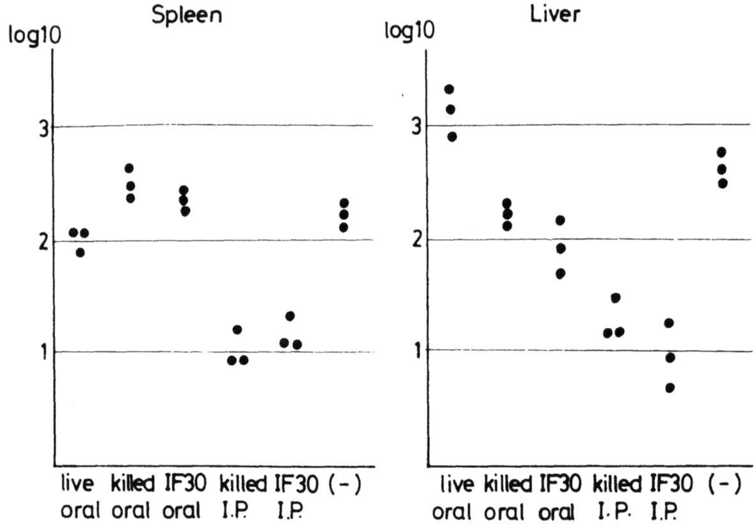

Fig. 8. Distribution of vibrios in spleen and liver after sensitization.

As shown in Fig. 1, vibrios do not persist long in the intestine but, as shown in Fig. 4, induction of IgE antibody was depressed while induction of vibriocidal antibody was promoted when the organisms were given repeatedly. There is a possibility that the organisms are killed in the intestines and become antigenic, but the effect is quite opposite to the group in which killed organisms are given, therefore, it is conceivable that live vibrios stimulate antibody forming cells by some other mechanism than heat killed organisms or components of live organisms not shared by killed ones do so.

Owen has shown by electronmicrography that *Giardia muris* was phagocyted by macrophages in Peyer's patches (5). If vibrios were phagocyted by macrophages when the organisms are given orally, then the value of carbon clearance should be elevated, but, as shown in Fig. 6, the value stayed on the same level as in the control group. Pierce *et al.* have shown that immunologically potent cells were sensitized in Peyer's patches, when cholera toxin was given orally, and left there to go through the mesenteric lymph nodes and recirculate (6). Also Cooper *et al.* have shown that when vibrios were inoculated in the small intestines, a single pulse was given to the circulating antibody (7).

In our experiments, as shown in Figs. 2 and 5, when the first sensitization was given orally with live organisms, heat killed organisms or with IF30 and the second sensitization intraperitoneally with IF30, induction of IgE antibody was depressed. In contrast, when the second sensitization was given intraperitoneally with IF30, induction of IgE antibody was depressed whereas a second sensitization given intraperitoneally with heat killed organism did not depress the induction.

These results, together with other experiments, indicate that cells of vibrio do not reach Peyer's patches in an intact form and some components of the organism prime immunologically potent cells in such a way that the cells react to the second sensitization in a positive or negative way according to the kind of the antigen. Therefore, it is important to select the most suitable combination of antigens for priming and immunization to obtain the maximum protection for cholera.

REFERENCES

1. Komogata, Y., Okudaira, H. and Ghoda, A. 1976. Production of Antihaptenic IgE Antibody by Somatic Components of *Vibrio cholerae.* Proceeding of the 12th Joint Conference, U. S.-Japan Cooperative Medical Science Program, Cholera Panel. 110
2. Tada, T. and Okumura, K. 1971. Regulation of Homocytotropic Antibody Formation in the Rat. I. Feed-Back Regulation by Passively Administered Antibody. J. Immunol. **106**:1002
3. Rappaport, R. S., B. A. Rubin and H. Tint. 1974. Development of a purified cholera toxoid. I. Purification of toxin. Infect. Immun. **9**: 294-303.
4. Komagata, Y. and Ghoda, A. 1980. Inhibition of Antihaptenic IgE Antibody Production and the Susceptibility of Mice to *Vibrio cholerae.* Proceeding of the 16th Joint Conference, U.S.-Japan Cooperative Medical Science Program, Cholera Panel, in press.
5. Robert L. Owen, C. Lennell Allen and David P. Stevens. 1981. Phagocytosis of *Giardia muris* by Macrophages in Peyer's Patch Epithelium in Mice. Infection and Immunity, Vol. 33, No. 2, 591-601.
6. Pierce, N. F. and Gowans, J. L. 1975. Cellular kinetics of the intestinal immune responses to cholera toxoid in rats. J. Exp. Med. **142**: 1550-1563.
7. G. N. Cooper and G. D. F. Jackson. 1981. Immune responses of rats to live *Vibrio cholerae*: Antibodies in serum and intestinal secretions. Parasite Immunology **3**, 57-68.

Advances in Research on Cholera and Related Diarrheas, eds., S. Kuwahara, N. F. Pierce, 29–33.

PROTECTION OF NEONATAL PIGLETS AGAINST COLIBACILLOSIS BY IMMUNIZATION OF DAMS WITH PROCHOLERAGENOID

E. Fürer, S.J. Cryz, Jr., F. Dorner and R. Germanier

Swiss Serum and Vaccine Institute Berne

Lethal *Escherichia coli*-induced diarrhea (enteric colibacillosis) results in major worldwide economic losses (8). In order to produce disease, strains of *E. coli* must be able to first colonize the small intestine and then elaborate enterotoxin(s) (5, 7). The heat-labile enterotoxin (LT) has been shown to elicit massive fluid outpouring in piglets (2). LT is structurally, functionally and immunologically related to cholera toxin (CT) (1). In addition, cross-neutralization and cross-protection have been deomonstrated between CT and LT (2, 6).

Attemps to protect neonatal piglets against colibacillosis have centered around immunization of dams and the passive transfer of colostral antibody to suckling piglets. To date, the most promising results have been achieved employing vaccines directed against colonization factors.

The purpose of the current investigation was to determine whether protection against colibacillosis could be obtained by evoking antitoxic immunity against LT. Procholeragenoid was selected as an immunizing agent in place of LT because CT can be obtained in much greater amounts than LT and procholeragenoid has been shown to be a good immunogen (4).

Procholeragenoid is a high molecular weight aggregate of CT (3). CT was converted to procholeragenoid in an almost quantitative manner by heating at 60°C in a Tris-EDTA buffer (6). The product formed during this process was found to be heterogeneous upon analysis by chromatography on Sepharose 4BCL (Peak I, Figure 1). Heating of CT in phosphate-buffered saline (PBS) (pH 7.4) for 30 minutes at 60°C produced a much more heterogeneous product (Peak II, Figure 1). Present in both procholeragenoid preparations was a peak of lower molecular weight (Peak III, Figure 1). The biological activities of the various peaks from both progenoid preparations were determined in the rabbit ileal loop, the Y-1 adrenal cell and in the skin permeability assay, and was found to be roughly 1% that of native CT.

When Peak III was analyzed by SDS-polyacrylamide gel electrophoresis, only a single band was observed which comigrated with choleragenoid (data not shown). We interpret these results to indicate that Peak III is composed primarily of choleragenoid but also contains small quantities of choleragen which account for the toxicity observed. Removal of Peak III did not measurally decrease the toxicity of the procholeragenoid

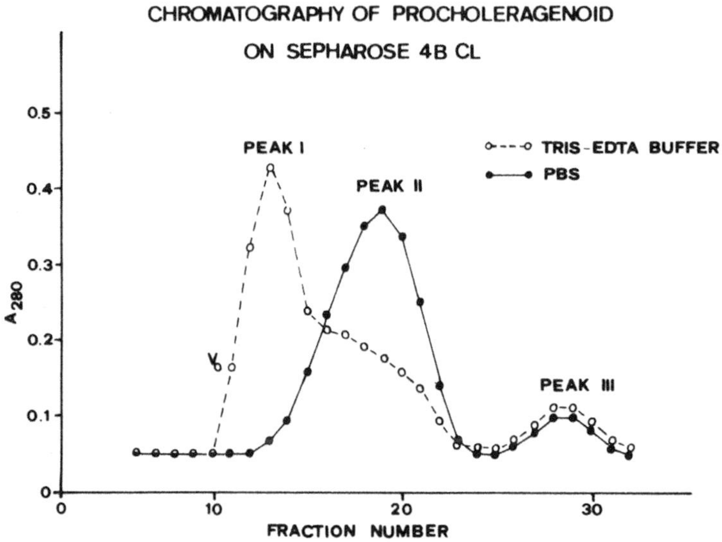

Figure 1

preparations. Therefore, procholeragenoid produced in PBS was used without further purification for all following experiments.

The immunogenicity of procholeragenoid was determined in dams by intramuscular immunization with either 50 μg or 100 μg 5 and 2 weeks prior to the expected delivery date. The antibody response in the sera and colostra was quantitated at the delivery date. Both doses of procholeragenoid were capable of eliciting high antitoxic-IgG and toxin-neutralizing titers (Tables 1 and 2). Although the antibody titers tended to be higher with the higher immunizing dose, this difference was not found to be statistically significant ($p > 0.5$). In the following experiments 50 μg of procholeragenoid were used as the immunizing dose.

Most deaths due to colibacillosis in neonatal piglets occur within 72 hours post parturition. Protective antibody during this period would be expected to be acquired from colostrum since there is little transplacental transfer of antibody in swine. Antibody titers in the serum and colostra of immunized dams were followed during the first week

Table 1. Antitoxic-IgG titers in immunized dams at day of parturition.

No. of dams	Dosage (μg)	Antitoxic-IgG titers*	
		Colostra	Sera
13	100	440 (150-880)	230 (80-640)
10	50	250 (50-640)	140 (50-250)

* Determined in ELISA.

Table 2. Toxin-neutralizing titers in immunized dams at day of parturition.

		Toxin-neutralizing titers*	
No. of dams	Dosage (μg)	Colostra	Sera
7	100	1250 (800-1,600)	280 (200-400)
8	50	/25 (200-1,600)	360 (200-800)

* Determined in Y-1 adrenal cell assay. Colostra and sera were titrated against LT.

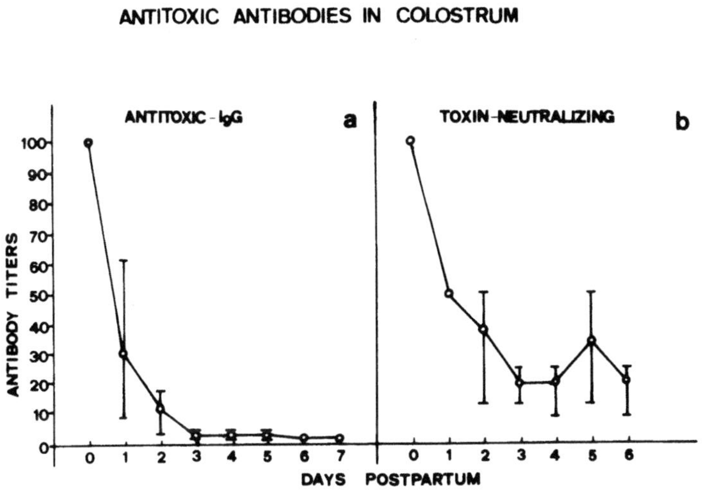

Figure 2

post partum (Figure 2). A sharp drop-off in antitoxic-IgG titers was observed during the first 3 days post partum, reaching levels of less than 5 % of those at day 0 (day of birth). Toxin-neutralizing titers also decreased during this period, but remained elevated throughout this time-period (roughtly 20 % of the titers present at day 0). These results would indicate that the majority of colostral toxin-neutralizing antibody is not IgG but most likely IgA.

Protection of piglets against colibacillosis by immunization of dams with procholeragenoid was evaluated in 3 independent field trials, each conducted at a different breeding facility. Dams were again immunized 5 and 2 weeks prior to delivery. A total of 229 dams and 2,331 piglets were involved in these trials (Table 3). More than 70 % of the control group had episodes of *E. coli*-induced diarrhea with approximately a 5 % mortality rate (Table 3). Bacteriological examination of stools from both groups presenting with diarrhea showed large numbers of *E. coli* serotype 0149. These strains were found to be toxinogenic (LT-producers) based on Y-1 adrenal cell assay results. A11 *E. coli* isolated from stools were found to be of the 0149 serotype.

Table 3. Incidence of death and diarrhea in piglets due to colibacillosis in immunized and non-immunized dams[1].

Group	No. of dams	No. of piglets	No. of piglets with diarrhea	No. of deaths
Non-immunized [2]	167	1,678	1,225 (73 %)	79 (4.7 %)
Immunized	62	653	74 (11 %)	5 (0.77%)

1) Dams were immunized intramuscularly with 50 μg of procholeragenoid approximately 5 weeks and again at 2 weeks before delivery.

2) All piglets in the non-immunized group which presented with diarrhea were immediately treated with antibiotics. No piglets in the immunized group received antibiotics.

These results demonstrated that a substantial degree of protection against colibacillosis in piglets could be attained by immunization of dams with procholeragenoid late in the gestation period. It was of interest to determine what levels of antibody could be obtained in the following gestation period by reimmunization with procholeragenoid. Dams which were immunized in the previous gestation period were given a single dose of procholeragenoid approximately 2 weeks prior to the expected second delivery. With such a booster injection, antitoxic-IgG and toxin-neutralizing titers (380 and 600, respectively) (Table 4) were comparable to those seen during the first gestation period with 2 doses of procholoeragenoid (250 and 725, respectively) (Tables 1 and 2). The death rate in piglets due to colibacillosis was also comparable, 0.77 % following the first delivery and 0.86 % after the second.

These results demonstrate that substantial protection of neonatal piglets against colibacillosis can be obtained by immunization of dams with procholeragenoid. Protection appeared to be based solely on antitoxic immunity.

Table 4. Effects of reimmunization of dams during following gestation period on colostral antibody levels and death due to colibacillosis.

No. of dams	No. of piglets	Colostrum antibody titers [1]		No. of piglets with diarrhea	No. of deaths
		Antitoxic-IgG [2]	Toxin-neutralizing [3]		
11	116	380 (160-880)	600 (200-1,000)	1 (0.86%)	1 (0.86%)

1) At day of delivery. Expressed as geometrical mean (range).

2) Determined in ELISA.

3) Determined in Y-1 adrenal cell assay. Colostra were titrated against LT.

Piglets were observed for 21 days post partum before compilation of data.

REFERENCES

1. Clements, J. D. and R. A. Finkelstein. 1978. Demonstration of shared immunological determinants in enterotoxins from *Vibrio cholerae* and *Escherichia coli*. Infect. Immun. **22**:709-713.
2. Dorner, F., P. Mayer and R. Leskova. 1980. Immunity to *Escherichia coli* in piglets: the role of colostral antibodies directed against heat-labile enterotoxin in experimental neonatal diarrhea. Zbl. Vet. Med. **27**:207-221.
3. Finkelstein, R. A., K. Fugita and J. J. LoSpalluto. 1971. Procholeragenoid: an aggregated intermediate in the formation of choleragenoid. J. Immunol. **107**:1043-1051.
4. Germanier, R., E. Fürer, S. Varallyay and T. M. Inderbitzin. 1976. Preparation of a purified antigenic cholera toxoid. Infect. Immun. **13**:1692-1698.
5. Gyles, C. L. and D. A. Barnum. 1969. A heat-labile enterotoxin from strains of *Escherichia coli* enteropathogenic for pigs. J. Infect. Dis **120**:419-426.
6. Holmgren, J., O. Soderlind and T. Wadström. 1973. Cross-reactivity between heat-labile enterotoxins of *Vibrio cholerae* and *Escherichia coli* in neutralization test in rabbit ileum and skin. Acta Pathol. Microbiol. Scand. **81**:757-762.
7. Jones, G. W. and J. M. Rutter. 1972. Role of the K88 antigen in the pathogenesis of neonatal diarrhea caused by *Escherichia coli* in piglets. Infect. Immun. **6**:918-927.
8. Kohler, E. M. 1972. Pathogenesis of neonatal enteric colibacillosis in pigs. J. Am. Vet. Med. Assoc. **160**:574-582.

Advances in Research on Cholera and Related Diarrheas, eds., S. Kuwahara, N. F. Pierce, 35–40.

EFFICACIOUS CARRIERS FOR MULTI-SPECIFIC PRIMING OF A MUCOSAL IgA RESPONSE

Juliet A. Fuhrman and John J. Cebra

University of Pennsylvania, Philadelphia 19104

1. Introduction

Small rodent models have been successful in demonstrating that cholera toxin can prime effectively by the intestinal route for an anti-toxic secretory IgA response (1-3). Secretory antibodies in the intestinal lumen have been shown to protect the gut from a toxin challenge by the enteric route (3,4). Thus, cholera toxin is fairly unique among non-replicating antigens in being able to prime effectively by the mucosal route for protective immunity. The studies presented here characterize this mucosal priming process, in particular the memory B cell component which is generated, in order to understand the superiority of cholera toxin over other non-living antigens in priming by the gut route. Our findings in the cholera toxin system are then applied to evaluating non-toxic substitutes as mucosal priming agents.

These studies use a mouse model of intestinal priming with cholera toxin and other purified proteins to analyze the effect of this priming on the antigen-specific B cell population both at the site of priming and at distant sites. One aspect of effective mucosal priming with cholera toxin, as demonstrated by these studies, is the generation of a high frequency of memory B cells, the plasma cell progeny of which will secrete only IgA. However, such an IgA-committed memory population can also be generated by priming with non-toxic substitutes, and it can be extended to antigenic specificites beyond those of the toxin molecule.

The Klinman clonal precursor assay (5) was adapted to study the frequency and isotype potential of antigen-specific B cells generated in various lymphoid compartments by different priming regimens. This assay entails an adoptive transfer of the donor lymphoid cells to be studied into a previously primed, lethally irradiated host. Eighteen hours after transfer, the recipient's spleen, in which donor cells have randomly lodged, is sliced into 50 fragments. These fragments are stimulated with antigen in organ culture, and the donor B cells which are seeded in the splenic fragments undergo division and maturation to plasma cells in response to the stimulating antigen. If the original adoptive transfer is performed as a limiting dilution, then each splenic fragment can be shown to contain zero or one donor B cell specific for the antigen used to drive the culture. By this method, then, the clonal progeny of a single antigen-sensitive B cell, or clonal precursor, can be isolated in order to study the individual monoclonal responses to the secondary antigenic challenge. By screening the supernatants for antibody activity, one can enumerate, by extrapolation, the antigen-specific clonal precursors which existed in the original donor tissue. Furthermore, since each antibody-producing fragment represents the clonal progeny of a single antigen-sensitive B cell, representative donor B cells can be characterized on a single cell basis, according to the isotype potential of their daughter plasma cells. Since the recipient has been antigen primed and lethally irradiated it supplies the donor inoculum with maximal antigen specific T cell help; so, the complete antibody potential of the donor B cell can be assessed under conditions of maximal help, and the effects of accompanying donor T cells are negligible.

Our original work in this system (6) compared donor tissues derived either from animals immunized intraduodenally (id) with toxin or from animals primed intraperitoneally (ip) with toxoid and adjuvant. These tissues were adoptively transferred into toxoid primed recipients, and the splenic fragment cultures were driven in vitro with purified toxoid. The culture supernatants were assayed for anti-toxoid antibodies using a solid phase RIA, and the products of positive fragments were further analyzed for the isotypes of the anti-toxoid antibodies.

Tables 1 and 2 show several key features of mucosal priming. First, the frequency of antigen-sensitive B cells is increased, compared to unprimed tissues, in PP and spleen as a result of priming by either mucosal or parenteral routes. However, mucosal priming with toxin is distinguished by its ability to generate a high frequency of antigen-sensitive cells which are committed to the exclusive expression of IgA through their daughter plasma cells. This IgA-committed class is generated in both PP and spleen after id priming.

In subsequent studies, then, we have looked for two key features to evaluate mucosal priming. First we looked for the rise in frequency of antigen-sensitive B cells, and second, we looked for development of the class of clonal precursors committed to exclusive IgA production.

Table 1. Isotype profile of PP-derived antitoxoid clones°.

	B cell donors						
Clonal product	Week after i.d. priming*					Week after i.p. priming	
	0	2	4	6	12	2	12
	Antitoxoid clones expressing product (%)						
μ only	5	0	0	0	0	0	0
Some μ	75	4	11	15	75	61	5
$\gamma \pm \alpha$, no μ	10	45	55	62	8	28	90
Some α	20	77	72	85	100	50	42
α only	10	50	33	23	17	11	10
Number of clones analyzed	20	22	18	13	12	18	19
Freq. per 10^6 B cells	<1	20	80	100	120	20	80

* 10 μg purified cholera toxin injected intraduodenally (i.d.).
\+ 100 μg cholera toxoid injected intraperitoneally (i.p.) with CFA.
°Adapted from (6).

Table 2. Isotype profile of spleen-derived antitoxoid clones°.

Clonal product	B cell donors					
	Week after i.d. priming *				Week after i.p. priming+	
	0	2-4	6	12	2	12
	Antitoxoid clones expressing product					
	%					
μ only	10	14	9	9	19	6
Some μ	58	38	42	30	75	12
$\gamma \pm \alpha$, no μ	36	23	39	52	25	82
Some α	21	62	69	56	38	18
α only	5	38	18	17	0	0
Number of clones analyzed	19	13	33	23	16	17
Freq. per 10^6 B cells	1	20	50	60	10	50

*Intraduodenal
+Intraperitoneal
°Adapted from (6)

Using this method we next asked if cholera toxin could be used to deliver a specific haptenic determinant to the mucosal B cell compartment in a way which would specifically prime anti-hapten B cells. One such determinant which we have used is TNP. Lonnroth and Holmgren (7) showed that low coupling ratios of TNBS could be used to create a haptenated toxin which maintained both its toxicity and its ganglioside binding function. We prepared a TNP-toxin conjugate by this method and then analyzed it to be certain that GMl binding functions remained intact on the same molecules which bore the hapten. Using an RIA which selected for molecules which could bind to GMl-bearing red blood cells while scoring for TNP determinants with an anti-TNP antibody, we could show that at least some molecules in our conjugate preparation displayed both binding and substitution with hapten.

This TNP-toxin preparation was then used as an id priming agent, and the anti-TNP response of the primed animals was analyzed to determine if TNP-specific B cells were increased in frequency or driven to IgA commitment. In order to score anti-TNP specific B cells independent of other specificites which the conjugate might prime, we modified the Klinman assay as follows: donor lymphoid tissues derived from TNP-toxin primed animals were transferred into recipients primed with hemocyanin; the splenic fragment cultures were driven with TNP-hemocyanin; and the culture supernatants were assayed for anti-TNP antibodies on TNP-BSA bound to a solid support. Using this protocol, we could demonstrate that TNP-toxin delivered id caused an expansion of the TNP-sensitive B cell pool in PP, and an increased commitment to IgA expression in the anti-TNP response (Table 3). We also observed, however, a less dramatic, but nevertheless significant, priming effect of the TNP-specific B cell pool when toxin alone was used to prime by the intestinal route. In conclusion, intestinal priming with cholera toxin seems to exert some

Table 3. Isotype profile of PP-derived anti-TNP clones.

% of clones expressing	Unprimed	B cell donors: 2 WK post TXN ID	2 WK post TNP-TXN ID	4 WK post TNP-TXN ID
μ only	16	18	25	9
Some μ	64	36	29	27
$\gamma \pm \alpha$, no μ	36	9	14	27
Some α	62	55	61	81
α only	11	45	58	45
Number of clones analyzed	44	11	28	11
Freq. per 10^6 B cells	50	110	210	100

non-specific or perhaps polyclonal activation of the PP B cell compartment, but the use of a hapten conjugate can show further specific priming of anti-hapten B cells above this non-specific priming.

Our next concern was to determine whether toxicity was a critical function in mucosal B cell priming by cholera toxin. Table 4 contrasts the priming of anti-toxoid B cells in animals primed id with holotoxin vs. purified B subunit. Both forms of antigen result in comparable increases in the frequency of toxoid-sensitive B cells of 1-2 orders of magnitude. However, on an equal weight basis, the B subunit is inferior to intact toxin, but with an increased dose of B subunit, the same level of priming, as judged by the

Table 4. Comparison of isotype profiles of anti-toxoid clones resulting from intraduodenal priming with holotoxin or B subunit.

Clonal Product	B cell source: PP			Spl	
	Tox, 10 μg	B Sub, 10 μg	B Sub, 40 μg	Tox, 10 μg	B Sub, 40 μg
	Anti-toxoid clones expressing product (%)				
μ only	0	0	0	14	5
Some μ	4	54	25	38	50
$\gamma \pm \alpha$, no μ	45	45	33	23	20
Some α	77	41	92	62	70
α only	50	0	42	38	30
Number of clones analyzed	22	22	12	13	20
Freq per 10^6 B cells	30-50	40-50	50	30	60

Table 5. Adoptive transfer of PP cells from PNA (id) primed donors generates antigen-specific plasma cells in recipient spleens.

PP cell donor	$\frac{\text{anti-PNA}^+}{\text{cIgA}^+}$ x 100%*
Control	2.5
PNA, 100 μg id+	6.2

*Percentage of cells which stain for donor cytoplasmic IgA allotype which also stain fluorescein-PNA by binding in the presence of 0.5 *M* galactose. Recipient spleens were scored 12 days post transfer.

+Immunization at 2 wks prior to transfer.

percentage of antigen-sensitive cells committed to IgA, can be achieved. The difference in dose required to drive this priming process likely reflects a decreased avidity on the part of the B subunit for the cell surface receptors. However, in order to eliminate the possibility that residual toxicity in this preparation accounts for the dose-dependent effect, we are repeating these studies with Texas Star choleragenoid (the gift of Dr. R. Finkelstein, Univ. of Missouri - Columbia).

Last, in an attempt to circumvent the toxicity question entirely, we have attempted to substitute in this mucosal priming regimen a purified protein which might exhibit similar binding properties in the complete absence of toxicity. One such molecule which we have worked with is a plant lectin, peanut agglutinin, which displays a binding specificity for terminal galactosyl-N-acetylgalactosaminyl carbohydrate residues. Our initial studies with PNA (Table 5) employed an adoptive transfer of unprimed or id primed PP tissues into sublethally irradiated recipients. At the time of transfer the recipients were challenged ip with 100 μg PNA, and 12 days after transfer their spleens were scored for antigen-specific plasma cells by direct fluorescent staining. The transfer used a congenic system which distinguishes donor derived IgA plasma cells, so we could score for the percentage of such cells which were anti-PNA producers. Table 5 shows that mucosal priming with PNA can increase this antigen-specific plasma cell class above background levels from unprimed animals. Preliminary studies using the clonal precursor assay have also indicated successful priming by the gut route with PNA. Unprimed animals show precursor frequencies below 1 per million B cells, but primed animals show frequencies between 5 and 8 per million B cells, and these precursors generate clones which are enriched for IgA committed cells (Table 6).

In conclusion we have shown that one component of effective mucosal priming is the generation of a high frequency of antigen-sensitive B cells which are committed to generating only IgA-producing plasma cell progeny upon secondary challenge. We have used intestinal priming with cholera toxin to elicit such a population, and we find that haptenic determinants coupled to toxin can prime hapten-specific B cells in the same manner upon mucosal delivery. Furthermore, we have indications that the binding properties, and not the toxicity of cholera toxin may account for its efficacy in mucosal B cell priming, since B subunit and PNA can be shown to prime the mucosal B cell compartment upon intestinal administration.

Table 6. Isotype profile of anti-PNA clones.

% of clones expressing	Donors	
	PP, id*	SPL, ip+
μ only	0	0
Some μ	0	40
$\gamma \pm \alpha$, no μ	55	60
Some α	44	60
α only	44	0

*Intraduodenally primed with 100 μg PNA at 2 wk prior to transfer.

+Intraperitoneally primed with 100 μg PNA and adjuvant at 2 wk prior to transfer.

REFERENCES

1. Pierce, N. F. 1978. The role of antigen form and function in the primary and secondary intestinal immune responses to cholera toxin and toxoid in rats. J. Exp. Med. **148**:195-206.
2. Lange, S. and J. Holmgren. 1978. Protective antitoxic cholera immunity in mice: Influence of route and number of immunizations and mode of action of protective antibodies. Acta Pathol. Microbiol. Scand. **86**:145-152.
3. Fujita, K. and R. A. Finkelstein. 1972. Antitoxic immunity in experimental cholera: Comparison of immunity induced perorally and parenterally in mice. J. Infect. Dis. **125**:647-655.
4. Lange, S., H. A. Hanson, S. O. Molin, and H. Nygren. 1979. Local cholera immunity in mice: Intestinal antitoxin-containing cells and their correlation with protective immunity. Infect. Immun. **23**: 743-750.
5. Klinman, N. R. 1969. Antibody with homogeneous antigen binding produced by splenic foci in organ culture. Immunochem. **6**:757-759.
6. Fuhrman, J. A. and J. J. Cebra. 1981. Special features of the priming process for a secretory IgA response J. Exp. Med. **153**:534-544.

Advances in Research on Cholera and Related Diarrheas, eds., S. Kuwahara, N. F. Pierce, 41–48.

ORAL IMMUNIZATION FOR CHOLERA: MUCOSAL ANTITOXIC IMMUNITY IS IMPORTANT AND CAN PROBABLY BE SAFELY ACHIEVED

Nathaniel F. Pierce, William C. Cray, Jr., and John B. Sacci, Jr.

Baltimore City Hospitals and Johns Hopkins University School of Medicine, Baltimore, Maryland 21224, USA and René Germanier, Swiss Serum and Vaccine Institute, Berne, Switzerland

There is now much evidence to support the notions that secretory IgA antibody is the first line of immunologic defense of the intestinal mucosa and that a mucosal IgA response is best stimulated by antigens applied to the mucosal surface. On this basis, it has been argued that immunization against cholera, a superficial mucosal infection, should be given orally with the aim of evoking a protective mucosal IgA response (1). Some progress in this direction has been made using either live avirulent mutants of *V. cholerae* or nonliving antigens derived from this organism (2, 3).

Among the latter, cholera toxin (CT) has been most extensively studied. It has proven to be an especially potent mucosal immunogen in a variety of experimental animals (3, 4, 5). Small amounts applied to the intestinal mucosa have reliably evoked vigorous local secretory IgA antitoxin reponses, and dogs immunized by oral dosing with purified CT, or a crude, CT-rich culture filtrate, have been protected against disease induced by oral challenge with live virulent *V. cholerae* (3, 4, 5). These observations demonstrated a protective role for mucosal antitoxin and suggested that cholera toxin might have practical value as a component of a multi–antigen oral vaccine.

One obstacle to the use of CT in an oral vaccine is the side effect of diarrhea. In our previously reported studies, oral doses of CT that evoked protection also caused transient diarrhea in a majority of dogs (3). We have, therefore, conducted further studies aimed at 1) developing a safe and effective means of oral immunization with CT or CT–derived antigens, 2) assessing the role of antitoxic immunity in multi–antigen immunization against experimental cholera, and 3) determining the duration of immunity induced by oral immunization. The results reported here support the view that antitoxic immunity contributes substantially to protection against cholera and suggest that effective and lasting antitoxic immunity can be achieved without the side effect of diarrhea.

Oral Immunization of Dogs with Purified and Crude CT. In initial studies mongrel dogs were immunized orally with either highly purified CT (NIH lot 0972) or crude CT (NIH lot 001). The latter is a nondialyzed culture filtrate of *V. cholerae* Ogawa B1307. For immunization, fasting dogs were given 50 ml of 6% $NaHCO_3$ by gastric tube followed by 100 ml of 2% casamino acids containing the toxin (3). The mucosal antitoxin response was assessed in jejunal biopsies usually taken 7 days after the final oral immunization. Antitoxin–containing plasma cells (ACC) in the lamina propria were enumerated by a highly specific fluorescent antibody method (6). Protection was determined by oral challenge of immunized and control dogs with 10^{11} *V. cholerae*, Ogawa 395, usually 3 weeks after immunization.

Results in dogs immunized orally with purified CT are in Figure 1. Protection is expressed as percent protection against severe or lethal diarrhea *and* as the percent *reduction* in stool output during the first 18 hours after challenge, both compared to concurrently challenged nonimmune controls. Significant protection followed oral immunization with 12 or 3 100 μg doses of CT (given over 54 or 42 days, respectively). However, a 16–fold reduction in CT dose, to 6 μg given 3 times, was nonprotective. It is apparent that protection closely paralleled the peak mucosal antitoxic response, even though challenge was 2 weeks after the peak. In fact, protection lasted at least 3 months after immunization, as indicated in the second columns from the left, even though the antitoxin response in prechallenge biopsies had declined by 96% compared to the peak response on day 7 after immunization.

In further studies, dogs were immunized orally with crude CT to determine whether this multi–antigen material might promote synergistically protective mucosal immune responses and thus permit immunization with a reduced dose of CT. Evidence suggesting synergistic protection is shown in Table 1. This table compares the mucosal antitoxin responses and protection in dogs immunized orally with purified CT, a comparable dose

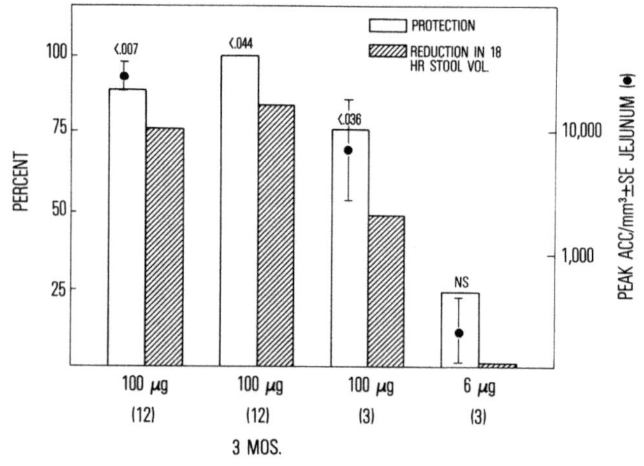

Fig. 1. Protection of dogs by oral immunization with purified cholera toxin. Individual toxin doses, and the number of doses given (parentheses), are shown. Immunization schedules are in the text. Challenge with 10^{11} *V. cholerae* Ogawa 395 was three weeks after the final oral dose of toxin, except in the group labelled 3 mos., in which it was three months after immunization. Percent protection against severe or lethal disease is shown in open bars; percent reduction in stool volume during the first 18 hours after challenge is in hatched bars; each value is obtained by comparison with concurrently challenged nonimmune controls. P values for protection are indicated above open bars. Antitoxin-containing plasma cells (ACC) were enumerated in jejunal biopsies taken 6-7 days after completion of immunization. Each immunization group contained 10-18 dogs.

Table 1. Comparison of crude and purified toxins as oral immunogens in dogs.

Antigen	Dose	Jejunal ACC/mm^{3} [a]	Percent Protection[b]	P
Pure toxin	6 μg X 3	250 (1.8)	29	NS
Crude toxin	6 μg X 2[c]	280 (1.5)	100	0.003
Toxin-depleted crude toxin	100 μg X 2[c]	138 (1.7)	16	NS

[a] Geometric mean antitoxin-containing plasma cells ($\bar{x}$ ± SE) in biopsies taken 6 days after last antigen dose.

[b] Protection against lethal diarrhea after challenge with 10^{11} *V. cholerae*, Ogawa 395, compared with concurrently challenged nonimmune controls. Antigen doses were at 21 day intervals and challenge was three weeks after final dose.

[c] Expressed as equivalent dose of purified toxin in antigen or in crude filtrate from which antigen was derived. Actual dose of undialyzed crude toxin was 63 mg, and dose of toxin-depleted dialyzed crude toxin was 250 mg.

of crude CT, or a 16–fold greater dose of crude CT from which CT was selectively removed by affinity chromatography using antitoxin immobilized on sepharose as the solid phase. It can be seen that only the crude CT was protective. This protection was not due solely to antitoxin, because comparable ACC responses were evoked by purified CT, which was nonprotective. Nor was it, apparently, due solely to antibodies evoked by nontoxin antigens, because the larger doses of toxin–free culture filtrate were nonprotective. From this observation we conclude that crude CT evokes synergistically protective immune responses and that antitoxin is an important participant in this synergy. Synergistic protection by antitoxic and antibacterial antibodies has also been observed by Svennerholm and Holmgren in parenterally immunized rabbits (7).

These results showed that the dose of CT required for protection was lower when crude CT was used as the immunogen rather than purified CT. This suggested that the side effect of diarrhea might be avoided by using crude CT in appropriately reduced dosage. Table 2 shows that this goal was partly achieved, but that the lowest protective dose of crude CT still caused very mild diarrhea in 21% of dogs. Although crude CT proved a safer immunogen than did purified CT, which was protective only in a dosage that caused diarrhea in a majority of dogs, it was not possible to achieve protection without some risk of mild diarrhea.

Oral Immunization with Cholera Toxoid or B Subunit. Because of the preceeding results, further studies were aimed at determining whether antigenic, but nontoxic, derivatives of CT could be used to safely promote a protective mucosal antitoxic response. Two materials were studied : 1) a nontoxic toxoid made by treatment of purified CT with glutaraldehyde (8), and 2) purified B subunit of CT, provided by Dr. Richard Finkelstein (9). These were given orally to dogs in doses of 50 μg of glutaraldehyde toxoid, or up to 1 mg of B subunit, using the methods described for oral

Table 2. Oral immunization: risk of diarrhea and protection achieved.

Immunization[a]	Diarrhea during immunization (%): mild	severe	Percent protection[b]
Pure toxin			
100 μg X 3	59	13	76
6 μg X 3	6	0	24
Crude filtrate			
1 gm X 3	16	54	100
63 mg X 2	21	0	90
16 mg X 3	11	0	31
Control (no antigen)	4	0	–

a Doses were given at 21 day intervals.
b Protection against the combined risk of severe or lethal diarrhea compared with concurrently challenged nonimmune control dogs.

immunization with CT. Neither of these materials caused diarrhea. However, as shown in Figure 2, the level of protection achieved was disappointing. Thus, 20 50 μg doses of glutaraldehyde toxoid given over 50 days evoked no detectable mucosal antitoxin response and insignificant protection against live vibrio challenge. Similarly, 3 100 μg or 1

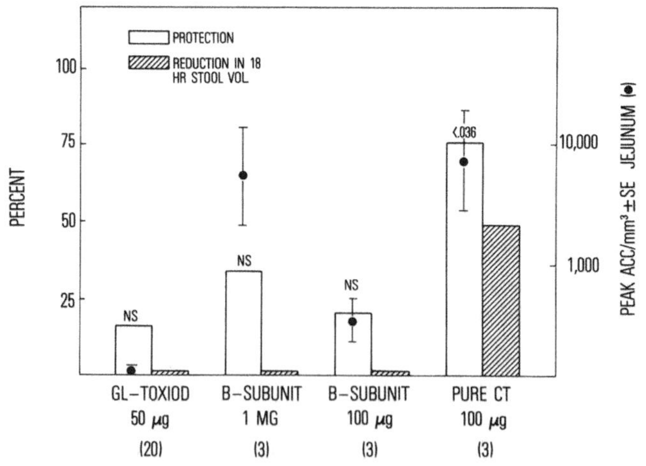

Fig. 2. Protection of dogs by oral immunization with glutaraldehyde toxoid (Gl-toxoid), B subunit, or purified cholera toxin (CT). Individual antigen doses, and the number of doses given (parentheses), are shown. Immunization schedules are in the text. Challenge with 10^{11} *V. cholerae* Ogawa 395 was three weeks after the final oral dose of antigen. Protection is expressed as explained in legend of Figure 1. Biopsies for enumeration of ACC were taken as explained in Figure 1. Each immunization group contained 16-18 dogs.

mg oral doses of B subunit were not significantly protective even though the larger dose evoked substantial mucosal antitoxin responses. Although other studies have shown that B subunit is an effective mucosal immunogen (4), these results suggest it is inferior to CT in at least two respoects. First, on a dose for dose basis it evokes much smaller mucosal antitoxin responses; e.g. the response to 3 100 μg doses of B subunit was only 5 % of that induced by equal doses of CT. And second, protection associated with antitoxin evoked by B subunit appears inferior to that associated with a comparable antitoxin response evoked by CT; e.g. 100 μg doses of CT and 1 mg doses of B subunit evoked similar mucosal antitoxin responses, but only CT caused significant protection. There are several possible explanations for these differences. But whatever the actual explanation, it is apparent that B subunit is markedly inferior to CT as an oral immunogen, at least in this animal model. Further studies with this antigen have not been pursued.

Oral Immunization with Heat Aggregated Cholera Toxin: The final series of studies in this report involved evaluation of heat aggregated cholera toxin (procholeragenoid; abbreviated HACT) as a possible oral immunogen. Earlier studies by Fujita and Finkelstein and by Peterson have suggested that HACT is immunogenic given orally (10, 11). HACT was made by heating purified CT at 60°C for 20 minutes in Tris–EDTA buffer. The resultant product consisted mostly of aggregated CT with a small residue of B subunit. HACT was minimally toxic. Measured in the rabbit skin vascular permeability assay by Dr. John Craig it had 1.2 % of the toxic activity of purified CT. However, when compared with CT for its ability to evoke fluid accumulation in rabbit intestinal segments, it was even less toxic (Figure 3). This figure compares CT with 100 fold greater doses of HACT; thus, residual toxicity at a 1 % level should produce similar dose/response curves for intestinal fluid accumulation. It is apparent that HACT has much less than 1 % of the secretion-inducing potency of CT. Moreover, the shallower dose/response curve

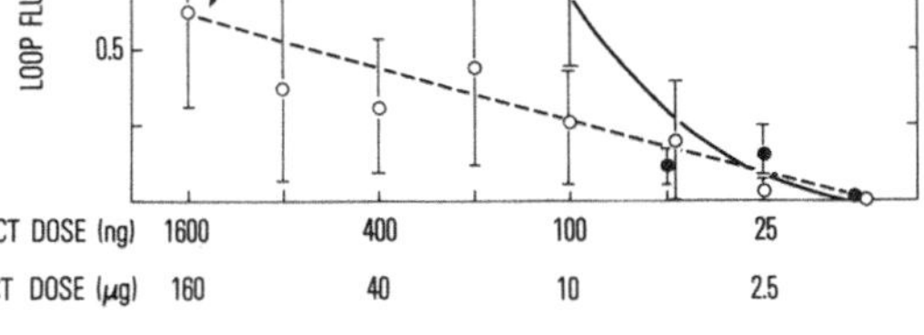

Fig. 3. Fluid accumulation in rabbit intestinal segments challenged with purified cholera toxin (CT) or heat-aggregated cholera toxin (HACT). Indicated doses of CT or 100-fold greater doses of HACT were injected into ligated segments of rabbit small bowel. The bowel was replaced in the abdominal cavity and the skin wound closed. Fluid accumulation was measured after 18 hours. Each point represents data from 4 rabbits.

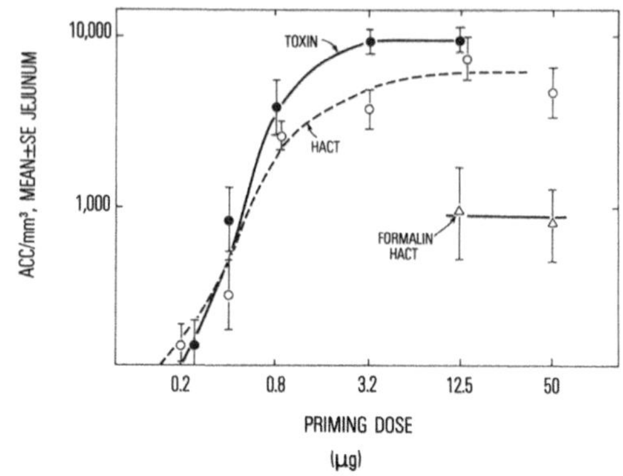

Fig. 4. Immunogenicity of purified cholera toxin, heat-aggregated cholera toxin (HACT), and formalin-treated HACT. Rats were given an intraduodenal priming dose of antigen as indicated. Two weeks later all rats were boosted intraduodenally with 12.5 µg CT. Jejunal biopsies were taken 5 days later and scored for ACC. Each point represents data from 6-7 rats.

suggests that residual "toxin" in HACT is less efficient at causing fluid secretion, perhaps due to competition for mucosal binding sites by B subunit. Whatever the explanation, these results suggest that HACT may be a safe oral immunogen.

HACT was first tested as a mucosal immunogen in rats. Varying amounts of HACT or CT were used for intraduodenal priming. Fourteen days later all rats were boosted intraduodenally with a standard dose of CT and jejunal biopsies were obtained 5 days later. The results (Figure 4) thus compare the ability of these antigens to prime for a mucosal antitoxin response. It is apparent that HACT was only slightly less effective than

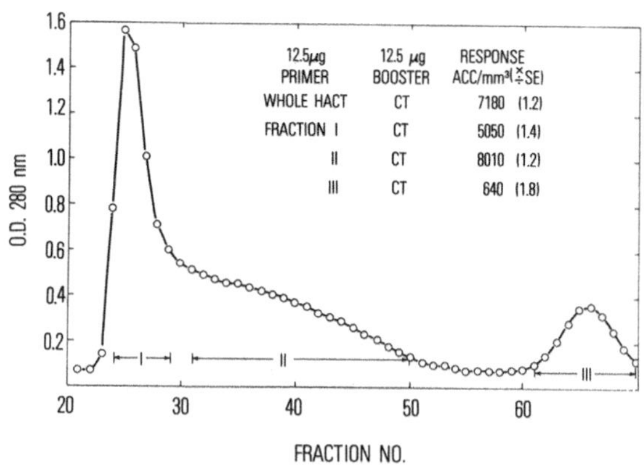

Fig. 5. Immunogenicity of chromatographically separated fractions of heat-aggregated cholera toxin (HACT). HACT was chromatographed on Sepharose 4BCL. The resultant chromatographic pattern is shown. Three fraction pools were prepared. Rats were primed intraduodenally with 12.5 µg of purified CT or one of the pools. Two weeks later all rats were boosted intraduodenally with 12.5 µg CT. Jejunal biopsies were taken 5 days later and scored for ACC. Geometric mean ACC responses are shown. Each mean represents data from 6-7 rats.

CT as a primary mucosal immunogen. In contrast, formalinized HACT, which had no residual toxic activity, was much less effective.

Because HACT contains a mixture of heat-induced aggregates of CT plus small amounts of B subunit, it was of interest to know which molecular species accounted for its ability to evoke a mucosal immune response. Figure 5 shows the chromatographic pattern obtained by filtration of HACT through sepharose 4BCL. The major peak and shoulder on the left represent various aggregated forms of CT and the smaller peak on the right contains B subunit. The immunogenicity of these differing materials was tested by creating 3 fraction pools as shown and using similar doses of each for primary intraduodenal immunization of rats. The mucosal antitoxin responses obtained after intraduodenal boosting with CT on day 14 are sown in the box. It is apparent that fractions I and II, containing aggregated CT, were equally effective and accounted for the immunogenicity of HACT. In contrast, fraction III was less than 10 % as effective and probably contributed little to the immunogenicity of HACT. Although previous studies have suggested that membrane binding and adenylate cyclase activation contribute substantially to the immunogenicity of CT (3), this observation suggests that molecular aggregation also promotes mucosal immunogenicity.

Finally, we have studied HACT as an oral immunogen in dogs. In this study dogs were given 500 μg oral doses of HACT over a 56 day period. Results in Table 3 show that 3 % of dogs had a small diarrheal stool during the 18 hours after oral immunization. This does not differ from the 4 % incidence observed in dogs given only casamino acids and $NaHCO_3$ orally (Table 2). Jejunal biopsies taken 7 days after immunization showed

Table 3. Oral immunization with heat aggregated cholera toxin: outcome of challenge.

	Control Dogs		Immunized Dogs[a]
ACC/mm^3, Jejunum[b] mean ($\bar{x}$ SE)	–		11,000 (1.2)
Challenge outcome:[c]			
No diarrhea	5		11
Mild-moderate diarrhea	3		1
Severe-lethal diarrhea	5		1
		P = 0.05	
First 18 hr stool volume mean, ml/kg	29		6.9

a 500 μg HACT by mouth on days 0, 21, 42, 49, 56.
b Biopsies taken on day 62.
c Challenge = 10^{11} Ogawa 395, Day 77.

vigorous mucosal antitoxin responses that compared favorably with those observed after oral immunization with the largest doses of purified or crude CT. And challenge with live vibrios 3 weeks after immunization showed 75–80 % protection against diarrhea which was statistically significant at the 0.05 level (Table 3).

These results show that HACT is both safe and highly effective as an oral immunogen in dogs. Among the various toxin-related antigens studied, it is the only one that has *both* of these qualities. Although antitoxic immunity alone is not likely to provide optimal protection against cholera, the present results suggest it makes an important contribution to synergistic protection. The evidence that antitoxic immunity can be safely and efficiently evoked using HACT suggests that this antigen combined with other nontoxic antigens of *V. cholerae* may constitute a simple, effective and safe means of oral immunization against cholera. Although the use of a nonliving vaccine is only one of the currently studied approaches to oral immunization against cholera, these studies suggest this approach may be both practical and provide substantial, lasting protection.

This work was supported by research grant 1 PO1 AI 14480 and research contract NO1 AI 92601, both from the National institute of Allergy and Infectious Disease, NIH. Research facilities were provided by the Gerontology Research Center, National Institute of Aging, NIH, under its Guest Scientist Program.

REFERENCES

1. Pierce, N. F. The experimental basis for oral immunization against cholera. In: Current Topics in Veterinary Medicine and Animal Science, Vol 12., The mucosal Immune System, F. J. Bourne (Editor), Martinus Nijhoff Publishers, The Hague, Netherlands, 1981, pp. 461-484.
2. Levine, M. M., Black, R. E., Clements, M. L., Young, C. R., Honda, T. and Finkelstein, R. A. Texas Star - SR. Attenuated *Vibrio cholerae* oral vaccine candidate. In: New Perspectives in Clinical Microbiology, Advances in Research on Cholera and Related Diarrheas, S. Kuwahara and N. F. Pierce (Editors), KTK Scientific Publishers, Tokyo/Martinus Nijhoff Publishers, The Hague, 1983.
3. Pierce, N. F., Cray, W. C. Jr., Engel, P. F. 1980. Antitoxic immunity to cholera in dogs immunized orally with cholera toxin. Infect. and Immun. **27**:632-637.
4. Pierce, N. F. 1978. The role of antigen form and function in the primary and secondary intestinal immune responses to cholera toxin and toxoid in rats. J. Exp. Med. **148**:195-206.
5. Fuhrman, J. A., Cebra, J. J. 1981. Special features of the priming process for a secretory IgA response. B cell priming with cholera toxin. J. Exp. Med. **153**:534-544.
6. Pierce, N. F., Gowans, J. L. 1975. Cellular kinetics of the intestinal immune response to cholera toxoid in rats. J. Exp. Med. **142**:1550-1563.
7. Svennerholm, A-M., Holmgren, J. 1976. Synergistic protective effect in rabbits of immunization with *Vibrio cholerae* lipopolysaccharide and toxin/toxoid. Infect. and Immun. **13**:735-740.
8. Rappaport, R. S., Bonde, G., McCann, T., Rubin, B. A., and Tint, H. 1974. Development of a purified cholera toxoid. II. Preparation of a stable, antigenic toxoid by reaction of purified toxin with glutaraldehyde. Infect. and Immun. **9**:304-317.
9. Finkelstein, R. A., LoSpalluto, J. J. 1969. Pathogenesis of experimental cholera. Preparation and isolation of choleragen and choleragenoid. J. Exp. Med. **130**:185-202.
10. Fujita, K., Finkelstein, R. A. 1972. Antitoxic immunity in experimental cholera: Comparison of immunity induced perorally and parenterally in mice. J. Infect. Dis. **125**:647-655.
11. Peterson, J. W. 1979. Protection against experimental cholera by oral or parenteral immunization. Infect. and Immun. **26**:594-598.

Advances in Research on Cholera and Related Diarrheas, eds., S. Kuwahara, N. F. Pierce, 49–55.

TEXAS STAR-SR: ATTENUATED VIBRIO CHOLERAE ORAL VACCINE CANDIDATE

Myron M. Levine,[1] Robert E. Black,[1] Mary Lou Clements,[1] Charles R. Young,[1] Takeshi Honda,[2] and Richard Finkelstein[3]

The Center for Vaccine Development,[1] University of Maryland School of Medicine, Baltimore, Maryland, The Research Institute for Microbial Disease,[2] Osaka, Japan, The Department of Microbiology, University of Missouri School of Medicine, Columbia, Missouri[3]

The search continues for a cholera vaccine that is both safe and highly protective for a long duration. Experimental cholera challenge studies in volunteers with *Vibrio cholerae* Ogawa and Inaba strains of the classical biotype have demonstrated that an initial clinical cholera infection provides solid clinical and bacteriologic protection against re-challenge with either the homologous or heterologous serotype.[1–4] Significant protection was found to persist for at least three years, the longest interval tested.[4] The rare isolation of vibrios from stool or jejunal fluid cultures of re-challenged volunteers and the infrequency of significant rises in serum or intestinal fluid antitoxin infer that antibacterial immune mechanisms limited proliferation of vibrios before they could produce enterotoxin.[2–4] These observations suggest that one promising approch toward immunologic control of cholera could be by way of development of attenuated, non-enterotoxinogenic *V. cholerae* strains employed as oral vaccines.

An ideal oral attenuated vaccine strain would be : 1) non-reactogenic; 2) genetically stable; 3) proliferative and adhesive in the proximal small bowel; 4) inductive of local antibody of both anti-colonizing and anti-subunit B activity; 5) stimulative of long-term protection after only one or two doses.

No naturally-occurring or laboratory-derived *V. cholerae* stain yet identified fulfills all these criteria. However, Texas Star-SR, the attenuated mutant prepared by Honda and Finkelstein,[5] exhibits many of the aforementioned qualities and has therefore served an invaluable role as a prototype in our studies of immunity to cholera. Texas Star-SR was obtained by nitrosoguanidine mutagenesis of El Tor Ogawa strain 3083.[5] Clones were painstakingly assayed until a stable clone was identified that produced copious amounts of B subunit but undetectable quantities of A Subunit. Texas Star-SR was shown to be negative in a number of assays for holotoxin.

Volunteers who participated in these clinical studies included college students and other community adults. The study was explained in detail and in order to ensure the informed nature of consent volunteers were required to pass a written examination covering all aspects of the clinical protocol. The studies were carried out under quarantine in our 22 bed Isolation Ward within the Univeristy of Maryland Hospital. All volunteers

Table 1. Clinical response of volunteers following ingestion of attenuated *Vibrio cholerae* el tor Ogawa strain Texas star-sr.

Dose (with $NAHCO_3$)	No. Volunteers	No. with Diarrhea (%)	Mean No. Diarrheal Stools per Ill volunteer	Mean Diarrheal Stool Volume (ML,)
10^5	14	3 (21)	4.7 (2-6)*	871 (340-1464)*
10^6	8	0	0	0
10^8	5	2 (40)	4.0 (3-5)	349 (339-358)
10^{10}	6	1 (17)	2.0	310
$5x10^{10}$	9	2 (22)	3.0 (2-4)	536 (413-659)
10^9 (Two doses one week apart)	8	2^+(25)	2.0	268 (261-275)
Totals	50	10 (20%)	3.1 (2-6)	523 (261-1464)

*(Range) +Diarrhea followed the first dose only

received a five day course of tetracycline and had negative stool cultures for *V. cholerae* prior to discharge.

Single doses of 10^5, 10^6, 10^8, 10^{10} or $5X10^{10}$ Texas Star-SR organisms with $NaHCO_3$ were ingested by a total of 42 volunteers (Table 1); eight others ingested two doses of 10^9 organisms one week apart (Table 1). Ten of the 50 vaccinees manifested loose stools meeting our definition of diarrhea. We define diarrhea as either: 1) three or more loose stools within 48 hours irrespective of volume; 2) two or more loose stools within 48 hours surpassing 200 ml in total volume; 3) or one loose stool if greater than 300 ml in volume. Each stool passed by each volunteer is examined, weighed and graded by consistency. Grades 3-5 comprise variants of loose stools.

Diarrhea was found to be unrelated to the dose of vaccine organisms ingested and was not accompanied by cramps, malaise, nausea, fever or anorexia. In only one instance did the total diarrheal stool volume exceed 1.0 liter (Table 2); this individual passed six loose stools over a two day period. In most instances the diarrheal response consisted of two loose stools rarely exceeding 400 ml in total volume (Table 2). When measured by the highly sensitive IgG-ELISA technique, significant rises in serum antitoxin occurred at the same rate in vaccinees with diarrhea (4/10) as in those who did not manifest diarrhea (11/40).

Texas Star-SR was recovered from stool cultures in only 22% of those who ingested 10^5 or 10^6 vibrios but in at least 60% of those who ingested 10^8 or more vibrios (Table 3); 10^2-10^3 vibrios per gm of stool were usually found. Jejunal fluid for culture was obtained 20 and 44 hours post-ingestion in volunteers who received higher doses of vaccine, i.e. 10^8 or greater. Texas Star was isolated from 70% of these vaccinees (Table 3). It is of interest that in the eight volunteers who ingested two 10^9 organism doses of Texas Star one week apart, the strain was recovered from 6/8 following the initial dose but from 0/8 following the second dose (p=0.05), suggesting that the first dose had already stimulated an antibacterial mechanism. Quantitative cultures of jejunal fluids revealed 10^2-10^6 vibrios per ml. Hundreds of clones recovered from jejunal fluid and

Table 2. Clinical pattern in nine vaccinees who developed diarrhea following ingestion of attenuated *Vibrio cholerae* Texas star-sr.

Vaccine dose	Incubation period (HRS.)	Total diarrheal stool volume (ML)	No. loose stools	Loose stools per day of observation 0	+1	+2	+3	+4	Significant rise in serum antitoxin (ELISA)
10^5	46	1464	6	0	2	4	0	0	+
10^5	24	808	6	1	1	0	2	2	–
$5x10^{10}$	42.5	659	4	0	2	1	0	1	–
$5x10^{10}$	17	413	2	2	0	0	0	0	+
10^8	21	358	5	2	2	1	0	0	+
10^5	67	340	2	0	0	1	1	0	–
10^8	48	339	4	0	0	3	0	1	–
10^{10}	44	310	2	0	1	0	1	0	–
10^9*	92	275	2	0	0	0	1	1	+
10^9*	99	261	2	0	0	0	0	2	–

*Diarrhea followed the first of two doses

coprocultures have been examined for the presence of cholera enterotoxin by Y-1 adrenal cell assay; all clones were negative.

At all dosage levels, Texas Star stimulated prominent vibriocidal antibody responses in 90% of vaccinees (Table 4); resultant titers were as high as those seen following clinical cholera. In contrast, while almost all volunteers manifest significant rises in circulating antitoxin following infection with pathogenic *V. cholerae*, such rises were seen in only 11 of 42 recipients of one dose of Texas Star and in only 4 of 8 recipients of two doses (Table 4). Furthermore, the levels of antitoxin attained were low. Samples of jejunal fluid obtained from 18 volunteers prior to and eight days following ingestion of Texas Star were tested for SIgA antitoxin; 5 of 18 (28%) manifested significant rises (Table 4).

Three challenge studies have been carried out so far in recipients of Texas Star-SR:

Table 3. Bacteriologic results in recipients of low and high doses of attenuated *Vibrio cholerae* el tor Ogawa Texas star-sr.

Vaccine dose (with $NAHCO_3$)	No. Immunized	Stool cultures: No. positive(%)	Stool cultures: Vibrios PER GM	Jejunal fluid cultures: No. positive (%)	Jejunal fluid cultures: Vibrios pER GM
10^5, 10^6	22	4 (22)			
10^8, 10^{10}, $5x10^{10}$	20	12 (60)	10^2-10^3	14 (70)	10^2-10^5
		Dose #1 Dose #2		Dose #1 Dose #2	
10^9 (Two doses one week apart)	8	5 (63) 1 (13)	10^2-10^6	6 (75) 0	10^2-10^5
				p=0.05	

Table 4. Immunologic response of volunteers following ingestion of varying doses of attenuated *Vibrio cholerae* strain Texas star-sr.

Vaccine dose (with $NAHCO_3$)	No. Inoculated	No. with significant rises in antibody (%): Serum Vibriocidal	Serum antitoxin ELISA	Intestinal SIGA antitoxin ELISA
10^5, 10^6	22	19 (86)	5 (23)	NA*
10^8, 10^{10}, $5x10^{10}$	20	18 (90)	6 (30)	5/18 (28)
10^9 (Two doses one week apart)	8	8 (100)	4 (50)	

*Intestinal fluids not available for testing

Challenge Study #1

Four to six weeks following ingestion of a single dose of 10^8 or 10^{10} Texas Star vibrios, eight vaccinees and four controls ingested 10^6 organisms of El Tor Ogawa strain 3083, the toxigenic, presumably pathogenic, strain from which Texas Star had been derived. Surprisingly, although all controls excreted *V. cholerae* and had rises in serum vibriocidal and antitoxic antibody, none developed diarrhea (Table 5). Among the Texas Star recipients 2 of 8 had positive coprocultures and one of eight had a rise in antibody. These observations show that the parent strain was of diminished pathogenicity although it produced complete cholera toxin. Further studies with 3083 will be necessary to clarify this point.

Challenge Study #2

In the second challenge study seven vaccinees who ingested a single $5X10^{10}$ organism dose of Texas Star two months earlier were challenged with known pathogenic El Tor Ogawa strain E7946 (Table 6). Diarrhea occurred in 7 of 10 controls but in only 2 of 7 vaccinees. Despite significant clinical protection, *V. cholerae* were isolated from coprocultures of six of seven vaccinees, although the mean level of excretion was three logs lower than the controls (Table 6).

Table 5. Clinical, bacteriologic and immunologic response of texas star vaccinees and controls to challenge with 10^6 wild el tor Ogawa 3083.

			No. with positive cultures		Significant antibody rises	Circulating	
	N	No. with diarrhea	stool	Jejunal fluid	Vibrio cidal	Elisa anti-toxin	Adrenal cell anti-toxin
Controls	4	0/4	4/4	2/4	4/4	4/4	4/4
Vaccinees †	8	0/8	2/8	0/4	1/8	1/8	1/8

† 4-6 weeks post-immunization with one dose (10^8-10^{10}) texas star
* p=0.05 (2 tailed fisher's exact test)

Table 6. Clinical and bacteriologic response of texas star vaccinees and controls following ingestion of 10^6 pathogenic *Vibrio cholerae* el tor Ogawa E7946.

				Excretion of V. cholerae:			
Group	N	Clinical attack rate	Mean No. loose stools per ill volunteer	Mean diarrheal stool volume (leters)	Direct culture	Enrichment	Quantitative Corproculture (Vibrios per GM stool)
controls	10	7/10	14	2.1 (0.7-3.4)	9/10	9/10	10^7
vaccinees	7	2/7	2	0.3 (0.2-0.4)	8/10	9/10	10^4

Challenge Study #3

In the third challenge study six vaccinees who had received two 10^9 organism doses of Texas Star seven weeks earlier and eight unimmunized control volunteers were challenged with 10^6 *V. cholerae* El Tor Inaba Nl6961. In this heterologous challenge study diarrhea occurred in 6 of 8 controls but in only 2 of 6 vaccinees (Table 7); although a trend was clearly apparent, these differences in attack rate were not statistically significant. Rises in both antitoxin and vibriocidal antibody occurred more frequently in controls than in vaccinees.

In summary, attenuated *V. cholerae* strain Texas Star was found to be well tolerated by 80% of recipients, while 20% manifested mild diarrhea. The strain readily colonized the proximal small bowel and no enterotoxigenic vibrios were detected among hundreds of coproculture clones tested. Serum vibriocidal responses occurred at the same rate and magnitude as with infection due to pathogenic *V. cholerae*. Despite the ability of Texas Star to elaborate copious amounts of B subunit in vitro antitoxin responses were uncommon and meager. Even a single dose of Texas Star provided significant protection against challenge with the homologous (Ogawa) serotype. The vaccine, however, provided only 56% efficacy against challenge with the heterologous (Inaba) serotype.

Table 7. Clinical and bacteriologic response of texas star vaccinees and controls following ingestion of 10^6 *Vibrio cholerae* el tor Inaba N16961.

				Significant rises in circulating antibody:	
Group	Clinical attack rate	Mean diarrheal stool volume (liters)	Positive coprocultures	antitoxin	Vibriocidal
controls	6/8	4.8	8/8	7/8	8/8
		$P<0.10$			
vaccinees	2/6	1.1	6/6	3/6	3/6

Table 8. Clinical, bacteriologic and serologic response following ingestion of non-toxigenic CFA/II-positive *escherichia coli* vaccine candidate strain E1392/75 2A.

Vaccine Dose (with NAHCO3)	Diarrhea Attack rate	Positive cultures: Stool	Jejunal fluid	Circulating antibody: Anti-CFA/II	Anti-0
10^9	0/4	4/4	1/4	0/4	2/4
10^{10}	*1/4	4/4	2/4	2/4	3/4

*Four loose stools totalling 240 ML.

Three questions, in particular, arise from these initial studies:

1) What mechanism is responsible for the mild diarrhea seen in 20% of vaccine recipients? 2) How disappointed should we be that vaccine efficacy was only 56% in the heterologous challenge? 3) What is the role of the B subunit in contributing to the protection observed?

We believe that the mild diarrhea encountered in 20% of Texas Star recipients is due to colonization of the proximal small bowel by a highly adhesive organism and has nothing to do with toxin. Some years ago British workers studying *E. coli* in pigs reported similar observations.[6] Mild but definite diarrhea occurred when newborn piglets were fed an *E. coli* strain that lacked enterotoxin but possessed K88 antigen pili which allowed them to adhere to small bowel mucosa.[6] Similarly, we recently fed a non-enterotoxigenic *E. coli* strain that produces CFA/II pili; mild diarrhea occurred in 1 of 8 recipients (Table 8), similar to our experience with Texas Star. These observations suggest that mild diarrhea in a minority of recipients is the price we shall have to pay for immunizing orally with any vaccine strain that adheres well to proximal small bowel mucosa.

In order to put the protective efficacy of Texas Star into proper perspective we must compare it with the ability of pathogenic El Tor vibrios to protect against re-challenge with El Tor vibrios of the homologous and heterologous serotype. To date large cohort studies have not yet been carried out with El Tor as they have been with classical vibrios. However, sporadic re-challenges with El Tor involving a total of six volunteers

Table 9. Clinical and bacteriologic response in six volunteers following serotype homologous and heterologous re-challenge with *vibrio cholerae* el tor.

Initial challenge strain	Re-Challenge strain	Re-Challenge results: Clinical Attack rate	Positive Stool culture
Inaba N16961	Inaba N16961	0/2*	0/2
Inaba P27459	Inaba P27459	0/1	1/1
Inaba N16961	Inaba P27459	1/1	1/1
Ogawa N15870	Inaba P27459	0/2	0/2
	Tatal	1/6	2/6

*No. positive/No. volunteers challenged

have taken place.[3] Among these six persons who experienced an initial episode of El Tor cholera and who were re-challenged, 2 of 6 had positive cultures and one had diarrhea (Table 9). Thus when viewed in this light, the occurrence of diarrhea in 2 of 6 Texas Star vaccinees following challenge with El Tor vibrios of the heterologous serotype is quite encouraging. Heretofore most attention has been directed toward lipopolysaccharide and toxin antigens in considering immunity to *V. cholerae*. Research should proceed to identify other anitgens of *V. cholerae* 01 that may differ from strain to strain and that may be important in protection. Such antigens may include outer membrane proteins, flagellar sheath material and lectins.

One way to determine the role of B subunit in protection is to feed two attenuated strains identical except for the presence of B subunit. Such strains are currently being prepared by Dr. James Kaper in our group. Dr. Kaper has recently cloned the genes for cholera enterotoxin as well as mapped the genes for the individual subunits.[7] Thus by application of recombinant DNA techniques we intend to prepare El Tor strains with and without B subunit that will allow us to study antibacterial immunity and the enhancing effect if any of B subunit.

In our studies of the feasibility of mimicking infection-derived immunity to cholera by use of attenuated strains as oral vaccines, Texas Star, the mutant strain prepared by Honda and Finkelstein, has played a pathfinding role as a prototype.

REFERENCES

1. Cash, R. A., Music, S. I., Libonati, J. P., Snyder, M. J., Wenzel, R. P., Hornick, R. B. 1974. Response of man to infection with *Vibrio cholerae*. II. Protection from illness afforded by previous disease and vaccine. J. Infect. Dis. **130**:325-333.
2. Levine, M M., Nalin, D. R., Craig, J. P., Hoover, D., Bergquist, E. J., Waterman, D., Holley, H. p., Hornick, R. B., Pierce, N. P., Libonati, J. P. 1979. Immunity to cholera in man: relative role of antibacterial versus antitoxic immunity. Trans. Roy. Soc. Trop Med. Hyg. **73**:3-9.
3. Levine, M. M. 1980. Immunity to cholera as evaluated in volunteers. *In* O. Ouchterlony and J. Holmgren (eds.). Cholera and related diarrheas. Karger, Basel, pp. 195-203.
4. Levine, M. M., Black, R. E., Clements, M. L., Cisneros, L., Nalin, D. R., Young, C. R. 1981. Duration of infection-derived immunity to cholera. J. Infect. Dis. **143**:818-820.
5. Honda, T., Finkelstein, R. A. 1979. Selection and characteristics of a *Vibrio cholerae* mutant lacking he A(ADP-ribosylating) portion of the cholera enterotoxin. Proc, Nat. Acad. Sci. USA **76**: 2052-2056.
6. Smith, H. W., Linggood, M. A. 1971. Observations on the pathogenic properties of the K88, Hly and Ent plasmids of *Escherichia coli* with particular reference to porcine diarrhoea. J. Med. Microbiol. **4**:467-486.
7. Kaper, J. B., Levine, M. M. 1981. Cloned cholera enterotoxin genes in study and prevention of cholera. Lancet **II**:1162-1163.

BACTERIOLOGY AND VIRULENCE FACTORS

Advances in Research on Cholera and Related Diarrheas, eds., S. Kuwahara, N. F. Pierce, 59–74.

SUGAR COMPOSITION OF LIPOPOLYSACCHARIDES OF FAMILY *VIBRIONACEAE* –ABSENCE OF 2-KETO-3-DEOXYOCTONATE (KDO) WITH THE EXCEPTION OF *VIBRIO PARAHAEMOLYTICUS* 06 AND *PLESIOMONAS SHIGELLOIDES*–

Kazuhito Hisatsune, Seiichi Kondo, Takehiro Iguchi, Masaaki Machida, Shinobu Asou, Makoto Inaguma and Fumihiro Yamamoto

Department of Microbiology, School of Pharmaceutical Sciences, Josai University, Sakado, Saitama 350-02, Japan

Extensive studies on the chemistry of 0-antigenic lipopolysaccharides (LPS) of *Enterobacteriaceae* have been made (52), and chemotaxonomy based on the sugar composition of LPS was subsequently established for *Salmonella* and *Escherichia coli* (22, 24). In contrast, very few studies have been reported with *Vibrionaceae* from the chemotaxonomical point of view on the basis of the sugar composition of LPS while the chemical properties of LPS from *V. cholerae* (14, 15, 16, 17, 18, 29, 30, 35, 37, 39, 40) have been relatively well documented. The sugar composition of 0-antigenic LPS from a representative strain of each of 12 0-serotypes of *V. parahaemolyticus* was elucidated recently by two research groups, Hisatsune and his colleagues (12) and Miwatani's group (26). Both groups divided *V. parahaemolyticus* in almost the same fashion, the former into nine and the latter into eight chemotypes. With regard to 0-antigenic LPS from members of *Vibrionaceae* other than *V. cholerae* as well as *V. parahaemolyticus*, two comparative studies of the sugar composition of LPS were recently carried out, one on group F vibrios and *Aeromonas* (19) and the other on *V. alginolyticus* and *V. parahaemolyticus* (13). Through the latter study, it was found that 2-keto-3-deoxyoctonate (KDO), known generally as a regular component sugar present in gram-negative bacterial LPS, is lacking in the LPS of both *V. alginolyticus* and *V. parahaemolyticus* with the exception of *V. parahaemolyticus* 06 LPS. Furthermore, some KDO-like thiobarbituric acid test-positive substances were shown to be present in LPS from *V. parahaemolyticus* 07 and 012, and also in three strains of *V. alginolyticus*.

According to Bergey's Manual of Determinative Bacteriology (8th edition) (5), the family *Vibrionaceae* consists of five genera, *Vibrio Aeromonas, Lucibacterium, Photobacterium* and *Plesiomonas.* The present study describes the results of a comparative study on the sugar composition of LPS isolated from representative strains of the members of *Vibrionaceae.* More than one hundred strains were examined, many of which are type or neotype strains or those recommended as working strains in Bergey's Manual of

Determinative Bacteriology (8th edition) (5). It was demonstrated for the first time that, except in LPS of *V. parahaemolyticus* 06 and *Pl. shigelloides*, KDO is lacking in LPS of all members of the *Vibrionaceae* so far examined. Instead, just as in LPS from *V. parahaemolyticus* 07 and 012 (12) and *V. alginolyticus* (13), some KDO-like thiobarbituric acid test-positive substances were found to be present in LPS from *Vibrio* ("*Beneckea*") (3) *nereida* and type strain (ATCC 14029) of *Plesiomonas shigelloides* examined. The present results are compatible with the interpretation that the absence of KDO in LPS is considered to be one of the taxonomical characteristics of *Vibrionaceae.*

Bacterial strains The sources of most of the bacterial strains employed in this study are listed in the footnote to Table 1. *Salmonella minnesota* R595 as a source of authentic 4-amino-4-deoxy-L-arabinose was provided by Dr. N. Kasai, Department of Microbiology, School of Pharmaceutical Sciences, Showa University, Tokyo, and *Pseudomonas fluorescense* (NCTC 10038) by the Type Culture Collection Center, Institute of Medical Sciences, Tokyo University, Tokyo.

Growth of cells The microbes were grown in liquid medium under vigorous shaking for 16-32 hr at temperature appropriate for each strain as listed in Tables 1 and 2. The cultures, with the exception of those of *V. parahaemolyticus* and *V. alginolyticus*, were killed, before being harvested, by exposure to a final concentration of 0.5% phenol (w/v) at room temperature for 2 hr, and then the harvested cells were acetone-dried. In the case of *V. parahaemolyticus* as well as *V. alginolyticus*, the cultures were heated at 100°C for 2 hr, before being extracted with phenol-water, as described in our previous papers (12, 13) according to Shimouchi's method (42) to avoid contamination of LPS by K-antigens. However, no difference was virtually found in the sugar composition between purified LPS from the phenol-killed and heat-killed cells, even in the cases of *V. parahaemolyticus* and *V. alginolyticus* when LPS was purified as described in this paper. Since dilute phenol-treatment of the cultures at room temperature was considered to be much milder than the heat-treatment and, therefore, much more adequate in order to avoid or minimize the probable loss or destruction of heat-labile components or linkages in LPS molecule, if any, the phenol-killed cells without the heat-treatment were used for extraction of LPS in this study. The following media were used: broth medium (pH 8.0) for *V. cholerae* (01 and non-01 groups and R-mutants); broth medium (pH 7.2-7.4) for *V. proteus* (NCTC 8563), *V. metchnikovii* (NCTC 2443), *V. albensis* (NCMB41), *A. hydrophila* and *A. punctata*; broth medium (pH 7.2-7.4) containing 2% NaCl for *A. salmonicida*, *V. anguillarum*, *V. fischeri* (NCMB 1143), *V. costicola* (NCMB 701), *V. harveyi* (ATCC 14126), group F vibrios (*V. fluvialis*), lactose-positive vibrios (*V. vulnificus*) and *Vibrio* ("*Beneckea*") *nereida*; and broth medium (pH 7.4) containing 3% NaCl for *V. parahaemolyticus*, and *V. alginolyticus. Plesiomonas shigelloides* strains were grown in a liquid medium (pH 6.0) containing heart infusion (0.5%), yeast extract (1.5%), peptone (1.5%) and NaCl (2%).

Preparation of LPS LPS was isolated from the acetone-dried cells by the phenol-water technique of Westphal et al. (48) and purified by repeated ultracentrifugation (105,000 x g, 3 hr, 6 times) and treatment with ribonuclease (20 μg/ml in 25 mM Tris-HCl buffer, pH 7.4) (9, 49). LPS of rough mutants was prepared from the acetone-dried cells by the phenol-chloroform-petroleum ether method of Galanos et al. (11) and purified as described above. The LPS preparations from *V. parahaemolyticus* and *V. alginolyticus* were examined for contamination of K-antigen by the double diffusion gel-precipitation technique, with K-antisera (Toshiba Chemical Co., Tokyo). No contamination of K-antigens was found.

Analytical methods Neutral sugars except fructose were determined after hydrolysis in 2 N trifluoroacetic acid at 120°C for 1 hr by gas-liquid chromatography as alditol acetates according to the method of Laine et al. (21) (column: 3% ECNSS-M coated on Chromosorb W, 3 mm x 2 m) with xylose used as an internal standard. Fructose was determined after hydrolysis in 0.2 M acetic acid at 100°C for 8 hr by gas-liquid chromatography as 0-acetylated-0-methyloxime derivatives prepared according to the method of Mawhinney et al. (25), on the ECNSS-M column. For amino sugar determination, LPS was hydrolyzed in 4 N HCl at 100°C for 8 hr, and the hydrolysates were fractionated on a Dowex 50 (X8, H^+) column according to the method of Wheat (50). The amino sugar fraction thus separated was N-acetylated according to the method of Hakomori (21). Amino sugars were then determined as N-acetyl-alditol acetates by gas-liquid chromatography (column: TABSORB (Regis Chemical Co., Morton Grove, Illinois, U.S.A.), 3 mm x 2 m). The identities of the neutral and amino sugars were based on retention time values and mass spectra compared to those of the derivatives of authentic standards. Gas-liquid chromatography/mass spectrometry was performed on an LKB model 9000S instrument (LKB Instrument Inc., Uppsala, Sweden) with the same column as described above.

Heptose was determined either by the method of Osborn (27) or by gasliquid chromatography. Standard L-glycero-D-mannoheptose and D-glycero-D-mannoheptose were prepared as described by Bagdian et al. (2). KDO and the KDO-like substances were estimated by the method of Weissbach and Hurwitz (47). KDO purchased from Sigma Chemical Co. (St. Louis, Missouri, U.S.A.) was used as a standard.

For high-voltage paper electrophoresis of KDO and the KDO-like substance, LPS was hydrolyzed in 5% acetic acid at 100°C for 2 hr. After centrifugation of the hydrolysates, the supernatants were dried under reduced pressure and dissolved in small amounts of water. Electrophoresis was performed on Whatman No. 1 paper with the solvent system pyridine/acetic acid/water, 10:4:86 (v/v/v), pH 5.3, at 45 v/cm for 40 min. On paper electrophoregrams and thin-layer chromatograms, KDO and the KDO-like substances were detected with a thiobarbituric acid reagent (46).

The results of the sugar analyses are presented in Tables 1 and 2. The list of strains in Table 1 represents the classification of the family *Vibrionaceae* in Bergey's Manual of Determinative Bacteriology (8th edition) (5) except some strains listed.

Absence of KDO and presence of KDO-like substances. A striking feature was demonstrated with the sugar composition of *Vibrionaceae* LPS. KDO, a regular component sugar of gram-negative bacterial LPS, was virtually absent from LPS of all of the *Vibrionaceae* strains tested, except in LPS of *V. parahaemolyticus* 06 and *Pl. shigelloides.* This finding was confirmed by gas-liquid chromatographic analysis on a TABSORB column. KDO is generally released from LPS of gram-negative bacteria by heating with mild acetic acid (0.1 M, 100°C for 2 hr). When an authentic KDO standard or the KDO--containing fraction thus isolated from LPS of *V. parahaemolyticus* 06 and *Pl. shigelloides* was reduced with $NaBH_4$, and then peracetylated according to the method of preparation of an alditol acetates of neutral sugars, both resultant acetates yielded, in gas-liquid chromatography, the identical peaks whose $Rt_{mannose}$ (retention time relative to mannose) were 7.13 and 8.87. In contrast, however, no acetate derivative yielding the correspond-

Table 1. Sugar composition of lipopolysaccharides isolated from *Vibrionaceae*.

Strain	Carbohydrate																	Unknown amino sugar				Obtained from[f]	Growth temperature (°C)
	Glc	Gal	Man	Fru	Rha	Ara	Fuc	Hep L-D	Hep D-D	KDO	KDO-like	GlcN	GalN	ManN	FucN	QuiN	PerN	P1	P2	P3	Y		
Vibrio																							
1. V. cholerae																							
1a. biotype cholerae																							
Inaba 35A3[a]	+	-	-	+	-	-	-	+	-	-	-	+	-	-	-	+	+	-	-	-	-	(1)	37
569B	+	-	-	+	-	-	-	+	-	-	-	+	-	-	-	+	+	-	-	-	-	(2)	37
P1418-UV401	+	-	-	+	-	-	-	+	-	-	-	+	-	-	-	+	+	-	-	-	-	(3)	37
Ogawa NIH 41[a]	+	-	-	+	-	-	-	+	-	-	-	+	-	-	-	+	+	-	-	-	-	(4)	37
NIH 90	+	-	-	+	-	-	-	+	-	-	-	+	-	-	-	+	+	-	-	-	-	(4)	37
P1418	+	-	-	+	-	-	-	+	-	-	-	+	-	-	-	+	+	-	-	-	-	(3)	37
NAG 03 4715[b]	+	+	-	+	-	-	-	+	+	-	-	+	-	-	-	-	-	-	-	-	+	(5)	37
722-75	+	+	-	+	-	-	-	+	+	-	-	+	-	-	-	-	-	-	-	-	+	(5)	37
05	+	-	-	+	-	-	-	+	-	-	-	+	-	-	-	-	-	-	-	-	-	(5)	37
07	+	+	-	+	-	-	-	+	-	-	-	+	-	-	-	-	-	-	-	-	-	(5)	37
08	+	-	-	+	-	-	-	+	-	-	-	+	-	-	-	-	-	-	-	-	-	(5)	37
R-mutant 35A3-R[a]	+	-	-	+	-	-	-	+	-	-	-	+	-	-	-	-	-	-	-	-	-	(5)	37
NIH 41-R	+	-	-	+	-	-	-	+	-	-	-	+	-	-	-	-	-	-	-	-	-	(5)	37
P1418-R	+	-	-	+	-	-	-	+	-	-	-	+	-	-	-	-	-	-	-	-	-	(3)	37
CA 385	+	-	-	+	-	-	-	+	-	-	-	+	-	-	-	-	-	-	-	-	-	(5)	37

	4715-R	+	+	-	+	-	-	-	+	-	-	-	+	-	-	-	-	-	-	-	-	-	(5)	37
	05-R	+	-	-	+	-	-	-	+	-	-	-	+	-	-	-	-	-	-	-	-	-	(5)	37
	07-R	+	-	-	+	-	-	-	+	-	-	-	+	-	-	-	-	-	-	-	-	-	(5)	37
	08-R	+	-	-	+	-	-	-	+	-	-	-	+	-	-	-	-	-	-	-	-	-	(5)	37
1b. biotype <u>eltor</u>	ATCC 14013	+	-	-	+	-	-	-	+	-	-	-	+	-	-	-	+	+	-	-	-	-	(4)	37
	SLH 22	+	-	-	+	-	-	-	+	-	-	-	+	-	-	-	+	+	-	-	-	-	(4)	37
	PE 1	+	-	-	+	-	-	-	+	-	-	-	+	-	-	-	+	+	-	-	-	-	(4)	37
	Ubon 13	+	-	-	+	-	-	-	+	-	-	-	+	-	-	-	+	+	-	-	-	-	(4)	37
1c. biotype <u>proteus</u>																								
<u>V. proteus</u> NCTC 8563		+	-	-	-	-	-	-	+	-	-	-	+	-	-	-	+	-	-	-	-	-	(5)	37
<u>V. metschnikovii</u> NCTC 8443		+	-	-	-	-	-	-	+	-	-	-	+	-	-	-	+	-	-	-	-	-	(5)	37
1d. biotype <u>albensis</u>																								
<u>V. albensis</u> NCMB 41		+	+	-	-	-	-	-	+	-	-	-	+	-	-	-	-	-	-	-	-	-	(5)	25
2. <u>V. parahaemolyticus</u>[c]	01	+	+	-	-	-	-	-	+	-	-	-	+	+	-	-	-	-	-	-	+	-	(3)	37
(biotype 1	02	+	+	-	-	-	-	-	+	+	-	-	+	-	-	-	-	-	-	-	-	-	(3)	37
<u>parahaemolyticus</u>)	03	+	+	-	-	-	-	-	+	-	-	-	+	-	-	-	-	-	-	-	-	-	(3)	37
	04	+	+	-	-	-	+	+	+	-	-	-	+	+	-	-	-	-	+	-	-	-	(3)	37
	05	+	+	-	-	-	-	-	+	-	-	-	+	-	-	-	-	-	-	-	-	-	(3)	37
	06	+	+	-	-	-	-	-	+	-	+	-	+	-	-	-	-	-	-	-	-	-	(3)	37
	07	+	+	-	-	-	-	-	+	-	-	+	+	+	-	-	-	-	+	-	-	-	(3)	37
	08	+	+	-	-	-	-	-	+	-	-	-	+	-	-	-	-	-	-	+	-	-	(3)	37
	09	+	-	-	-	-	-	-	+	-	-	-	+	+	-	-	-	-	-	+	-	-	(3)	37
	010	+	+	-	-	-	-	-	+	-	-	-	+	+	-	-	-	-	+	-	-	-	(3)	37
	011	+	+	-	-	-	-	-	+	-	-	-	+	-	-	-	-	-	-	-	-	-	(3)	37
	012	+	+	-	-	-	-	-	+	-	-	+	+	+	-	-	-	-	+	-	-	-	(3)	37
<u>V. parahaemolyticus</u>[d]	505-78	+	+	-	-	-	-	-	+	-	-	+	+	+	-	-	-	-	+	-	-	-	(5)	37
(biotype 2	905-78	+	+	-	-	-	-	-	+	-	-	+	+	+	-	-	-	-	+	-	-	-	(5)	37

Table 1. Continued.

alginolyticus)	1013-79	+	+	-	-	-	-	-	+	-	-	+	+	+	-	-	-	-	+	-	-	-	(5)	37
	53-79	+	+	-	-	-	-	-	+	-	-	-	+	+	-	-	-	-	-	+	-	-	(5)	37
	1027-79	+	-	-	-	-	-	-	+	-	-	-	+	+	-	-	-	-	-	+	-	-	(5)	37
3. V. anguillarum	NCMB 6	+	-	-	-	+	-	-	+	-	-	-	+	-	+	-	-	-	-	-	-	-	(6)	27
	NCMB 828	+	-	-	-	+	-	-	+	-	-	-	+	-	+	-	-	-	-	-	-	-	(6)	27
4. V. fischeri	NCMB 1143	+	-	-	-	-	-	-	+	-	-	-	+	-	-	-	-	-	-	-	-	-	NCMB	15
5. V. costicola	NCMB 701	+	-	-	-	-	-	-	+	-	-	-	+	-	-	-	-	-	-	-	-	-	NCMB	27
6. Vibrio ("Beneckea")																								
V. nereida	ATCC 25917	+	-	-	-	-	-	-	+	-	-	+	+	-	-	-	-	-	-	-	-	-	(6)	27
V. campbelli	ATCC 25920	+	+	-	-	-	-	-	+	-	-	-	+	-	-	-	-	-	-	-	-	-	(6)	27
V. natrigens	ATCC 14018	+	+	-	-	+	-	-	+	-	-	-	+	-	-	-	-	-	-	-	-	-	(6)	27
Aeromonas																								
1. A. hydrophila																								
1a. subsp. hydrophila	ATCC 7966[e)]	+	-	-	-	-	-	-	+	-	-	-	+	-	-	-	-	-	-	-	-	-	(5)	37
1b. subsp. anaerogenes	ATCC 15467	+	-	+	-	-	-	-	+	-	-	-	+	+	-	-	-	-	-	-	-	-	(5)	27
1c. subsp. proteolytica	ATCC 15338	+	+	-	-	-	-	-	+	-	-	-	+	+	-	-	-	-	-	-	-	-	(6)	27
2. A. punctata																								
2a. subsp. punctata	NCMB 74	+	-	-	-	+	-	-	+	-	-	-	+	-	-	-	-	-	-	-	-	-	NCMB	37
2b. subsp. caviae	ATCC 15468[e)]	+	-	-	-	+	-	-	+	-	-	-	+	-	-	-	-	-	-	-	-	-	(5)	37
3. A. salmonicida																								
3a. subsp. salmonicida	NCMB 1102	+	+	-	-	+	-	-	+	-	-	-	+	+	+	-	-	-	-	-	-	-	NCMB	20
3b. subsp. achromogenes	NCMB 1110	+	+	-	-	-	-	-	+	-	-	-	+	+	-	-	-	-	-	-	-	-	NCMB	25
3c. subsp. masoucida	ATCC 27013	+	+	-	-	+	-	-	+	-	-	-	+	+	+	-	-	-	-	-	-	-	ATCC	26
A. sobria	CIP 202	+	-	-	-	-	-	-	+	+	-	-	+	-	-	-	-	-	+	-	-	-	(5)	37
	CIP 210	+	-	-	-	-	-	-	+	+	-	-	+	-	-	+	-	-	-	-	-	-	(5)	15

	CIP 208	+	+	-	-	-	-	-	+	-	-	-	+	-	-	-	-	-	+	-	-	-	(5)	25
	CIP 217	+	+	-	-	+	-	-	+	-	-	-	+	-	-	+	-	-	+	-	-	-	(5)	20
Plesiomonas																								
1. P. shigelloides	ATCC 14029	+	+	-	-	-	-	-	+	-	+	+	+	-	-	-	-	-	-	-	-	-	ATCC	30
	011	+	+	-	-	-	-	-	+	-	+	?	+	+	-	-	-	-	-	-	-	-	(5)	30
	017	+	+	-	-	-	-	-	+	-	+	?	+	-	-	-	-	-	-	-	-	-	(5)	30
	022	+	+	-	-	-	-	-	+	-	+	?	+	+	-	-	-	-	-	-	-	-	(5)	30
Photobacterium																								
1. P. phosphoreum	NCMB 844	+	+	-	+	-	-	-	+	+	-	-	+	-	-	-	-	-	-	-	-	-	NCMB	25
2. P. mandapamensis	NCMB 391	+	+	-	-	-	-	-	+	-	-	-	+	-	-	-	-	-	-	-	-	-	NCMB	26
Lucibacterium																								
1. V. harveyi	ATCC 14126	+	+	-	-	-	-	-	+	-	-	-	+	+	-	-	-	-	-	-	-	-	(6)	27

a) Data are quoted from the previous report (14).
b) Data are quoted from the previous report (15)
c) Data are quoted from the previous report (12).
d) Data are quoted from the previous report (13).
e) Data are quoted from the previous report (19).
f) Bacterial strains were obtained from (1) Dr. N. Ohtomo, Chemo-Sero-Therapeutic Institute, Kumamoto, (2) Dr.R. A. Finkelstein, Department of Microbiology, School of Medicine, University of Missouri-Columbia, Columbia, (3) Dr. M. Ohashi and Dr. K. Ohta, Tokyo Metroporitan Research Laboratory for Public Health, Tokyo, (4) Dr. S. Shimodori and Dr. K. Takeya, Department of Bacteriology, School of Medicine, Kyushu University, Fukuoka, (5) Dr. T. Shimada and Dr. R. Sakazaki, National Institute of Health, Tokyo, (6) Dr. S. Shinoda, Department of Environmental Hygiene, School of Pharmaceutical Sciences, Okayama University, Okayama, (7) Dr. E. Yabuuchi, Department of Bacteriology, Kansai Medical College, Moriguchi.
Abbreviation: Glc, glucose; Gal, galactose; Man, mannose; Fru, fructose; Rha, rhamnose; Ara, arabinose; Fuc, fucose Hep L-D, L-glycero-D-manno-heptose; Hep D-D, D-glycero-D-mannoheptose; KDO, 2-keto-3-deoxyoctonic acid; GlcN, glucosamine; GalN, galactosamine; ManN, mannosamine; FucN, fucosamine, QuiN, quinovosamine; PerN, perosamine; ATCC, American Type Culture Collection; NCMB, National Collection of Marine Bacteria.

Table 2. Sugar composition of lipopolysaccharides isolated from group F vibrio (*V. fluvialis*) and lactose-positive vibrio (*V. vulnificus*).

Strain		Carbohydrate																					Obtained from	Growth temperature (°C)
																			Unknown amino sugar					
		Glc	Gal	Man	Fru	Rha	Ara	Fuc	Hep L-D	Hep D-D	KDO	KDO-like	GlcN	GalN	ManN	FucN	QuiN	QerN	P1	P2	P3	Y		
Group F vibrio[a)]	308-77	+	+	-	-	-	-	-	+	+	-	-	+	-	+	-	+	-	-	-	-	-	(5)	37
(V. fluvialis)	210-73	+	-	-	-	-	-	-	+	+	-	-	+	-	+	-	+	-	-	-	-	-	(5)	37
	305-77	+	+	-	-	+	-	-	+	+	-	-	+	+	-	-	-	-	-	-	-	-	(5)	37
	306-77	+	+	-	-	+	-	-	+	+	-	-	+	+	-	-	-	-	-	-	-	-	(5)	37
Lactose (+) vibrio	ATCC 27562	+	-	-	-	-	-	-	+	-	-	-	+	-	-	-	-	-	-	-	-	-	ATCC	37
(V. vulnificus)	C4123	+	-	-	-	-	-	-	+	-	-	-	+	-	-	-	-	-	-	-	-	-	(7)	37

Abbreviations and sources of the strains are the same as described in the footnote to Table 1.
a) Data for group F vibrio are quoted from previous report (19).

ing peaks was obtained from the acetic acid hydrolysates of LPS isolated from *Vibrionaceae* with the exception of *V. parahaemolyticus* 06 and *Pl. shigelloides.* The absence of KDO in LPS was confirmed further with 17 strains of *V. anguillarum* and more than 30 strains of 01 *V. cholerae* isolated from patients, in addition to the strains listed in Tables 1 and 2.

Instead of KDO, however, some periodate-thiobarbituric acid test-positive KDO-like substances were found in LPS isolated from *Vibrio* ("*Beneckea*") (3) *nereida* (ATCC 25917) and *Plesiomonas shigelloides*, as was the case with LPS from *V. parahaemolyticus* 07 and 012 and the three strains of *V. alginolyticus* as reported in our previous papers (12, 13). As seen in Table 3, the KDO-like substances were not identical to KDO in behavior, at least in high-voltage paper electrophoresis and thin-layer chromatography. In our previous papers (12, 13) we reported that the three KDO-like substances from LPS of *V. parahaemolyticus* 07 and 012 and *V. alginolyticus* were identical because they showed identical mobility in high-voltage paper electrophoresis, the mobility relative to KDO being 1.21. However, it was disclosed in this study that, as seen in the data presented in Table 3, each of these three KDO-like substances isolated from various sources exhibited different bahavior in thin-layer chromatography, Rf values relative to KDO being 1.31, 1.58 and 1.17, respectively, (solvent system pyridine/ethyl acetate/acetic acid/water, 36:36:7:21, v/v/v/v, Avicel plate), an indication that these three substances are not identical. The KDO-like substances found in LPS from *Vibrio* ("*Beneckea*") *nereida* (ATCC 25917)

Table 3. Behaviors of KDO and KDO-like substances in high-voltage paper electrophoresis and thin-layer chromatography.

	Absorption maximum of color (nm)[a]	High-voltage paper[b] electrophoresis	Thin-layer[c] chromatography
KDO	549	1.00	1.00
KDO from V. parahaemolyticus 06 LPS	549	1.00	1.00
KDO-like substances present in LPS from			
V. parahaemolyticus 07	549	1.21	1.31
012	549	1.21	1.58
V. alginolyticus 905-78	549	1.21	1.17
V. nereida ATCC 25917	549	0.81	0.68
P. shigelloides ATCC 14029	549	1.00	0.81

a) Absorption maximum in periodate-thiobarbituric acid test.
b) Electrophoresis was performed with the solvent system pyridine / acetic acid / water, 10:4:86, v/v/v, at 45 v/cm for 40 min.
c) Thin-layer chromatography was performed on Avicel plates (Funakoshi Chemical Co., Tokyo) with the solvent system pyridine/ethyl acetate/acetic acid/water, 36:36:7:21, v/v/v/v.

and *Plesiomonas shigelloides* were also different in their behavior in either high-voltage paper electrophoresis or thin-layer chromatography (Table 3).

Neutral and amino sugar composition Glucose, L-glycero-D-manno-heptose and glucosamine were found as component sugar in common in the LPS of all of the *Vibrionaceae* strains examined. The first two sugars are known to be regular sugar constituents of the core region of gram-negative bacterial LPS, while glucosamine is known as a basic structural unit consisting of the β-1,6-N-acetyl-glucosaminyl-N-acetyl-glucosamine disaccharide backbone of lipid A (4, 38). It was particularly noticed that mannose was not found in *Vibrionaceae* LPS with the exception of only one strain, *Aeromonas hydrophila* subsp. *anaerogenes* ATCC 15467. This strain is, however, presently not regarded as a member of genus *Aseromonas* because of its (G+C) content, DNA homology and other taxonomical characteristics that are not consistent with those for this genus (unpublished data of Shimada and Sakazaki, National Institute of Health, Tokyo). Furthermore, rhamnose was rarely present; only eight strains contained this sugar in their LPS. As far as *Vibrio cholerae* (01 and non-01 groups) are concerned, neither mannose nor rhamnose was detected in their LPS, although the presence of mannose of both sugars in LPS from 01 *V. cholerae* has been reported in a number of papers (16,17,29,30,31,32,33,34,40,41). By gas-liquid chromatographic sugar analysis, a mannose-like component was definitely detected in the hydrolysates of LPS from 01 *V. cholerae* and *V. parahaemolyticus*, because the alditol acetate derivative of this component yielded a peak whose retention time value was identical to that of the same derivative of authentic mannose (Rt value relative to xylose 1.48). However, the mass-spectrometric fragmentation pattern obtained in combined gas-liquid chromatography/ mass spectrometry for this peak was not identical with that obtained for the alditol acetate derivative of authentic mannose as a standard. Furthermore, this peak was totally eliminated when the hydrolysates were passed through a Dowex 50 (H^+) column and then subjected to gas-liquid chromatographic sugar analysis, an evidence that it is not mannose but some kind of basic substance, most probably an amino compound.

D-glycero-D-mannoheptose, which has been rarely reported as a component of gram-negative bacterial LPS (52), was found in LPS from *A. sobria* CIP 202 and 210, *Photobacterium phosphoreum* NCMB 844, all four strains of *V. fluvialis* (group F vibrios) and *V. cholerae* NAG 4715 and NAG 722-75 (both 03 group).

A chemotaxonomically interesting feature was disclosed with the sugar composition of LPS isolated from *Vibrio cholerae.* Fructose was present exclusively in LPS of *V. cholerae* (both 01 and non-01 groups and both classical and eltor biotypes) with the exception of one strain, *Photobacterium phosphoreum* NCMB 844. Furthermore, a pair of rarely occurring amino sugars, perosamine and quinovosamine were found only in LPS from 01 group *V. cholerae* regardless of either the biotype (classical or eltor) or the serotype (Inaba or Ogawa), whereas this pair is not present in non-01 group *V. cholerae* (the so-called NAG vibrios). This feature was confirmed with LPS from more than 30 additional strains of 01 group *V. cholerae* isolated from patients. In contrast, neither perosamine nor quinovosamine was present in LPS isolated from R mutants of 01 *V. cholerae* regardless of the biotype (classical or eltor) or serotype (Inaba or Ogawa), whereas they contain fructose.

With regard to amino sugars other than glucosamine, perosamine and quinovosamine, mannosamine was found in LPS from only a limited number of strains, i.e., *V. anguillarum* NCMB 6 and 828, *A. salmonicida* subsp. *salmonicida* NCMB 1102, and two strains of *V. fluvialis*. In addition, at least four unidentified amino sugars were found in LPS, tentatively designated here as P1, P2, P3 and Y; P1 in *V. parahaemolyticus* 04, 07, 010 and 012, *A. sobria* CIP 202, 208 and 217; P2 in *V. parahaemolyticus* 08 and 09; P3 in *V. parahaemolyticus* 01; and Y in 03 *V. cholerae* (NAG) 4715 and 722-75. A positive reaction was obtained with either N-acetylated P1 and P3 in the colorimetric method of Ashwell et al. (1) for the determination of N-acetyl-3-amino hexose. Our preliminary results obtained by combined gas-liquid chromatographic/mass spectrometric analysis showed that, in both the retention time and mass fragmentation pattern, N-acetyl-alditol acetate derivatives of P1 and P3 are identical to the corresponding derivatives of 3-amino-3, 6-dideoxy-D-glucose isolated from *Citrobacter freundii* ATCC 8090 LPS (23) and 3-amino-3, 6-dideoxy-D-galactose isolated from *Pseudomonas fluorescense* NCTC 10038 LPS (51), respectively. However, their absolute configurations were not yet determined. Their identities as 3-amino-3, 6-dideoxy-D-mannose were fully excluded using an authentic standard of this amino sugar isolated from amphotericin B (8). The presence of 4-amino-4-deoxy-L-arabinose was reported for LPS from Ogawa serotype strains of 01 *V. cholerae* (36). In this study, however, no evidence for the presence of this amino sugar was obtained for LPS from not only Inaba serotype strains but also Ogawa serotype strains of 01 *V. cholerae*.

The absence of KDO in LPS from the genus *Vibrio* was first pointed out by Jackson and Redmond (16) with *V. cholerae* 569B (Inaba), and then it was confirmed in various laboratories with the same strain as well as other strains of 01 *V. cholerae* (17). Our laboratory demonstrated the lack of KDO in LPS not only from 01 *V. cholerae* (14), but also from non-01 *V. cholerae* (NAG vibrios) (15), *V. parahaemolyticus* (12), *V. alginolyticus* (13), group F vibrios (19), *Aeromonas hydrophila* (ATCC 7966) and *A. punctata* (ATCC 15468) (19). Furthermore, it was speculated by the author's group (19) that the absence of KDO in LPS may be one of the characteristics possessed by the genus *Vibrio* and related bacteria including *Aeromonas* and thus of taxonomical significance. In the present study, it was demonstrated for the first time that KDO, known generally as a regular constituent sugar of the core region of gram-negative bacterial LPS, is totally lacking in LPS of not only the genus *Vibrio* but also all members of the family *Vibrionaceae* so far tested with the exception of *V. parahaemolyticus* 06 and *Pl. shigelloides*. This finding was confirmed in the acetic acid hydrolysates of LPS not only by the periodate-thiobarbituric acid test (45) in combination with high-voltage paper electrophoresis and thin-layer chromatography, but also by gas-liquid chromatographic analysis, a method different, in principle, from the color test of the thiobarbituric acid reaction. Thus, it was revealed that the absence of KDO in LPS is of taxonomical importance for the family *Vibrionaceae*, although it was reported with a small number of strains belonging to other families (10, 52). Furthermore, it was particularly noticeable that mannose is also lacking in LPS of the *Vibrionaceae* with the exception of *A. hydrophila* subsp. *anaerogenes* (ATCC 15467). However, this strain is now pending taxonomically with respect to its identity as *Aeromonas*, or further as a member of the family *Vibrionaceae* (unpublished data of Shimada and Sakazaki, National Institute of Health, Tokyo).

L-glycero-D-mannoheptose, glucose and glucosamine were present as the component sugar in common in the LPS of all of the *Vibrionaceae* strains examined. The first two sugars are well doccumented as regular sugar constituents of the core polysaccharide of usual gram-negative bacterial LPS, while glucosamine is known as a basic structural unit constituting of the glucosamine-disaccharide backbone of lipid A (4, 38). Furthermore, the yields of LPS from the corresponding acetone-dried cells of the S-form strains ranged from 1.3% to 6.0% and the total lipid content of LPS from 13% to 32%, both of which are considered to be compatible with the reported data of those for other gram-negative bacterial LPS. These facts indicate that the Westphal's phenol-water technique (48, 49) is relevant for extraction and purification of LPS from the family *Vibrionaceae* strains. Neither ribose nor deoxyribose was detected in the gas-liquid chromatographic analysis for all LPS studied here, a proof for used LPS to be free from contamination by nucleic acids. In our previous works on the LPS of *V. parahaemolyticus* (12) and *V. alginolyticus* (13), the cells were heated at 100°C for 2 hr prior to phenol-water extraction. This was done with the aim of eliminating contamination of LPS by K-antigens on the basis of the Shimouchi's description (42). However, as mentioned before, it was revealed during this study that there was no virtual difference in the sugar composition between LPS prepared from the phenol-treated and heat-killed cells. Moreover, no contamination by K-antigens was found with LPS purified from the phenol-treated but not heat-killed cells of *V. parahaemolyticus* when examined by the double diffusion technique using K-antisera (Toshiba Chemical Co., Tokyo). These facts indicate that the purification procedures of LPS employed in this study including 6 times repeated washings by ultracentrifugation (105,000 x g, 3 hr) as well as ribonuclease treatment, eliminate contamination of even *V. parahaemolyticus* LPS by K-antigens, and consequently other polysaccharide, if any. These combined data seem to support a contention that this situation with the *V. parahaemolyticus* LPS is also the case perhaps with those prepared from the phenoltreated cells of the other strains of *Vibrionaceae* employed in the present study.

In our previous study (12, 13), the periodate-thiobarbituric acid test-positive KDO-like substances were found in LPS from *V. parahaemolyticus* 07 and 012, and *V. alginolyticus.* In the present study, two other kinds of KDO-like substances were found in LPS, one in *Vibrio* ("*Beneckea*") *nereida* (ATCC 25917) and the other in *Plesiomonas shigelloides.* These components were strongly positive in the thiobarbituric acid test, yielding a color with maximal absorption at 549 nm. The spectra were identical to that of KDO, whereas neither electrophoretic mobilities or Rf values in thin-layer chromatography were identical to those of KDO. The color with the maximal absorption at 549 nm is not always specific to KDO in the thiobarbituric acid test (43). The test as conducted by Weissbach's periodate-thiobarbituric acid method yields two kinds of chromophores with different absorption maxima, depending on the chromogens produced by the periodation of the sample. Malonaldehyde is formed from 2-deoxy sugar (44), 3-deoxy hexose, and 3, 6-dideoxy hexose (6) by the periodation. This chromogen yields, upon reaction with 2-thiobarbituric acid, the chromophore with maximal absorption at 532 nm. On the other hand, an alkali-labile chromophore with an absorption maximum at 549 nm is produced by the same test on a number of compounds. This is characteristic for β-formylpyruvate which is formed from 2-keto-3-deoxy aldonic acids including KDO (47), 4-deoxy-5-keto-uronic acid (7), galactal (28), 4-deoxy5-keto-glucaric acid (7) and sialic acid (45). Characterization of these components is now under investigation in our laboratory.

A feature of particular interest from the chemotaxonomical point of view revealed in this work is the exclusive presence of the pair perosamine and quinovosamine in LPS from cholera vibrios, i.e., 01 group of *V. cholerae*, regardless of either the biotype (classical or eltor) or the serotype (Inaba or Ogawa), and, in addition, the exclusive presence of fructose in both 01 and non-01 groups of *V. cholerae* with the exception of only one other strain, *Photobacterium phosphoreum* (NCMB 844). Neither fructose nor the pair perosamine and quinovosamine was found in LPS from *V. metschnikovii, V. proteus* or *V. albensis*, the former two being presently classified under the species *V. cholerae* as biotype *proteus* and the latter as biotype *albensis* by Shewan and Veron in Bergey's Manual of Determinative Bacteriology, 8th edition (5). It should be kept in mind that, however, since R mutants of 01 *V. cholerae* lack both perosamine and quinovosamine in their LPS (14), the presence of this pair in LPS is limited only to the S form of 01 *V. cholerae.*

In general, the molecules of gram-negative bacterial LPS are composed of a polysaccharide portion (0-specific side chain + the core) and lipid A portion, and the di- or tri-saccharide of KDO connects the two parts (52). The lack of KDO in *Vibrionaceae* LPS indicates that the structure of the core region, in particular the inner core region, of LPS of this family might be fundamentally different from that of usual gram-negative bacteria. *V. parahaemolyticus* 06 LPS was found to be the only one which contains KDO. Chemical and immunochemical characterization of LPS of this strain is now in progress in our laboratory in order to determine whether or not the KDO residue present in this strain is located between the heptose residue of the core polysaccharide and lipid A, connecting these two portions as in the usual gram-negative bacterial LPS, or in a different portion, for instance, in the 0-antigenic polysaccharide region as an immunodominant sugar as is the case with the KDO residue found in *Shigella sonnei* Phase II LPS (20).

The absence of KDO in LPS of the *Vibrionaceae* was demonstrated for the first time in the present work. This is believed to be the first report of a comparative study, though qualitative, of the sugar composition of LPS isolated from *Vibrionaceae* including all of the constituting genera, i.e., *Vibrio, Aeromonas, Lucibacterium. Photobacterium* and *Plesiomonas.* Our results are compatible with the interpretation that the absence of KDO in LPS can be one of the taxonomical characteristics of *Vibrionaceae* in addition to those such as (G+C) content, DNA (or RNA) homology, numerical analysis data and other biological and biochemical properties. In the present report, only qualitative data on the sugar composition of LPS of *Vibrionaceae* are presented. Detailed quantitative analysis of the sugar composition will offer a further basis for a chemical method for differentiating members of this family. The results of a structural and immunochemical study as well as detailed quantitative data on the sugar composition of LPS isolated from individual members of *Vibrionaceae* will be published elsewhere. A gas-liquid chromatographic analysis of fatty acid components present in lipid A of LPS from the family *Vibrionaceae* strains is now under investigation in our laboratory from a chemotaxonomical point of view.

We thank, for providing us the bacterial strains used in this study, Dr. T. Shimada and Dr. R. Sakazaki, National Institute of Health, Tokyo; Dr. K. Ohta and Dr. M. Ohashi, Tokyo Metropolitan Research Laboratory, Tokyo; Dr. T. Miwatani and Dr. Y. Takeda, The Research Institute of Infectious Diseases, Osaka University, Osaka; Dr. S. Shimodori,

Department of Bacteriology, School of Medicine, Kyushu University, Fukuoka; Dr. N. Ohtomo, Chemo-Sero-Therapeutic Institute, Kumamoto; Dr. S. Shinoda, Department of Environmental Hygiene, School of Pharmaceutical Sciences, Okayama University, Okayama; Dr. E. Yabuuchi, Department of Bacteriology, Kansai Medical College, Moriguchi; Dr. M. Masui, Department of Bacterioloty, School of Medicine, Osaka City University, Osaka; and Dr. N. Kasai, Department of Microbiology, School of Pharmaceutical Sciences, Showa University, Tokyo. Professor K. Takeya, Department of Bacteriology, School of Medicine, Kyushu University, Fukuoka, is particularly acknowledged for the support and encouragement. This investigation was partly supported by a Government Research Grant from the Ministry of Education of Japan.

REFERENCES

1. Ashwell, G., Brown, N. C., and Volk, W. A. 1965 A colorimetric procedure for the determination of N-acetylated-3-amino hexoses. Arch. Biochem. Biophys., **112**:648-652
2. Bagdian, G., Dröge, W., Kotelko, K., Lüderitz, O., and Westphal, 0. 1966 Vorkommen zweier Heptosen in Lipopolysacchariden enterobacterieller Zellwände: L-glycero- und D-glycero-D-mannoheptose. Biochem. Z., **344**:197-211
3. Baumann, P., Baumann, L., Bang, S. S., and Woolkalis, M. J. 1980 Reevaluation of the taxonomy of *Vibrio, Beneckea,* and *Photobacterium*: Abolition of the genus *Beneckea.* Current Microbiol., **4**:127-132
4. Broady, K. W., Rietschel, E. T., and Lüderitz, 0. 1981 The chemical structure of the lipid A component of lipopolysaccharides from *Vibrio cholerae.* Eur. J. Biochem., **115**:463-468
5. Buchanan, R. E., and Gibbons, N. E. 1974 Family II. *Vibrionaceae* Veron 1965, 5245. p340. *In* R. E. Buchanan and Gibbons, N. E. (eds.), Bergey's Manual of Determinative Bacteriology, 8th ed. The Williams and Wilkins Co., Baltimore.
6. Cynkin, M. A., and Ashwell, G. 1960 Estimation of 3-deoxy sugars by means of the malonaldehyde-thiobarbituric acid reaction, Nature, **186**: 144-156
7. Dagley, S., and Trudgill, P. W. 1965 The metabolism of galactarate, D-glucarate and various pentoses by species of *Pseudomonas.* J. Biochem., **95**:48-58
8. Dutcher, J. D. 1963 Chemistry of amino sugars derived from antibiotic substances. Adv. Carbohyd. Chem., **18**:259-308
9. Fensom, A. H., and Gray, G. W. 1969 The chemical composition of the lipopolysaccharide of *Pseudomonas aeruginosa.* Biochem. J., **114**:185-196
10. Galanos, C., Lüderitz, O., Rietschel, E. T., and Westphal, O. 1977 Newer aspects of the chemistry and biology of bacterial lipopolysaccharides, with special reference to their lipid A component. p.239-335. *In* Goodwin, T. W. (ed.), International Review of Biochemistry, vol. 14 Biochemistry of lipids II, University Park Press, Baltimore.
11. Galanos, C., Lüderitz, O., and Westphal, O. 1969 A new method for the extraction of R lipopolysaccharides. Eur. J. Biochem., **9**:245-249
12. Hisatsune, K., Kiuye, A., and Kondo, S. 1980 Sugar composition of 0-antigenic lipopolysaccharides isolated from *Vibrio parahaemolyticus.* Microbiol. Immunol., **24**:691-701
13. Hisatsune, K., Kiuye, A., and Kondo, S. 1981 A comparative study of the sugar composition of 0-antigenic lipopolysaccharides isolated from *Vibrio alginolyticus* and *Vibrio parahaemolyticus.* Microbiol. Immunol., **25**:127-136
14. Hisatsune, K., and Kondo, S. 1980 Lipopolysaccharides of R mutants isolated from *Vibrio cholerae.* Biochem. J., **185**:77-81
15. Hisatsune, K., Kondo, S., Nozaki, S., and Kawata, T. 1978 Glycine containing lipopolysaccharide isolated from *Vibrio cholerae* 4715 (NAG). Chem. Pharm. Bull., **26**:3597-3599.
16. Jackson, G. D. F., and Redmond J. W. 1971 Immunochemical studies of the 0-antigens of *Vibrio cholerae.* The constitution of a lipopolysaccharide from *V. cholerae* 569B (Inaba). FEBS Lett., **13**:117-120

17. Jann, B., Jann, K., and Beyaert, G. O. 1973 2-amino-2, 6-dideoxy-D-glucose (D-quinovosamine) : a constituent of the lipopolysaccharides of *Vibrio cholerae*. Eur. J. Biochem., **37**:531-534
18. Kenne, L., Lindberg, B., Unger, P., Holme, T., and Holmgren, J. 1979 Structural studies of the *Vibrio cholerae* 0-antigen. Carbohyd. Res., **68**:C14-C16
19. Kondo, S., Iguchi, T., and Hisatsune, K. 1980 Lipopolysaccharides of group F, a new group of vibrios. Biochem. Biophys. Res. Commun., **97**:437-442
20. Kontrohr, T., and Kocsis, B. 1978 Structure of the hexose region of *Shigella sonnei* Phase II lipopolysaccharide with 3-deoxy-D-manno-octurosonic acid as possible immunodeterminant and its relation to *Escherichia coli* RI core. Eur. J. Biochem., **88**:267-273
21. Laine, R. A., Stelner, K., and Hakomori, S. 1974 Isolation and characterization of membrane glycolipids. p.228-244. *In* Korn, E. E. (ed.), Methods in Membrane Biology, vol. 2, Plenum Press, New York.
22. Lüderitz, O., Jann, K., and Wheat, R. 1968 Somatic and capsular antigens of gram-negative bacteria. p. 105-228. *In* Flokin, M., and Stortz, E. H. (eds.), Comprehensive Biochemistry, vol. 26A, Elsvier, Amsterdam.
23. Lüderitz, O., Ruschmann, E., Westphal, O., Raff, R., and Wheat, R. 1967 Occurrence of 3-amino-3, 6-dideoxyhexoses in *Salmonella* and related bacteria. J. Bacteriol., **93**:1681-1687
24. Lüderitz, O., Westphal, O. Staub, A. M., and Nikaido, H. 1971 Isolation and chemical and immunological characterization of bacterial lipopolysaccharides. p. 145-233. *In* Weinbaum, G., Kadis, S., and Ajl, S. J. (eds.), Microbial Toxins, vol. 4, Academic Press, New York.
25. Mawhinney, T., Feather, M., Martinetz, R. R., and Barbero, G. J. 1979 A rapid, convenient method for the detemination of hexosamines as 0-acetylated-0-methyloximes by gas-liquid chromatography. Carbohyd. Res., **75**:C21-C23
26. Miyano, K., Ishibashi, M., Kunita, N., Takeda, Y., and Miwatani, T. 1980 Chemotypes of *Vibrio parahaemolyticus* lipopolysaccharides. FEMS Microbiol. Lett., **8**:23-28
27. Osborn, M. J. 1963 Studies of the gram-negative cell walls. I. Evidence for the role of 2-keto-3-deoxyoctonate in the lipopolysaccharide of *Salmonella typhimurium*. Proc. Natl. Acad. Sci. U.S.A. **50**:499-506
28. Preiss, J., and Ashwell, G. 1962 Alginic acid metabolism in bacteria. J. Biol. Chem., **237**:309-316
29. Raziuddin, S., and Kawasaki, T. 1976 Biochemical studies on the cell wall lipopolysaccharides (0-antigens) of *Vibrio cholerae* 569B (Inaba) and eltor (Inaba). Biochem. Biophys. Acta, **431**: 116-126
30. Raziuddin, S. 1977 Characterization of lipid A and polysaccharide moieties of the lipopolysaccharides from *Vibrio cholerae*. Biochem. J., **167**:147-154
31. Raziuddin, S. 1977 Studies of the polysaccharide fraction from the cell wall lipopolysaccharides (0-antigens) of *Vibrio cholerae*. Indian J. Biochem. Biophys., **14**:262-263
32. Raziuddin, S. 1978 Toxic and immunological properties of the lipopolysaccharides (0-antigens) from *Vibrio eltor*. Immunochemistry, **15**: 611-614
33. Raziuddin, S. 1979 Structure-function relationship: biological activities of the lipopolysaccharides and lipid A from *Vibrio cholerae*. J. Infect. Dis., **140**:590-595
34. Raziuddin, S. 1980 Immunochemical studies of the lipopolysaccharides of *Vibrio cholerae*: constitution of 0-specific side chain and core polysaccharide. Infect. Immun., **27**:211-215
35. Redmond, J. W. 1975 4-Amino-4, 6-dideoxy-D-mannose (D-perosamine): a component of the lipopolysaccharide of *Vibrio cholerae* 569B (Inaba). FEBS LETTER, **50**:147-149
36. Redmond, J. W. 1978 The 4-amino sugars present in the lipopolysaccharides of *Vibrio cholerae* and related vibrios. Biochim. Biophys. Acta, **542**:378-384
37. Redmond, J. W. 1979 The structure of the 0-antigenic side chain of the lipopolysaccharide of *Vibrio cholerae* 569B (Inaba). Biochim. Biophys. Acta, **584**:346-352
38. Rietschel, E. T., Hase, S., King, M. T., Redmond, J. W., and Lehmann, V. 1977 Chemical structure of lipid A, p. 262-268. *In* Schlessinger, D. (ed.), Microbiology-1977, American Society for Microbiology, Washington, D.C.
39. Sen, A. K., and Mukherjee, A. K. 1978 Structural studies of a specific polysaccharide isolated from non-agglutinable *Vibrio*. Carbohyd. Res., **64**:215-223
40. Sen, A. K., and Mukherjee, A. K. 1979 Structural investigations on the lipopolysaccharide

isolated from *Vibrio cholerae*, Inaba 569B. Carbohyd. Res., **72**:191-199

41. Sen, A. K., Mukherjee, A. K., Guhathakurta, B., Dutta, A., and Sasmal, S. 1980 Studies on the partial structure of the 0-antigen of *Vibrio cholerae*, Inaba 569B. Carbohyd. Res. **86**:113-121
42. Shimouchi, H. 1972 Purification and immunochemical properties of 0- and K-antigens of *Vibrio parahaemolyticus*. J. Osaka City Med. Center, **21**:65-78
43. Unger, F. M. 1981 The chemistry and biological significance of 3-deoxy-D-manno-2-octulosonic acid (KDO), p.323-388. *In* Tipson, R. S., and Horton, D. (eds.), Advances in Carbohydrate Chemistry and Biochemistry, vol. 38, Academic Press, New York.
44. Waravdekar, V. S., and Saslaw, L. D. 1959 A sensitive colorimetric method for the estimation of 2-deoxy sugars with the use of the malon-aldehyde-thiobarbituric acid reaction. J. Biol. Chem., **234**:1945-1950
45. Warren, L. 1959 The thiobarbituric acid assay of sialic acids. J. Biol. Chem. **234**:1971-1975
46. Warren, L. 1960 Thiobarbituric acid spray reagent for deoxy sugars and sialic acid. Nature, **186**: 237
47. Weissbach, A., and Hurwitz, J. 1959 The formation of 2-keto-3-deoxy-heptonic acid in extracts of *Escherichia coli* B. J. Biol. Chem., **234**:705-709
48. Westphal, O., Lüderitz, O., and Bister, R. 1952 Über die Extraction von Bakterien mit Phenol/ Wasser. Z. Naturforsch., **7b**:148-155
49. Westphal, O., and Jann, K. 1965 Bacterial lipopolysaccharides. Extraction with phenol-water and further applications of the procedure. p.83-91. *In* Whistler, L. (ed.), Methods in Carbohydrate Chemistry, vol. 5, Academic Press, New York.
50. Wheat, R. W. 1966 Analysis of hexosamines in bacterial polysaccharide by chromatographic procedures, p. 60-75. *In* Neufeld, E. F., and Ginsburg, V. (eds.), Methods in Enzymology, vol. 8, Academic Press, New York.
51. Wilkinson, S. G. 1972 Amino sugars in the wall of *Pseudomonas fluorescens*. J. Gen. Microbiol., **70**: 365-369
52. Wilkinson, S. G. 1977 Composition and structure of bacterial lipopolysaccharides, p. 97-175. *In* Sutherland I. W. (ed.), Surface Carbohydrates of The Prokaryotic Cell, Academic Press, New York.

Advances in Research on Cholera and Related Diarrheas, eds., S. Kuwahara, N. F. Pierce, 75–86.

ENTEROPATHOGENICITY AND SOME BIOLOGICAL FEATURES OF GROUP F (EF–6) VIBRIO ISOLATES

Yasuo Kudoh, Masaaki Tsuno, Shigeru Matsushita, Sumio Yamada, Kenji Ohta, Senzo Sakai and Makoto Ohashi

Department of Microbiology, Tokyo Metropolitan Research Laboratory of Public Health, Tokyo 160

The organism now referred to as group F or EF-6 vibrio had probably been put together with *Aeromonas* species in the past without drawing any special attention from the standpoint of gastrointestinal diseases.

However, following the report by Dr. Furniss *et al.*[1)] and Brenner *et al.*[2)], who first described this organism independently as having an intermediate nature between *Vibrio* and *Aeromonas*, the organism was isolated not only environment but also from human diarrheal cases in Bangladesh[3)] and other areas,[4,5)] and this aroused much interest in its relation to the diarrheal diseases.

Being led by interest in its possible enteropathogenicity, the authors have, since 1979, also been looking for its diarrheal cases in Japan. Although no domestic cases with strict sense has been encountered as yet many cases with this vibrio have been observed among travellers to Asian countries or people in Thailand [6,7)].

These epidemiological findings are very suggestive of its close relation to diarrheal diseases, but information are missing about its enteropathogenicity. Pathogenic factors of the organism are not yet clearly understood[3,8)]. On the contrary, its taxonomical position is almost firmly established owing to exaustive studies recently conducted by Lee *et al.*[9)] who proposed a species name *Vibrio fluvialis* for this organism, which they believe should belong to Genus *Vibrio* and be classified into 2 biotypes.

However, its serological classification is not yet established, and its biotypes suggested by Lee *et al.* and the relation between biotypes and enteropathogenicity may need further elucidation.

The purpose of this study, which involved 116 strains of group F vibrio from various origins, was to confirm its biological characteristics and at the same time to try some approaches of biotyping and serotyping, and furthermore to derive some information suggestive of its enteropathogenicity from experimental results in several biological assay systems.

Table 1 provides sources of those strains tested in this study. One-hundred sixteen strains were examined in total, out of which 105 were of human origin including travellers' diarrheal cases, diarrheal cases in Thailand, Singapore and India, as well as healthy individuals. Nine strains were isolates from environment including 7 from esturine water and 2 from shellfish. As reference strains, 1 anaerogenic and 1 aerogenic strains were kindly provided by Dr. Brenner of CDC.

Table 1. Group F vibrio strains used in the experiment.

Source	No. of strains	Note
Human	105	Travellers' diarrhea
		Diarrheal cases in Thailand, Singapore and India
		Healthy individuals
		Unknown
Environment	7	Esturine waters
Food	2	Shellfishes
Reference strain	2	Dr. Brenner, CDC
Total	116	

The identification was based on the following definition:
- yellowish colony on TCBS agar
- motility and oxidase positive
- arginine dihydrolase positive, but lysine and ornithine decarboxylase negative
- Voges-Proskauer negative
- acid from glucose, sucrose, arabinose and mannitol positive, but negative from lactose and inositol
- sensitive to 0/129, 150 μg
- no growth in peptone water without NaCl, but growth in 3,7 and 9% NaCl.

The results of biochemical characterization study are summarized in Table 2 for 116 strains of group F vibrio including 2 reference strains.

As shown in the table, fairly good agreement was observed in major characteristics studied including those applied for identification, except those proposed by Lee *et al.* as being useful for biotyping such as gas production from glucose, utilization or fermentation of cellobiose, aesculin hydrolysis and citrullin utilization, and mannose fermentation, indole production and growth in 1% peptone water without NaCl.

Among those characteristics with exception, almost all the previous results were indole negative and many of them had positive growth in 1% peptone water without NaCl. However, all our strains with the exception of one were weakly positive in indole when tested in Lysine-Indole-Motility(LIM) medium at 37 C for 1 or 2 days. Also growth in peptone water without NaCl was negative for all our strains except one, when tested in 1% peptone water at 37 C for 4 days. We do not know with any certainty the reason why we saw these differences, but they could probably be attributed to the difference of types of medium or cultural conditions adopted in these tests.

In this study, we also wanted to look at the hemolytic activity of the organism because of its possible relation to the pathogenicity to be mentioned later, and found all our strains β-hemolytic positive against horse and sheep red blood cells.

Table 2. Biochemical characteristics of group F vibrio strains.

Characteristic	Reference strains		Isolate (n=114)	
	9554-78	9552-78	Sign	% +
Oxidase	+	+	+	100
Nitrate reduction	+	+	+	100
H_2S (TSI)	–	–	–	0
Indole	+	+	+	99
Gelatinase	+	+	+	100
Voges-Proskauer	–	–	–	0
Lysine	–	–	–	0
Ornithine	–	–	–	0
Arginine	+	+	+	100
Glucose: Gas	–	+	d	11
Acid from:				
Glucose	+	+	+	100
Sucrose	+	+	+	100
Arabinose	+	+	+	100
Lactose	–	–	–	0
Mannose	+	–	+	99
Cellobiose	–	+	d	17
Mannitol	+	+	+	100
Inositol	–	–	–	0
Aesculin	+	–	d	84
Sole carbon source:				
Cellobiose	–	+	d	17
Citrullin	+	–	d	88
β-galactosidase	+	+	+	100
Catalase	+	+	+	100
0/129 (150 μg)	+	+	+	100
Motility	+	+	+	100
NaCl: 0 %	–	–	–	1
: 3 %	+	+	+	100
: 7 %	+	+	+	100
: 9 %	+	+	+	100
:11 %	–	–	–	0
Hemolysis: Sheep	+	+	+	100
: Horse	+	+	+	100

In addition to the sensitivity to vibrio static agent 0/129, antibiotic sensitivity was also examined with streptomycin, chrolamphenicol, tetracycline, kanamycin and ampicillin by the plate agar dilution method. Ninty-nine strains were subjected to the test and results are shown in Table 3. Except the fairly high frequency of moderate to intensive resistance seen with streptomycin, a majority of the strains were distributed in a susceptible range with other antibiotics regardless of their biotypes.

Table 4 summarizes the results of 116 strains as to their biotyping characterization. Lee *et al.* proposed in addition to gas production from glucose, several other characters of the organism as useful for biotyping. In order to see if his results were reproducible, we have included 3 characters in his report, namely aesculin hydrolysis, and utilization of citrullin and cellobiose as a sole carbon source.

Table 3. Antibiotic sensitivity of group F vibrio strains.

Antibiotic	Minimal inhibitory concentration (μg/ml)									
	100	50	25	12.5	6.25	3.12	0.56	0.78	0.39	0.20
Streptomycin	5	3	80	11	–	–	–	–	–	–
Chloramphenicol	–	2	1	–	1	2	12	70	11	–
Tetracycline	–	2	1	2	–	4	70	20	–	–
Kanamycin	–	–	1	38	55	5	–	–	–	–
Ampicillin	–	4	15	16	23	38	2	1	–	–

No. of strains tested: 99(including 10 strains of biotype II).

As can be seen in the table, gas production alone or with aesculin or citrullin could type 85% or more into either typical type I or typical type II, whereas by combination with gas and cellobiose or gas, cellobiose and others only 16 to 24% were typed, leaving a majority of the strains typed as being intermediate due to the failure to meet the criteria for any type. In other words, aesculin and citrullin were found to be useful for biotyping due to fairly good agreement with gas production from glucose. On the other hand, cellobiose seemed inappropriate in our results, contrary to the results of Lee *at al.*, due to the absence of specific correlation to these characteristics.

However, both aesculin and citrullin, in combination with gas production, were unable to type approximately 11% of the strains, and the latter in particular is a rather cumbersome procedure for typing and somewhat difficult to evaluate the results, reducing its practical value significantly. Based on those observations, we finally decided that it was most practical under the present circumstances to apply the gas production from glucose for biotyping, tentatively definiting biotype I as anaerogenic and biotype II as aerogenic strain.

The relationship between the biotypes determined by this system and the sources of 114 strains is shown in Table 5. The majority of our strains or 101 out of 114 strains were gas negative and typed as type I. Both human -derived and environment-derived strains had the same frequency of biotype I, 89%, revealing no difference in biotype distribution related to the source of isolation.

Table 4. Biotyping of group F vibrio strains.

Character used for biotyping	Number of strains typed as :		
	Biotype I	Biotype II	Intermediate
Gas from glucose (Gas)	102 (88%)	14 (12%)	–
Gas + Aesculin (Aes)	93 (80)	10 (9)	13 (11%)
Gas + Citrullin (Cit)	97 (84)	9 (8)	10 (8)
Gas + Cellobiose (Cel)	17 (15)	11 (9)	88 (76)
Gas + Aes + Cit	89 (77)	9 (8)	18 (15)
Gas + Aes + Cit + Cel	11 (9)	7 (6)	98 (84)

Number of strains tested: 116.

Table 5. Biotypes of group F vibrio strains.

Source	No. of strains	Biotype I	Biotype II
Human	105 (100%)	93 (89%)	12 (11%)
Environment and food	9 (100%)	8 (89%)	1 (11%)
Total	114 (100%)	101 (89%)	13 (11%)

We then tried to establish a system of serological typing based on O antigen of this organism, hoping that it will become a useful tool in epidemiological study.

Antisera were prepared by immunizing rabbits with cells killed by heating at 121 C for 60 minutes or formalinized cells as antigens. Immunological heterogenicity was examined by a cross agglutination test between the antisera thus obtained and heated antigens.

The results indicate that the O antigen of this organism is not immunologically uniform, and by cross agglutination test at least 12 types have so far been identified, although some weak cross reactions were observed between certain serotypes (Table 6). This finding strongly suggests that the agglutination test based on O antigen will be a useful system for serotyping of this bacteria, and thus we introduced it to a routine test in our laboratory.

Table 7 shows results of serotyping by this system performed with 116 strains. Fifty-six out of 102 strains or 55% of biotype I fell into one of the 12 types, which were found to vary considerably in frequency. However, based on this system, it was unable to type approximately 45% of biotype I and almost all strains of biotype II, suggesting that more than 12 O-serotypes may exist in this organism and some of them may be specific to either biotype I or biotype II only.

Next, we attempted to elucidate the enteropathogenicity of this organism by testing culture filtrate of each strain to see if there are any extracellular pathogenic factor(s) present in the organism.

Materials and biological assays used in this study are outlined in Table 8. Strains were incubated at 37 C for 24 hours in BHI broth containing 1% NaCl with constant shaking. Sterile culture filtrate was obtained after centrifugation and membrane filtration, and submitted for biological assays. As far as biological assays are concerned, we wanted to know if the organism had any activities resembling those of Kanagawa hemolysin or cholera toxin, known as pathogenic factors of other members of the same genus *Vibrio* such as *V. parahaemolyticus* and *V. cholerae*, or other toxins such as *E. coli* LT/ST or *Aeromonas* cytotoxin, and therefore we have examined the hemolytic activity, mouse lethal toxicity, reactivities in CHO cells and fluid accumulation in the infant mouse intestine.

The result of 116 strains studied are summarized by the biotypes in Table 9. When hemolytic activity was tested by the agar plate method, approximately 80% of both biotypes were positive, giving similar results as the case of cultures previously described.

Table 6. O antigen analysis of group F vibrio by cross agglutination test.

Antigen (Strain No.)	Serotype No.	Agglutination titer against antiserum of:											
		TFO 1	TFO 2	TFO 3	TFO 4	TFO 5	TFO 6	TFO 7	TFO 8	TFO 9	TFO 10	TFO 11	TFO 12
FV-0036	TFO 1	800	–	–	–	–	–	–	–	–	–	–	100
FV-0004	TFO 2	–	400	–	–	–	–	–	–	–	–	–	100
FV-0007	TFO 3	–	–	800	–	–	–	–	–	–	–	–	–
FV-0015	TFO 4	–	–	–	400	–	–	–	–	–	–	–	–
FV-0024	TFO 5	–	–	–	–	400	–	–	–	–	–	–	–
FV-0043	TFO 6	–	–	–	–	–	800	–	–	–	–	–	100
FV-0005	TFO 7	–	–	–	–	–	–	400	–	–	–	–	–
FV-0011	TFO 8	–	–	–	–	–	–	–	1,600	–	–	–	–
FV-0017	TFO 9	–	–	–	–	–	–	–	–	800	–	–	–
FV-0009	TFO 10	–	–	–	–	–	–	–	–	–	800	–	–
FV-0013	TFO 11	–	–	–	–	–	–	–	–	–	–	1,600	–
FV-0032	TFO 12	100	100	–	–	–	100	–	–	–	–	–	800

Antiserum: Rabbit antiserum obtained by immunizing with formalin-killed cells.
Antigen: Heat-killed cells at 121 C for 60 minutes.
– = Less than X 100.

Table 7. O serotype of group F vibrio strains.

O serotype	Biotype I	Biotype II
TFO 1	16 (17%)	1
TFO 2	4 (4%)	–
TFO 3	3	–
TFO 4	4 (4%)	–
TFO 5	4 (4%)	–
TFO 6	3	–
TFO 7	1	–
TFO 8	2	–
TFO 9	2	–
TFO 10	1	–
TFO 11	2	–
TFO 12	12 (10%)	1
Untypable	46 (45%)	12 (86%)
Total	102 (100%)	14 (100%)

Table 8. Method used for biological assay with culture filtrate of group F vibrio.

Culture medium and condition:
BHI broth with 1% NaCl; shaking (120 rev/min) at 37 C for 24 hours

Biological assays in culture filtrates:

1. Hemolytic activity — Agar plate method using blood agar with 5% sheep erythrocytes(24 hours)
2. Mouse lethality ——— Intravenous inoculation(24 hours)
3. CHO-cell assay ——— Chamber slide method (24 hours)
4. Infant mouse assay — Direct intragastric inoculation(4 hours)

Table 9. Biological activities of group F vibrio strains.

Biotype	No. of strains	Number of positive strains in assay of: Hemolytic activity	Mouse lethality	Cytotoxicity in CHO cells	Infant mouse reactivity
I	96 (100%)	75 (78%)	54 (56%)	76 (79%)	32 (33%)
II	13 (100%)	10 (77%)	6 (46%)	10 (77%)	5 (38%)
Total	109 (100%)	85 (78%)	60 (55%)	86 (79%)	37 (34%)

The diameter of the hemolytic zone ranged between 4mm to 10mm. Thirty per cent of positives found in biotype I and 38% of positives found in biotype II were strongly hemolytic, revealing zones greater than 7mm in diameter. Some of those strains giving intense hemolytic reaction were further subjected to the RPHA test for detection of Kanagawa hemolysin in *V. parahaemolyticus* [10], and all gave negative results, suggesting that hemolysin produced by group F vibrio is immunologically different from Kanagawa hemolysin of *V. parahaemolyticus.*

Mouse leathality was defined by death of animals within 24 hours after intravenous inoculation of the test materials. Fifty-six per cent of biotype I and 46% of biotype II were found positive. Some animals reacted severely, and died within few minutes after exhibiting spasmodic movement.

In the CHO cell assay, most of the strains were found to give cytopathic effect. Elongation was absent even in the strains which demonstrated no cytotoxicity. When cytotoxicity was examined with the culture filtrates diluted 1:100, about 80% of both type I and II were found positive.

On the other hand, in the infant mouse assay, 3 mice were allocated for each material and the average intestine/body weight ratio fell into the range of 0.043 to 0.099. If positivity was defined as a ratio of 0.07 or greater when averaged from 3 mice, positives were found 32 out of 96 or at 32% in biotype I and 5 out of 13 strains (40%) in biotype II.

Furthermore, some of the hemolysis positive and negative strains were submitted to the guinea pig skin test, rabbit ileal loop test and RPHA test for choleratoxin and *E. coli* LT[11], but none of these results suggested the presence of any factor(s) similar to choleratoxin or *E. coli* LT.

Then we examined how these activities related to one another. Table 10 summarizes results based on the combination of these 4 activities for each biotype. The combination of 4 positives accounted for 27 strains(28%) in biotype I and 3 strains (23%) in biotype II. Thirty-one strains(32%) of biotype I and 4 strains(31%) of biotype II had 3 positive reactions while being negative for either the mouse lethality or infant mouse

Table 10. Patterns of biological activities observed in group F vibrio.

Reaction in assay of:				Number of strains		
Hemolytic activity	CHO Cells	Mouse lethality	Infant mouse	I	II	Total
+	+	+	+	27 (28 %)	3 (23 %)	30 (28 %)
+	+	+	–	27 (28)	3 (23)	30 (28)
+	+	–	+	4 (4)	1 (8)	5 (5)
+	+	–	–	10 (10)	2 (15)	12 (11)
+	–	–	–	7 (7)	1 (8)	8 (7)
–	+	–	+	1 (1)	–	1 (1)
–	+	–	–	7 (7)	1 (8)	8 (7)
–	–	–	–	13 (14)	2 (15)	15 (14)
Total				96 (100%)	13 (100%)	109(100%)

reactivity. In short, the majority of the strains of both types showed positive results in 3 or more assays. Twenty-five strains(26%) of biotype I and 4 strains (31%) of biotype II were positive in one or two tests. About 14% of both biotypes had negative results in all 4 assays. Again, no difference was observed between the 2 biotypes, either in the result of individual assays or in combination of different assays.

On the other hand, when we tried to analyze the interrelation between these activities, a fairly strong correlation was observed between the hemolytic activity and cytotoxicity in CHO cells, as well as between the mouse lethality and each of the other two. The hemolytic activity and infant mouse reactivity were also found to be related to each other, although the correlation was not so strong.

The relation between the hemolytic activity and mouse lethality is depicted in Fig. 1. As clearly indicated in the figure, all hemolysis negatives allowed the animals to survive, whereas the hemolysis positives revealed higher mouse mortality, the survival time being progressively shorter with increasing intensity of the hemolytic reaction. In other wards, the hemolytic activity and mouse lethality are well correlated.

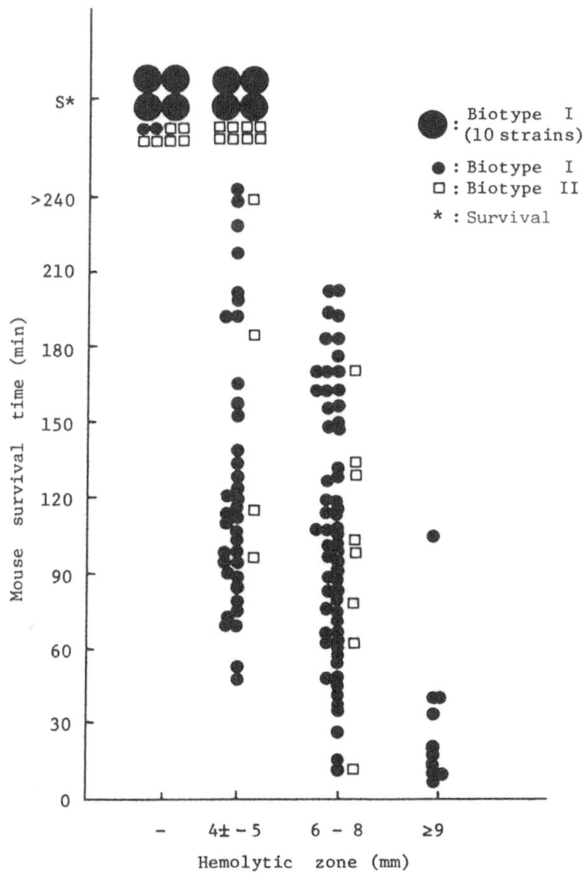

Fig. 1. The correlation between the hemolytic activity and mouse lethal toxicity of group F vibrio.

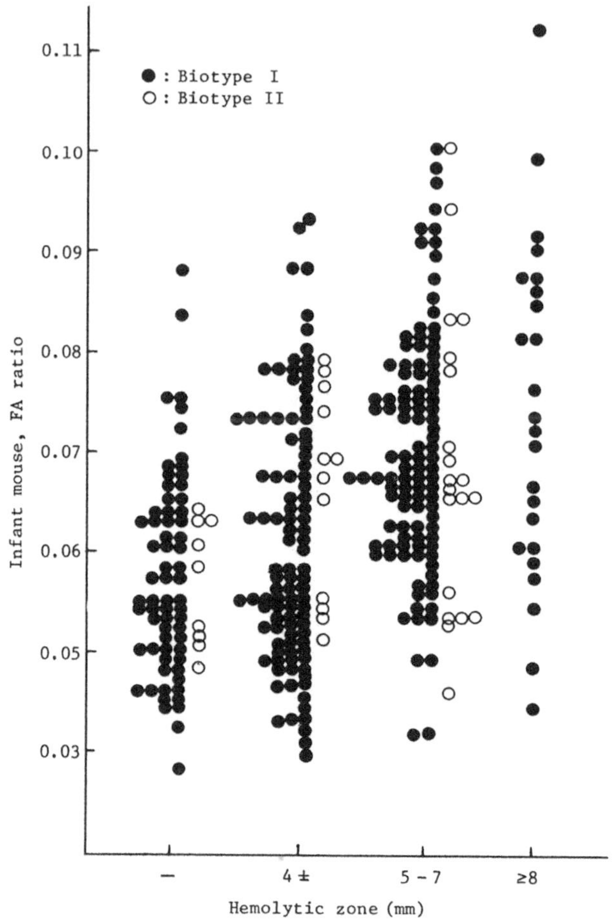

Fig. 2. The correlation between the hemolytic activity and infant mouse reactivity of group F vibrio.

Fig. 2 shows the relation between the hemolytic and infant mouse reactivity. Again, the fluid accumulation ratio seems to increase almost in parallel with the hemolytic activity increase, suggesting the existence of a certain level of correlation.

We have reported in this paper an outline of characterization of group F vibrio. As far as the major biochemical characters of this vibrio are concerned, our results basically agree quite well with the previously reported results.[1,2,9,12] However, our results differ significantly from the others with respect to indole reaction and growth in peptone water without NaCl. These characters are presently accepted as being useful for identification of this organism, and their description must be quickly corrected so that any confusion in identification should be avoided. Although we attempted to study biotyping of the organism proposed by Lee *et al.*,[9] our results are still unsatisfactory due to a limited number of test strains, and difference in biotype distribution is not yet fully understood. We also examined the value of these characters as criteria for biotyping and noticed that some were not suitable with the exception of gas from glucose. Application of these characteristics for differentiation must be carefully studied in future.

The serotyping system based on O antigen of this organism was experimented for the first time in our study and was confirmed as a useful system. In addition to the attempt to further develop this system, the relationship between the serotype and biotype and the serotype distribution remain to be elucidated in future.

In an attempt to elucidate the enteropathogenicity of vibrio, we have studied extracellular pathogenic factors. As already been mentioned, our results suggested absence of any substance similar to those commonly known pathogenic factors such as Kanagawa hemolytsin, choleratoxin or *E. coli* LT and ST. However, we were much interested in noting that a significant number of strains demonstrated hemolytic activity and cytotoxicity in CHO cells, and some showed lethal toxicity in mice and reactivity in infant mice, regardless of their origin or biotype.

We are in the process of trying to identify factors responsible for those activities. We are not certain whether they are induced by a single common factor or by different factors. However, the fact that the hemolytic activity correlated well with the other activities suggests that a certain kind of hemolysin(s) is playing an important role in these reactions. Enteropathogenicity of *V. parahaemolyticus* [13] or *Aeromonas* [14] has so far been attributed to a certain kind of hemolysin.

We hope that a better understanding of the factor(s) responsible for the hemolytic activity of this organism will provide many useful informations to help us elucidate the pathogenicity of this organism.

REFERENCES

1. Furniss, A. L., J. V. Lee, and T. J. Donovan. 1977. Group F: a new *Vibrio*? Lancet ii:565-566.
2. Brenner, D. J., R. E. Weaver, D. G. Hollis, and B. R. Davis. 1979. The EF-6 group of *Vibrio*-like bacteria. Abstracts of the Annual Meeting of the American Society for Microbiology, p. 35.
3. Huq, M. I., A.K.M.J. Alam, D. J. Brenner, and G. K. Morris. 1980. Isolation of *Vibrio* like group, EF-6, from patients with diarrhea. J. Clin. Microbiol. **11**: 621- 624.
4. WHO Scientific Working Group. 1980. Cholera and other vibrio-associated diarrhoeas. WHO Bull. **58**:353-374.
5. Blake, P. A., R.E. Weaver, and D. G. Hollis. 1980. Diseases of human (other than cholera) caused by vibrios. Ann. Rev. Microbiol. **34**:341-367.
6. Kudoh, Y., M. Tsuno, S. Matsushita, S. Yamada, K. Ohta, T. Itoh, S. Sakai, and M. Ohashi. 1981. Biochemical and serological chracteristics and enteropathogenicity of Group F vibrio. Japan. J. Bacteriol. **36**:242(Text in Japanese).
7. Itoh, T., T. Maruyama, M. Tsuno, S. Matsushita, S. Yamada, A. Kai, K. Saitoh, K. Ohta, Y. Kudoh, S. Sakai, M. Ohashi, S. Kumaoka, and R. Phan-Urai. 1981. Bacteriological survey on diarrheal diseases in a rural area in Thailand, Chanthaburi. Proc. 16th Jt. Conf. Cholera, U. S.-Japan Coop. Med. Sci. Prog., Gifu, p.29-45.
8. Sanyal, S. C., R. K. Agarwal, E. Annapurna, and J. V. Lee. 1980. Enterotoxicity of Group F vibrios. Japan. J. Med. Sci. Biol. **33**:217-222.
9. Lee, J. V., P. Shread,. L. Furniss, and T. N. Bryant. 1981. Taxonomy and description of *Vibrio fluvialis* sp. nov.(synonym group F vibrios, group EF6). J. Appl. Bacteriol. **50**:73-94.
10. Ohta, K., Y. Kudoh, M. Tsuno, S. Sakai, T. Maruyama, T. Itoh, and M. Ohashi. 1979. Development of a sensitive serological assay based on reversed passive hemagglutination for detection of enteropathogenic toxin(kanagawa hemolysin) of *Vibrio parahaemolyticus*, and re-evaluation of the toxin producibility of isolates from various sources. Japan. J. Bacteriol. **34**:837-846 (Text in Japanese).

11. Kudoh, Y., S. Yamada, S. Matsushita, K. Ohta, M. Tsuno, T. Muraoka, N. Ohtomo, and M. Ohashi. 1978. Detection of heat-labile enterotoxin of *Escherichia coli* by reversed passive hemagglutination test with specific immunoglobulin against choleratoxin. Proc. 14th Jt. Conf. Cholera, U. S.-Japan Coop. Med. Sci. Prog., Karatsu, p.266-273.
12. Jensen, M. J., P. Baumann, M. Mandel, and J. V. Lee. 1980. Characterization of facultatively anaerobic marine bacteria belonging to group F of Lee, Donovan, and Furniss. Curr. Microbiol. 3:373-376.
13. Zen-Yoji, H., Y. Kudoh, H. Igarashi, K. Ohta, K. Fukai, and T. Hoshino. 1976. Further studies on characterization and biological activities of an enteropathogenic toxin of *Vibrio parahaemolyticus.* p. 479-498. *In* A. Ohsaka, K. Hayashi and Y. Sawai(ed.), Animal, Plant, and Microbial Toxins, Vol. 1. Plenum Publ. Corp., New York.
14. Ljungh, Å., M. Popoff, and T. Wadström. 1977. *Aeromonas hydrophila* in acute diarrheal disease: Detection of enterotoxin and biotyping of strains. J. Clin. Microbiol. 6:96-100.

Advances in Research on Cholera and Related Diarrheas, eds., S. Kuwahara, N. F. Pierce, 87–99.

IN VITRO AND *IN VIVO* BIOLOGIC ACTIVITIES OF *VIBRIO FLUVIALIS* AND ITS TOXIC PRODUCTS

D. E. Lockwood, S. H. Richardson, A. S. Kreger, M. Aiken, and B. McCreedy

Bowman-Gray School of Medicine, Wake Forest University
Winston-Salem, N. C. 27103

Introduction

Vibrio fluvialis sp. nov. (15) is a halophilic bacterium which was originally isolated in 1975 from a patient with diarrhea from Bahrain from whom no other bacterial enteric pathogens could be isolated (8) and was first called group F (8, 11, 13, 14) or EF-6 (10). *V. fluvialis* is widely distributed in marine and estuarine environments and has been repeatedly isolated from humans exhibiting severe diarrheal disease (4, 8, 10, 15, 17, 19, 20). The clinical features of the disease closely resemble cholera, except that 75% of the patients examined during a *V. fluvialis*-associated diarrheal outbreak in Bangladesh in 1976-1977 had blood and mucus in their stools (10). Reports on the enteropathogenicity of this organism have yielded conflicting results ranging from negative reports of enterotoxin production (4, 10, 17, 20) to reports that whole cultures and sterile culture filtrates cause fluid accumulation in rabbit ileal loops as well as cytotoxic and cytotonic responses in tissue culture (1, 19). However, no toxin has been found to be associated with these effects. These observations prompted us to investigate the possibility that *V. fluvialis* produces toxin(s) which might contribute to the pathogenesis of the disease attributed to this organism.

Assays. (i) Activity against Chinese hamster ovary (CHO) cells. The ability to kill or to cause a change in the morphology of CHO cells (elongation or rounding) was estimated by the general methodology of Guerrant *et al.* (9). Serial two-fold dilutions of the preparations to be tested were made and 10 ul of each dilution were added to CHO cells plated in separate microtiter wells. The cells were examined (without staining) for necrosis, elongation, and rounding after incubation for 18 hrs. at 37 C. One unit of CHO cell killing (CK), CHO cell rounding (RF), and CHO cell elongation (CEF) activity was expressed as the reciprocal of the highest dilution that killed >10% of the cells or that caused >10% of the cells to exhibit a change in their characteristic epithelioid morphology, respectively.

(ii) Hemolytic activity. Hemolytic activity was determined by the method of Bernheimer and Schwartz (3). One hemolytic unit was defined as the reciprocal of the dilution that resulted in the release of 50% of the hemoglobin in a standardized (0.7%, v/v) rabbit erythrocyte suspension.

(iii) Protease activity. Protease activity was assayed by the azocasein substrate method described by Kreger and Gray (12). One unit of activity was defined as the reciprocal of the dilution that yielded a reaction mixture containing enough trichloroacetic acid-soluble, diazotized peptides to give an absorbance of 1 at 440 nm.

Toxin production by V. fluvialis strain 5439. Seed cultures were obtained from a slant streaked with one loopful of a rapidly thawed specimen of the bacterium and incubated for 6 h at 37 C. The bacteria were washed from the slant with heart infusion broth (HI, 3 ml) and the suspension was adjusted to an optical density at 640 nm of ca. 6. Two ml of the bacterial suspension were added to 1 liter of HI contained in a New Brunswick Multigen bench-top fermentor. The culture was maintained at 30 C, infused with 0.5 liters of air/min., and agitated at an impeller speed of 250 rpms. The growth of bacteria was monitored by plate counts every 2 hrs., and portions (2 ml) of the culture supernatant fluids were obtained by centrifugation. In addition, cell-free extracts were prepared from washed (5 ml of 0.85% NaCl) cell pellets suspended in 0.85% NaCl (5 ml) and sonically disrupted at 4 C until the suspension was clarified. Debris was removed by centrifugation. Culture supernatant fluids and cell-free extracts were stored at -60 C until assayed.

Isolation of crude concentrated preparations of toxins produced by V. fluvialis strain 5439. Culture conditions were the same as described before.

(i) CK. Growth was halted when the culture reached an optical density at 640 nm of ca. 5 (approximately 6 hrs.). Supernatant fluids obtained by centrifugation were filtered through a 0.8 u Millipore filter and precipitated by 50% saturation with ammonium sulfate at 4 C. The precipitate, removed by centrifugation, was resuspended in 10 ml of 5 mM Tris-HCl buffer (pH 7.5) and was dialyzed for ca. 18 hrs. against 4 liters of the same buffer at 4 C. The dialyzed preparation was clarified by centrifugation and stored at -60 C until assayed.

(ii) RF. A concentrated preparation containing RF activity was prepared as described for the isolation of CK except that the growth of the culture was continued for 18 hrs.

(iii) CEF. After 18 hrs. of growth, cells were removed by centrifugation and washed twice with 0.85% NaCl (200 ml). The cells were resuspended in 100 ml of cold (4 C) 5 mM Tris-HCl buffered saline (PB buffer; pH 7.1) containing 1 mg polymyxin B per ml. Cell-free extracts, containing CEF activity, were prepared by a modification of the polymyxin B extraction technique described by Evans *et al.* (6). Cells were shaken in a 37 C water bath for 2.5 min. after the temperature of the suspension reached 10 C. The cell suspension was cooled (<10 C) in an ice-water bath and cellular debris was removed by centrifugation. The cell-free extract was acidified to pH 2.0, precipitated cellular material was removed by centrifugation, and the supernatant fluid was adjusted to pH 7.1. Reneutralization of the pH resulted in additional precipitation of contaminating material which was removed by centrifugation. Soluble protein was precipitated by 70% saturation with ammonium sulfate at 4 C. The precipitate was dissolved in 5 ml 5 mM Tris-HCl buffer and dialyzed for ca. 18 hrs. against 4 liters of the same buffer at 4 C. The dialyzed cell extract was clarified by centrifugation and stored at –60 C until assayed.

Screening of clinical and environmental isolates of V. fluvialis for activity against CHO cells. Cultures of *V. fluvialis* isolates examined for CEF, CK or RF activities were prepared by inoculating HI (5ml in 50-ml erlenmeyer flasks) with 5 colonies from

Columbia agar-5% sheep blood cultures grown overnight at 37 C and incubating the broths at 30 C for 18 hrs. with gyratory agitation (220 cycles/min.). The culture supernatant fluids were obtained by centrifugation and were stored at –60 C until assayed. Cell-free extracts of washed (10 ml of 0.85% NaCl) bacteria were prepared by shaking the cells for 7 min. at 37 C in 1 ml of 5 mM Tris-HCl-buffered saline (pH 7.1) containing 1 mg of polymyxin B per ml, and removing debris and remaining cells by centrifugation. The extracts were stored at –60 C until assayed.

Infant mouse assay. Infant CFW mice employed in the experiments weighed 3.0 – 5.0 gr. (4–5 days old) and were starved 6 hrs. prior to inoculation. Viable cell inocula were prepared by washing 12–hr. HI agar slant cultures (grown at 37 C) with HI (1 ml). Serial dilutions were made in HI plus 0.01% Evans blue dye (dissolved in 0.85% saline). Cholera toxin or *V. fluvialis* toxic products were diluted in PB buffer with 0.01% Evans blue dye. A 0.25 ml glass tuberculin syringe fitted with a 23-gauge needle tipped with 1 cm of intramedic polyethylene tubing was used to inoculate mice intragastrically with 50 ul of sample. After the desired time interval, mice were sacrificed by cervical dislocation and the fluid accumulation (FA) ratio was determined for each mouse as described by Baselski *et al.* (2). The FA ratio is defined as follows: weight of stomach and intestines/(total body weight–weight of stomach and intestines). FA ratios are interpreted as follows: (–), <0.064; (±), 0.065–0.069; (+), 0.070–0.099; (strong +), >0.100.

Results and Discussion

A prototype *V. fluvialis* organism, strain 5439, originally isolated from a patient with diarrhea in Bangladesh was grown at 30 C with agitation in HI for 24 hrs. Because of our past experience with the isolation of cell-bound *E. coli* heat–labile toxin, both culture supernatant fluids and sonicated cell-free extracts from washed cells at various stages of growth were tested for hemolytic activity against rabbit erythrocytes, protease activity using an azocasein substrate and activity in CHO cells. The results of these experiments are shown in Fig. 1. Figure 1A shows a growth curve (triangles) expressed as colony forming units (CFU)/ml as well as titers of two products found in *cell-free extracts* of the organism. A factor which caused CHO cell elongation (CEF) similar to that produced by *V. cholerae* toxin and *E. coli* heat-labile enterotoxin was first detected after 8 hrs. of incubation and it continued to be produced maximally through 20 hrs. (closed circles). A CHO cell killing factor (open circles) reached maximum levels during log phase growth, 4 to 8 hrs. after inoculation, and decreased but persisted through 12 hrs., during which it interfered with the detection of the CEF at lower dilutions.

CEF was not detected in *supernatant fluids* because of two cytotoxic factors present. In Figure 1B, CHO cell killing activity (CK; closed circles) which caused complete lysis of the cells was detected in supernatant fluids after 4 hrs. of incubation. This activity then disappeared concomitant with the appearance of a factor that caused a rounding of the normally epithelioid-shaped CHO cells (RF; open circles). The kinetics of the appearance of CK and RF were similar to that of the appearance of hemolytic and protease activities found in supernatant fluids of this organism (Figure 1C). The loss of hemolytic activity (closed circles), which peaked 6 hrs. after inoculation, correlated with the appearance of protease activity (open circles). Neither hemolytic nor proteolytic activities were found in cell-free extracts. It is possible that the RF (Figure 1B) is a function of the protease (Figure 1C), due to their similar kinetics. However, the CK (Figure 1B) in supernatant fluids and the hemolysin (Figure 1C) may be different prod-

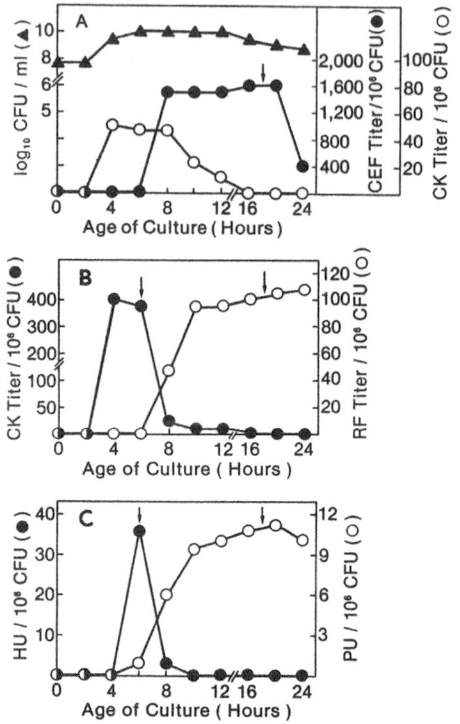

Figure 1. Detection of CEF, CK, RF, hemolytic and protease activities in cultures of *V. fluvialis* strain 5439. Arrows indicate the time at which each culture was harvested to provide concentrated preparations of each respective toxin. (A) Relationship between growth (▲) and the amount of intracellular CEF (●) and CK (○) activities. (B) Production of extracellular CK (●) and RF (○) activities. (C) Production of extracellular hemolysin(s) (●) and protease(s) (○).

ucts because of their slightly different kinetic curves; the CK being produced at 4 hrs. in the absence of any hemolytic activity.

The remaining studies were carried out using concentrated preparations of each toxin. Culture supernatant fluids were concentrated by ammonium sulfate precipitation after removal of cells either 6 hrs. after inoculation (for isolation of CK activity) or 18 hrs. after inoculation (for isolation of RF activity). Crude CEF was removed by polymyxin B extraction (6) from washed cells after 18 hrs. of growth and extensively purified by acid precipitation of contaminants followed by ammonium sulfate precipitation, flat-bed isoelectric focusing and gel filtration. This partially purified preparation was free of cytolytic activity but still formed several bands on polyacrylamide gel electrophoresis and was much less potent in CHO cells than purified cholera toxin; requiring 22 ng of material to produce CHO elongation compared to 11.6 pg of cholera toxin. (16)

Toxin-induced changes in CHO cell topography were further characterized by scanning electron microscopy. Figure 2 shows asynchronous cells after 2 hrs. of incubation. CHO cells vary in roundness and relative densities of microvilli and surface blebs depending on the stage of the cell cycle they happen to be in. Untreated cells (Figure 2A) contain numerous microvilli and few blebs, a majority of which are contained on the rounded central portions of the cells. Irregular cell peripheries are ruffled and flattened reflecting attachment. In contrast, cells treated with CK (Figure 2C) and RF (Figure 2D) show a definite retraction of their flattened peripheries, while CK-treated cells contain profuse microvilli and RF–treated cells contain abundant blebbing, apparently a manifestation of the different effects of these toxins on the cells. CHO cells treated with CEF (Figure 2B) are beginning to flatten, lose surface extensions and elongate.

After 12 hrs., when all apparent morphological changes are maximal (Figure 3), control cells (Figure 3A) are much more flattened out, reflecting increased adhesion to the surface and contain varying numbers of microvilli on more rounded cells and blebs on more flattened cells. CK-treated cells (Figure 3C) have degenerated to shrunken cell remnants resembling cells treated with the thermostable direct hemolysin of *V. parahemolyticus* (18). RF-treated cells (Figure 3D) are completely rounded with prominant blebbing and exhibit much reduced adhesion to the surface reminiscent of tissue culture cells treated with trypsin (21). Cells treated with CEF (Figure 3B) are fully elongated with no surface protrusions, like cells treated with cholera toxin or *E. coli* heat-labile enterotoxin. Other cells shown in Figure 3B that are not fully elongated may suggest that cells in a particular phase of their growth cycle are more sensitive to this cytotonic toxin.

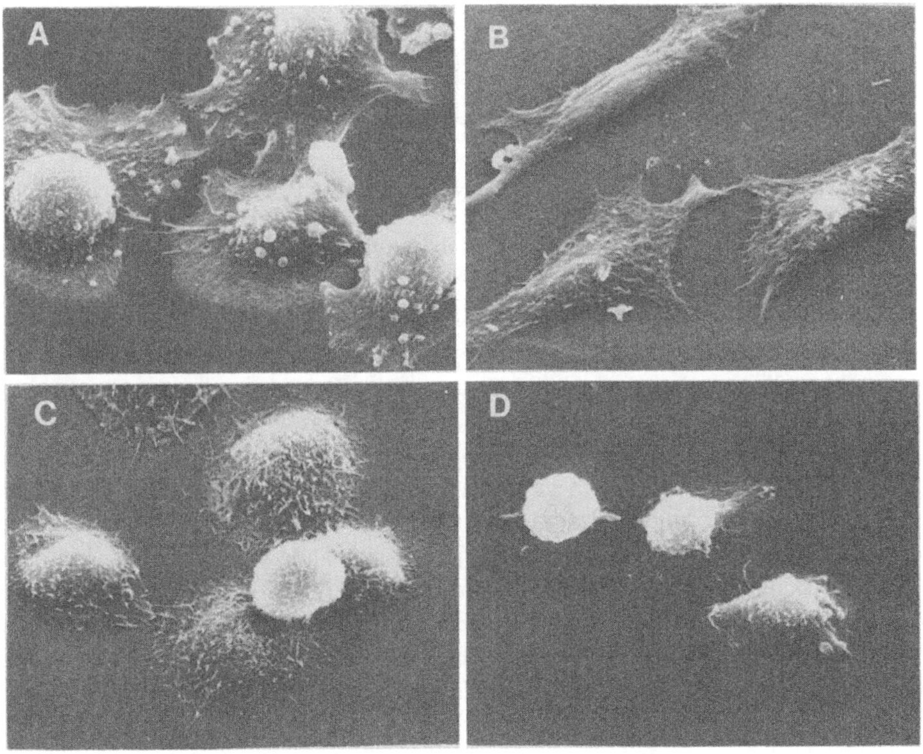

Figure 2. Scanning electron micrographs of asynchronous CHO cells exposed to *V. fluvialis* toxic products for 2 hrs. at 37 C. (A) Untreated cells. (B) Cells treated with cell-free extract containing 4 CEF units of activity. (C) Cells treated with culture supernatant fluid containing 40 CK units of activity. (D) Cells treated with culture supernatant fluid containing 20 RF units of activity.

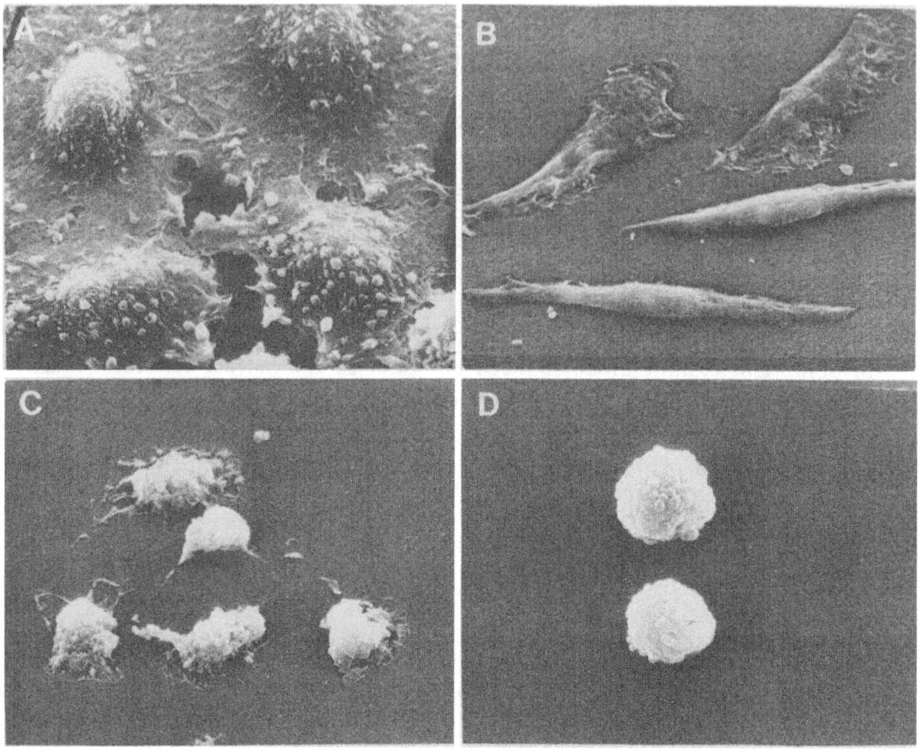

Figure 3. Scanning electron micrographs of asynchronous CHO cells exposed to *V. fluvialis* toxic products for 12 hrs. at 37 C. (A) Untreated cells. (B) Cells treated with cell-free extract containing 4 CEF units of activity. (C) Cells treated with culture supernatant fluid containing 40 units of CK activity. (D) Cells treated with culture supernatant fluid containing 20 units of RF activity.

The concentrated *V. fluvialis* toxin preparations were then tested by the rabbit ileal loop assay (5) and the permeability factor assay (7). The preparation containing RF activity produced a positive hemorrhagic ileal loop response while the preparations containing CEF or CK activity were negative in this model. Each toxin preparation was then tested for increased permeability activity in rabbit skin. The CEF preparation produced only trace amounts of blueing while the CK and RF preparations produced strong, atypical reactions, consisting of hemorrhaging and necrosis at the injection sites.

The skin and ligated loop assays constitute highly artificial systems not resembling the naturally occurring disease complex. Because cholera is a diarrheal disease, we were interested in employing a model where fluid secretion is used as an index of infection. For this we chose the orally inoculated infant mouse model reported in 1977 by Dr. Charlotte Parker's laboratory (2). In this system, resulting signs closely resemble human disease (severe diarrhea and subsequent death) and the mode of infection is that which occurs naturally.

Groups of mice (6 mice or greater) were therefore challenged with 10^9 viable organisms of *V. fluvialis* and *V. cholerae* 569 B, each washed from a 12-hr. HI agar slant with HI. HI was injected as a negative control and mice were examined 4, 8, 12, and 16 hrs. post challenge. The results expressed as means of FA ratios plus 1 standard error of the mean are shown in Figure 4. The positive FA ratios at 0 time are due to the weight of the fluid inoculated. The controls thereafter have uniformly negative FA ratios not statistically different than FA ratios from uninoculated animals. In contrast, 569B-infected animals demonstrated a steady increase in FA ratios from 4 until 16 hrs. post inoculation. By 8 hrs. post challenge the difference between control and 569 B-infected animals was significant. On the other hand, *V. fluvialis* challenged mice showed a significantly greater FA ratio after only 4 hrs. post challenge. This early response was referrable to viable organisms because mice injected with an equivalent number of heat-killed bacteria produced a negative FA ratio not statistically different from control mice. In this experiment, *V. fluvialis*-infected mice produced positive FA ratios throughout the 16-hr. time period. There was also noticeable hemorrhage in the 12 and 16-hr. infected mice. The FA ratios varied considerably at each time period, however. In some cases, beginning at 4 hrs. post challenge, the *V. fluvialis*-infected mice were actively purging to the extent that the FA ratios from these mice were very close to the negative value of 0.065. In order to more reproducibly quantitate the fluid produced by challenged mice, the system was closed by anally occluding infected mice with Elmer's Wonder Bond (cyanoacrylate ester glue).

To determine whether a bolus of 10^9 normal flora organisms could produce positive FA ratios non-specifically in this closed system, single mice were inoculated with 10^9 *V. fluvialis* or HI as shown in Table 1. After 4 hrs. the FA ratio was determined for each individual mouse, the intestines were homogenized in HI, and viable bacteria were quantitated. 10^9 *V. fluvialis* were recovered from a positive mouse while sham-infected mice yielded two logs less of viable *E. coli* and *S. epidermidis*. A culture of each of these organisms was grown up on HI agar, washed from the slant with HI and 10^9 bacteria of

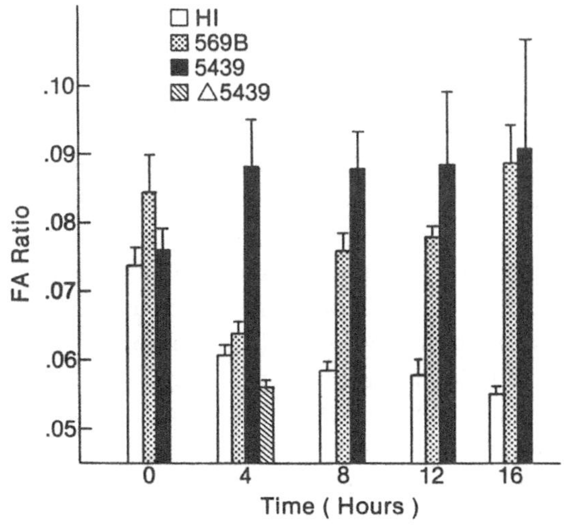

Figure 4. Time course of FA in CFW mice challenged with *V. fluvialis* strain 5439 or *V. cholerae* strain 569 B. Means of FA ratios plus 1 standard error of the mean are shown. Symbols: □, control animals given HI; ▩, test animals challenged with 1 x 10^9 CFU of *V. cholerae* strain 569 B; ■, test animals challenged with 1 x 10^9 CFU of *V. fluvialis* strain 5439; ▧, test animals challenged with 1 x 10^9 heat-killed *V. fluvialis* organisms.

Table 1. Measurement of the pathogenicity of *V. Fluvialis, E. coli, S. Epidermidis*, during mouse passage.[a]

First passage			Second passage		
Inoculum/ID	Recovery/ID	FA[b]	Inoculum/ID[c]	Recovery/ID	FA[d]
1.2×10^9[e] *V. fluvialis*	1.67×10^9 *V. fluvialis*	.1065	1.38×10^9 *V. fluvialis*	1.37×10^9 *V. fluvialis* 1.9×10^8 *E. coli*	.0850 ±.0037 ($p<0.1$)
HI	2.1×10^7 *E. coli* 5.7×10^6 *S. epidermidis*	.0576	1.12×10^9 *S. epidermidis*	1.04×10^9 *S. epidermidis* 4.00×10^8 *E. coli*	.0621 ±.0020
HI	4.38×10^7 *E. coli* 1.31×10^7 *S. epidermidis*	.0573	1.07×10^9 *E. coli*	1.07×10^9 *E. coli*	.0605 ±.0020

[a]FA ratios determined 4 hrs. postchallenge.

[b]FA ratio determined on individual animals.

[c]Inoculum consisted of cultures derived from organisms recovered from first mouse passage.

[d]Mean FA ratio ±1 standard error of the mean of 6 mice challenged with each organism.

[e]CFU/animal.

each species were inoculated into 6 additional mice. 10^9 bacteria of each respective species were recovered from second passage mice along with accompanying normal flora in two cases. The mean positive FA ratio of *V. fluvialis*-infected mice was significantly greater than either *E. coli* or *S. epidermidis*-challenged mice. The *V. fluvialis* recovered from each challenged mouse had the same biotype as the inoculum, thereby satisfying Koch's postulates for this organism in this animal model.

Figure 5 demonstrates the appearance of occluded mice with positive or negative FA ratios. This figure shows a *V. fluvialis*-infected mouse on the left and a HI-inoculated animal on the right 4 hrs. post challenge. The distension of the gut of the mouse on the left reflects secretion of fluid into the intestinal lumen.

The relative virulence of *V. fluvialis* in this animal model was then compared to that of *V. cholerae* 569 B and *V. cholerae* CA 401, a classical Inaba strain isolated from a fatal case of diarrhea in Calcutta. Dr. Parker has used CA 401 as her prototype *V. cholerae* strain with this animal model. Dose response curves were determined at the time period post challenge at which maximal fluid accumulation first occurred. The end point of each dose response curve was the minimum number of organisms required to produce FA ratios significantly greater than the FA ratios of mice inoculated with HI. Table 2 indicates that 4.3×10^7 CFU of *V. fluvialis* 4 hrs. post challenge was required for a response significantly greater than controls. In experiments not shown, there was no significant

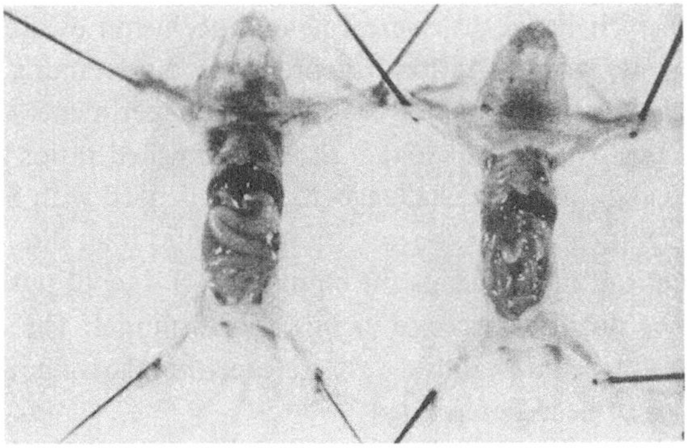

Figure 5. Intestines of occluded CFW mice challenged 4 hrs. previously with 1 x 10^9 CFU of *V. fluvialis* strain 5439(left) and heart infusion (HI) broth (right). The mouse challenged with viable *V. fluvialis* organisms contains intestines distended with clear fluid. The HI-inoculated mouse has an intestinal tract similar to that seen in uninoculated mice.

increase in FA ratios beyond 8 hrs. post challenge in 569 B-infected mice. Therefore, the dose response at 8 hrs. was determined for this organism and was found to be 2.9x 10^7 CFU. However, CA 401, which Dr. Parker has shown to be more virulent in this model than 569 B, required 6.8x10^6 organisms to produce a positive response at 8 hrs. post challenge, but only 7.9x10^5 CFU to produce positive FA ratios at 16 hrs. The dose response values of the *V. cholerae* strains in our experiments were similar to those obtained by Dr. Parker and reflect the greater virulence of CA 401 compared to 569 B in this model. However, we did find that *V. fluvialis* is at least as virulent in this animal model as 569 B, a strain used by many investigators because of its ability to produce unusually large amounts of cholera toxin *in vitro*.

The three toxin preparations isolated form *V. fluvialis* were then tested in the suckling mouse. Figure 6 shows the results of these experiments. Mean FA ratios plus 1 standard error of the mean are shown. Mice inoculated with diluent (5 mM Tris-buffered saline) showed positive FA ratios at 0 time and negative values at 4 and 8 hrs. Both the CK and RF-challenged mice showed FA ratio patterns similar at 4 hrs. post challenge to

Table 2. Smallest number of live vibrios that induces a significant fluid response.[a]

Strain	Time postchallenge (hr)	Dose[b]	*p*
5439	4	4.29 x 10^7	$p < .05$
569 B	8	2.88 x 10^7	$p < .05$
CA 401	8	6.77 x 10^6	$p < .01$
CA 401	16	7.94 x 10^5	$p < .01$

[a]Significance was determined by comparing FA ratios of vibrio-inoculated animals with controls given HI plus Evans blue dye.

[b]CFU/animal.

mice inoculated with viable *V. fluvialis* organisms. Fluid accumulation was abundant enough by 8 hrs. post challenge to overcome anal occlusion of most mice, resulting in extensive purging and negative FA ratios. The preparation containing CEF produced a FA ratio pattern similar to that of cholera toxin in this experiment. Mice inoculated with both toxins showed positive FA ratios at 0 time, diminished ratios at 4 hrs. and significantly positive ratios at 8 hrs. post challenge. Mice challenged with 8 ug of cholera toxin, however, showed a significantly greater response at 8 hrs. than did mice inoculated with 28 ug of CEF preparation. In our hands the equivalent of 4 ug of purified cholera toxin is necessary to produce a positive response in this animal model. The dose response of the CEF preparation has not been established, therefore the relative potency of this toxin in this animal model has not been determined.

To determine if production of these toxic products was limited to our prototype *V. fluvialis* strain, 22 human isolates and 21 environmental isolates of *V. fluvialis* from our collection were surveyed for production of CEF, CK, and RF activities. In each case, organisms were grown in HI for 18 hrs. at 30 C with agitation. Supernatant fluids and polymyxin B extracted cell-free extracts were tested for activities in CHO cells. The results are shown in Table 3. No significant difference was noted in the production of CEF and either CK or RF activities by the clinical and environmental strains. 82% of the clinical isolates and 71% of the environmental strains were found to have CEF activity associated with their cell-free extracts. In some cases CK activity was also found in cell-free extracts but was diluted out before reaching the end points of the CEF activity. CK and RF activities seemed to be mutually exclusive because in no case were the two toxins found together in supernatant fluids from either clinical or environmental isolates.

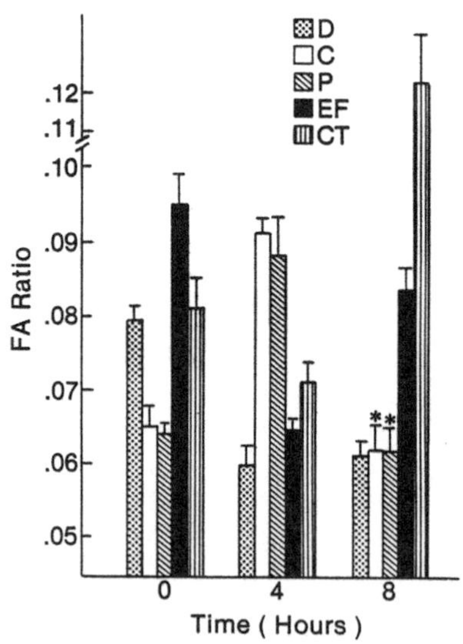

Figure 6. Time course of FA in CFW mice challenged with *V. fluvialis* toxic products. Means of FA ratios plus 1 standard error of the mean are depicted. Symbols: Mice inoculated with ▩,5 mM Tris-buffered saline (D); □, 640 units of CK activity (C); ▧,80 units of RF activity (P); ■,1,280 units (28 ug) of CEF activity (EF); ▥, 8ug of cholera toxin (CT).

Table 3. Screening of clinical and environmental isolates of *V. fluvialis* for production of CHO cell elongation Factor (CEF), CHO killing factor (CKF), and CHO rounding factor (CRF) activities.

Number of strains	Isolated from	Cult. Supt. Flds.		Cell-free extracts	
		CKF	CRF	CEF	CKF
4 (18)[a]	Human	+		+	
6 (27)	"	+		+	+[b]
2 (9)	"	+			+
1 (4.5)	"	+			
4 (18)	"		+	+	
1 (4.5)	"		+	+	+
1 (4.5)	"		+		
2 (9)	"			+	
1 (4.5)	"			+	+
		13(59)[c]	6(27)	18(82)	10(45)
5 (24)	Environment	+		+	+
1 (5)	"	+		+	
2 (9.5)	"	+			
7 (33)	"		+	+	+
1 (5)	"		+	+	
1 (5)	"		+		+
1 (5)	"		+		
1 (5)	"	CEF		+	+
2 (9.5)	"				
		8 (38)[c]	10 (48)	15 (71)	14 (67)

[a]Number in parentheses indicates the percentage of strains demonstrating activity pattern.
[b]CHO cell killing activity did not interfere with detection of CEF activity in cell-free extracts because the former was removed by dilution prior to reaching the titer of CEF activity.
[c]Number in parentheses indicates the percentage of strains demonstrating activity.

68% of the clinical isolates produced either CK or RF in combination with CEF and 67% of the environmental isolates showed like patterns of toxic activities. One strain isolated from the bottom water of Chesapeake Bay was unique in that CEF activity was detected both in the cell-free extract and in the supernatant fluid.

The results of this survey point to two important facts. First, environmental isolates show the same potential to produce the toxic products that clinical isolates elaborate, indicating that environmental strains may have similar pathogenic capabilities. In support of this theory, Seidler and coworkers (19) reported that anaerogenic environmental isolates from the Washington, D.C. area produced fluid accumulation in rabbit ileal loops and cytotoxic and cytotonic reactions in Y-1 adrenal cells. Also these environmental strains were indistinguishable on a molecular-genetic basis from anaerogenic isolates from cases of human diarrhea. Second, the observation that CEF activity usually was detected in cell-free extracts but not in supernatant fluids of *V. fluvialis* cultures, should not be interpreted as indicating that the toxin is not released into the organism's environment. The presence of high titers of CK and RF in the culture supernatant fluids may interfere with detection of CEF activity. This idea is supported by the observation that the only supernatant fluid in which CEF activity was detected did not possess CK or RF activity. Therefore, when surveying bacteria for cholera toxin-like or *E. coli* heat labile-like toxins one must not neglect cell-free extracts.

The public health significance of *V. fluvialis* is still uncertain, but at least three observations suggest that *V. fluvialis* and/or its toxic products play a role in the pathogenesis of enteric disease. First, oral challenge of infant mice with viable cells produces intestinal fluid accumulation, diarrhea, and death with accompanying hemorrhage in some cases, which is similar to the clinical symptoms of patients from whom *V. fluvialis* was isolated. Second, the prototype *V. fluvialis* strain is as virulent in this animal model as a *V. cholerae* 01 strain, although producing an earlier FA response like that seen with *E. coli* ST. Third, a partially purified preparation of CEF and crude concentrates of CK and RF, all heat-labile products, also elicit fluid accumulation and diarrhea in animal models used to test enteric toxins. Studies are in progress to obtain homogeneous preparations of these products, so that their roles in the pathogenesis of enteric disease attributed to this organism can be evaluated.

This investigation was supported by an Intramural Research Support grant from the Bowman Gray School of Medicine.

REFERENCES

1. Agarwal, R. K., S. C. Sanyal, E. Annapurna and J. V. Lee. 1979. Enterotoxicity of group F vibrios. Abstr. Suppl. 6th Inter. Symp. Animal, Plant and Microb. Tox., p. 1.
2. Baselski, V., R. Briggs, and C. Parker. 1977. Intestinal fluid accumulation induced by oral challenge with *Vibrio cholerae* or cholera toxin in infant mice. Infect. Immun. **15**:704-712.
3. Bernheimer, A. W. and L. L. Schwartz. 1963. Isolation and composition of staphylococcal alpha toxin. J. Gen. Microbiol. **30**:455-468.
4. Blake, P. A., R. E. Weaver and D. G. Hollis. 1980. Diseases of humans (other than cholera) caused by vibrios. Ann. Rev. Microbiol. **34**:341-367.
5. De, S. N. and D. N. Chatterje. 1953. An experimental study of the mechanism of action of *Vibrio cholerae* on the intestinal mucous membrane. J. Pathol. Bacteriol. **66**:559-562.
6. Evans, D. J., D. G. Evans, and S. L. Gorbach. 1974. Polymyxin B-induced release of low-molecular weight heat-labile enterotoxin from *Escherichia coli*. Infect. Immun. **10**:1010-1017.
7. Evans, D. J. JR., D. G. Evans and S. L. Gorbach. 1973. Production of vascular permeability factor by enterotoxigenic *Escherichia coli* isolated from man. Infect. Immun. **8**:725-730.
8. Furniss, A. L., J. V. Lee and T. J. Donovan. 1977. Group F, a new vibrio? Lancet **2**:565-566.
9. Guerrant, R. L., L. L. Brunton, T. C. Schnaitman, L. I. Rebhun, and A. C. Gilman. 1974. Cyclic adenosine monophosphate and alteration of Chinese hamster ovary cell morphology: a rapid, sensitive *in vitro* assay for the enterotoxins of *Vibrio cholerae* and *Escherichia coli*. Infect. Immun. **10**:320-327.
10. Huq, M. I., A. K. M. J. Alam, D. J. Brenner, and G. K. Morris. 1980. Isolation of vibrio-like group, EF-6, from patients with diarrhea. J. Clin. Microbiol. **11**:621-624.
11. Jensen, M. J., P. Baumann, M. Mandel and J. V. Lee. 1980. Characterization of facultatively anaerobic marine bacteria belonging to group F of Lee, Donovan and Furniss. Curr. Microbiol. **3**:373-376.
12. Kreger, A. S. and L. D. Gray. 1978. Purification of *Pseudomonas aeruginosa* proteases and micro-

scopic characterization of pseudomonal protease-induced rabbit corneal damage. Infect. Immun. **19**:630-648.

13. Lee, J. V., T. J. Donovan and A. L. Furniss. 1978. Characterization, taxonomy, and amended description of *Vibrio metschnikovii*. Inter. J. Sys. Bacteriol. **28**:99-111.
14. Lee, J. V., P. Shread and A. L. Furniss. 1978. The taxonomy of group F organisms: relationships to *Vibrio* and *Aeromonas*. J. Appl. Bacteriol. **45**:ix.
15. Lee, J. V., P. Shread and A. L. Furniss. 1981. Taxonomy and description of *Vibrio fluvialis* sp. nov. (synonym group F vibrios, group EF6). J. Appl. Bacteriol. **50**:73-94.
16. Lockwood, D. E., A. S. Kreger, and S. H. Richardson. 1982. Detection of Toxius produced by *Vibrio fluvialis*. Infect. Immun. **35**:702-708.
17. McNicol, L. A., J. B. Kaper, H. A. Lockman, E. F. Remmers, W. M. Spira, M. J. Voll, and R. R. Colwell. 1980. R-factor carriage in a group F vibrio isolated from Bangladesh. Antimicrob. Agents Chemother. **17**:512-515.
18. Sakurai, J., T. Honda, Y. Jinguji, M. Arita, and T. Miwatani. 1976. Cytotoxic effect of the thermostable direct hemolysin produced by *Vibrio parahemolyticus* on FL cells. Infect. Immun. **13**: 876-883.
19. Seidler, R. J., D. A. Allen, R. R. Colwell, S. W. Joseph, and O. P. Daily. 1980. Biochemical characteristics and virulence of environmental group F bacteria isolated in the United States. Appl. Environ. Microbiol. **40**:715-720.
20. Spira, W. M., R. R. Daniel, Q. S. Ahmed, A. Huq, A. Yusef and D. A. Sack. 1978. Clinical features and pathogenicity of 0 group 1 nonagglutinating *Vibrio cholerae* and other vibrios isolated from cases of diarrhea in Dacca, Bangladesh. p. 137-153. *In* K. Takeya and Y. Zinnaka (ed.), Symposium on cholera, Karatsu, 1978. Proceedings of the 14th Jt. Conf. of the U.S.-Jpn. Coop. Med. Sci. Prog. Fuji Printing Co., Ltd., Tokyo, Japan.
21. Vogel, K. G. 1978. Effects of hyaluronidase, trypsin, and EDTA on surface composition and topography during detachment of cells in culture. Exp. Cell Res. **113**:345-357.

Advances in Research on Cholera and Related Diarrheas, eds., S. Kuwahara, N. F. Pierce, 101–112.

INFLUENCE OF SALINITY, NUTRIENT CONCENTRATION AND TEMPERATURE ON GROWTH AND SURVIVAL OF *VIBRIO CHOLERAE* IN THE AQUATIC ENVIRONMENT

F.L. Singleton, R.W. Attwell, M.S. Jangi and R.R. Colwell

Department of Microbiology, University of Maryland,
College Park, Maryland 20742, U. S. A.

Although *Vibrio cholerae*, the causative agent of epidemic cholera, has been isolated from a variety of clinical and environmental samples (2-7, 9, 10, 16, 22), the majority of environmental isolates have been non-01 serovars (16, 23). However, isolation of 01 serovars has been reported in geographical areas free of epidemics of cholera (3). Such isolations indicate that *V. cholerae* 01 may be only sporadically distributed in the aquatic environment. To account for the distribution of 01 and non-01 serovars in estuarine waters, including the presence of *V. cholerae* in regions with no reported outbreaks of cholera, Colwell *et al.* (7) hypothesized that *V. cholerae* is a member of the autochthonous bacterial community of brackish waters and estuaries.

The influence of environmental parameters, viz. temperature, salinity, and nutrient concentration, on *V. cholerae* has not been extensively investigated due, no doubt, to the fact that investigations of the biology of *V. cholerae* have been approached from the viewpoint that this species is solely of clinical origin. However, as results of recent studies indicate, *V. cholerae* may, in fact, be an autochthonous estuarine bacterial species, an important consideration in the ecology of the organism (7).

Many problems are encountered in determining the influence of one or more environmental parameters on a single bacterial species. Although environmental surveys allow correlations to be made between selected environmental parameters and the distribution of a species, in general, surveys alone do not always provide good insight into the mechanism of interaction and effect on survival and growth of the species. To circumvent difficulties arising from a constantly changing environment *in situ*, laboratory microecosystems, i.e., microcosms, can be employed. Microcosms allow for simulation, but not complete duplication, of *in situ* conditions and replication of experiments designed to test conditions within and between experiments. The objective of the studies reported here was to evaluate the influence of selected environmental parameters on the survival and growth of *V. cholerae.*

Microcosms, consisting of 50 ml of a chemically-defined sea-salts solution (27) prepared to appropriate salinities and contained in acid-cleaned, 125-ml Erlenmeyer flasks, were amended with selected concentrations of an organic nutrient, i.e., tryptone, and inoculated with washed cell suspensions of strains of *V. cholerae.* All microcosms were incubated for appropriate intervals at designated temperatures, with constant agitation supplied by rotary shakers at 125 rpm.

Ten strains of *V. cholerae* were used in this study and these were selected from the stock culture collection at the University of Maryland. Fresh cultures of tryptic soy agar (Difco Laboratories, Detroit, MI) slants were prepared, as required, from stock cultures maintained under liquid nitrogen. Cells inoculated into microcosms were grown for 18 hr at 30 C in tryptic soy broth (Difco) and collected by centrifugation. Following five washings in sterile 0.85% NaCl solution, the cell concentration was determined by acridine orange direct counts (8, 11, 14) and appropriate dilutions prepared in 0.85% NaCl solution. Inoculum size was *ca.* 4 x 10^2 cells/ml. In experiments designed to quantify ionic requirements, rinse and diluent were a basal salts solution with no added NaCl.

Samples for viable, i.e., ''culturable'', counts were collected aseptically from microcosms, using sterile 1-ml pipets, and enumerated by spread plating onto tryptic soy agar. Samples for enumeration were diluted in sea-salts solution prepared to the same salinity as the microcosms being sampled. Inoculated plates were incubated for 7 days at 25 C, before colony-forming units (cfu) were counted. A statistically designed sampling regime was established, based on a principal component of variance analysis (18), to estimate accurately the mean number of culturable bacteria. For the experiments reported herein, a design employed consisted of three microcosms per treatment, one sample per microcosm and three culture plates per sample. For total bacterial counts, i.e., acridine orange direct counts, a 1-ml sample was collected from each microcosm and processed (8, 11, 14).

Heterotrophic activity of *V. cholerae* populations in the microcosms was measured by the method of Hobbie and Crawford (13). Sterile, acid-cleaned, serum vials, each containing 25 ml of sea-salts solution, with salinity or specific salt concentration adjusted appropriately, were inoculated with 25 μl or 50 μl samples collected from microcosms following incubation. In those experiments so indicated, washed-cell suspensions of *V. cholerae* were used as inoculum for heterotrophic activity assay. Each vial was amended with a ^{14}C-labelled amino acid mixture (57 milli Ci/mg-Atom carbon; Amersham Corp., Arlington Heights, IL) to a final concentration of 50 μg/l or 100 μg/l. Under the experimental conditions employed, these concentrations of amino acids did not result in substrate saturation. After addition of amino acids, the vials were sealed with serum stoppers fitted with a plastic cup containing a folded 1 cm^2 piece of filter paper (Whatman No. 1). All vials, including controls fixed with 0.2 ml of a solution of 30% (w/v) trichloroacetic acid and 0.05%(w/v) mercuric chloride in 40%(v/v) formalin, unless otherwise stated, were incubated at *ca.* 25 C for 2 hrs before the reaction was terminated by injecting the trichloroacetic acid-mercuric chloride-formalin solution. The filter paper wicks were saturated with 0.2 ml phenethylamine to absorb $^{14}CO_2$ evolved during an additional 1 hr incubation period. Following the second incubation period, the filter wicks were placed into scintillation vials and the sea-salts solution filtered through a 0.2 μm membrane filter (Gelman) and rinsed with 10 ml of sterile sea-salts solution. The membrane filters were air-dried and placed into scintillation vials. Ten ml of scintillation cocktail (ACS, Amersham Corp.) were added to each vial and radioactive counts made using a Beckman Liquid Scintillation Spectro-photometer model LS-3155T. Uptake of amino acids ($\mu g\ l^{-1} hr^{-1}$) was calculated according to the procedure of Hobbie and Crawford (13).

The influence of different concentrations of NaCl of growth and viability of *V. cholerae* was measured employing microcosms prepared with a salt solution consisting of (g/l) $MgSO_4$, 2.86; KBr, 0.07; H_3BO_3, 0.019; $MgCl_2 \cdot 6H_2O$, 7.74; $CaCl_2$, 0.82; $SrCl_2$, 0.017; K_2CO_3, 0.05; and amended with selected concentrations of NaCl. In order to minimize changes in total salinity, Cl^- and monovalent cation concentrations were conserved by substitution of molar equivalents of KC1 or LiCl for NaCl, as the latter was decreased. Also, microcosms, thusly prepared, allowed determination of the extent to which Na^+ requirement, if any, could be spared by K^+ or Li^+ (12, 19-21).

To investigate the ion requirements of *V. cholerae* in greater detail, a turbidimetric assay for growth in the presence of different ion concentrations and substrates was employed. Acid-cleaned culture tubes (18 mm) containing basal salts solution were supplemented with 1% (w/v) tryptone (Difco), 1% (w/v) glucose (Sigma Chemical Co., St. Louis, MO), or 1% (w/v) glucose plus 0.05% yeast extract (Difco). The culture tubes were amended with selected concentrations of NaCl, NaCl plus KCl or LiCl, inoculated with a washed-cell suspension of *V. cholerae* to an initial concentration of approximately 7 x 10^5 cells/ml, and incubated at 25 C. At 24 hr intervals, for a period of 14 days, culture tubes were examined for growth, indicated by visible turbidity. All tubes positive for growth were sampled to verify viability and purity of the culture by streaking onto tryptic soy agar (Difco) and thiosulfate citrate bile salts agar (Oxoid, Columbia, MD).

Studies were carried out to measure the effect of nutrient and salinity on growth of *V. cholerae*. The strain employed was *V. cholerae* LA 4808, a toxigenic 01 strain isolated from a patient in Louisiana who became ill following ingestion of improperly prepared seafood. Population size of *V. cholerae* developing in microcosms of salinities from 5 $^o/_{oo}$ to 45 $^o/_{oo}$ were influenced by organic nutrient, i.e. tryptone concentration (Figure 1). Regardless of tryptone concentration, optimum growth of *V. cholerae*, indicated by maximum population size, as measured by both culturable and total count, occurred in the presence of an intermediate salinity of 25$^o/_{oo}$. However, at lower tryptone concentrations, i.e. less than 500 μg/l, a pronounced salinity effect was evident. Not only were there differences in population sizes at given tryptone concentrations, but also lack of recoverability of cells at the extremes of high or low salinity, coupled with low tryptone concentration. Above 500 μg tryptone/1, however, the salinity effect was masked if larger concentrations of tryptone were present, indicating that the salinity requirement was spared by a high organic nutrient concentration.

Ca. 25$^o/_{oo}$ salinity was found to be optimum for growth of *V. cholerae* strain LA 4808. Also, 500 μg tryptone/1 was concluded not to mask salinity effects. Therefore, growth of other *V. cholerae* strains were compared. On average, all isolates, including clinical and environmental 01 serovars, grew to approximately the same population size (Table 1). Culturable bacterial counts were compared by Duncan's multiple comparison test (24) using $\log_{10}$-transformed counts and were not significantly different ($p \leqslant 0.05$). Since all strains tested developed to approximately the same cell concentration and behaved similarly in the experiments, data for strain LA4808 are discussed in detail herein.

Microcosms prepared to selected salinities and amended with 500 μg tryptone/1 were incubated at temperatures of 10, 15, 20 and 25 C to evaluate the influence of temperature of growth of *V. cholerae*. At 10 C, a decrease in culturable bacterial counts was detected for all salinities tested (Figure 2). There were, however, viable *V. cholerae* cells present in the microcosms throughout the 8-day incubation period, indicating

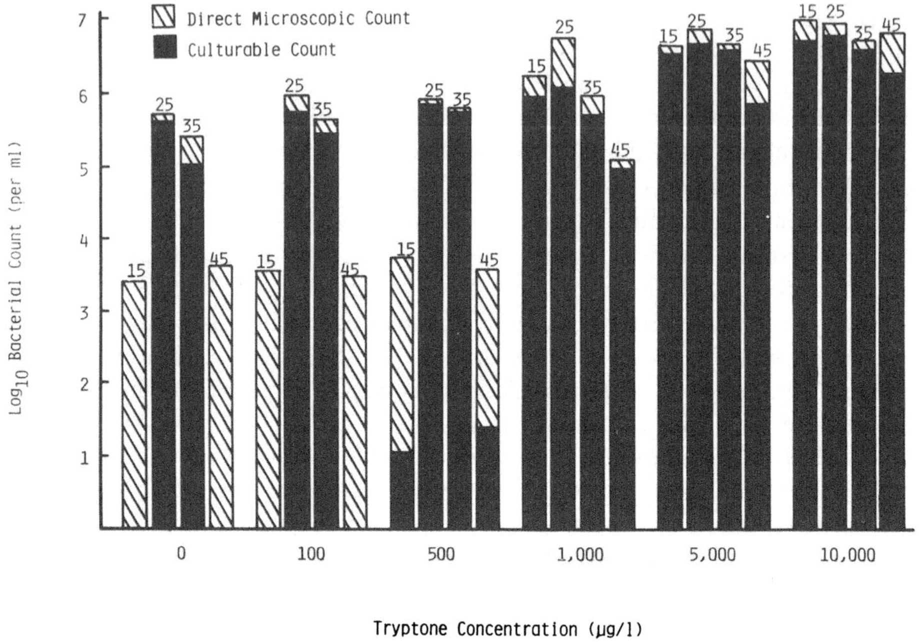

Figure 1. Comparison of direct microscopic and plate counts of *Vibrio cholerae* grown in a medium containing various concentrations of tryptone. Numbers represent salinities (°/oo) of the medium.

Table 1. Population sizes of *Vibrio cholerae* strains in microcosms adjusted to a salinity of 25 °/oo and trptone concentration of 500 µg/1[a].

Strain	Source	Mean Log_{10} Colony Count/ml	Mean Log_{10} Total Cell Count
V-69[b]	Environmental	5.788 ± 0.055[c]	5.806 ± 0.054
N-19	Environmental	5.780 ± 0.029	5.908 ± 0.016
N-17	Environmental	5.730 ± 0.018	5.763 ± 0.055
N-1400	Environmental	5.845 ± 0.022	5.857 ± 0.130
N-1403	Environmental	5.769 ± 0.048	5.869 ± 0.063
N-33	Environmental	5.571 ± 0.060	5.716 ± 0.080
N-999	Environmental	5.685 ± 0.025	5.732 ± 0.110
SGN-7677[b]	Environmental	5.768 ± 0.034	5.748 ± 0.175
LA-4808[b]	Clinical	5.840 ± 0.010	5.954 ± 0.044
CA-401[b]	Clinical	5.746 ± 0.035	5.792 ± 0.051

[a] No significant difference between the colony count, obtained by plating on a nutrient medium, and the total direct count, obtained by the AODC method (8, 11, 14), was detected using Duncan's multiple comparison (24).

[b] 01 serovar.

[c] Mean ± standard error.

extended survival at 10 C under the conditions employed.

An incubation period of 15 C yielded similar results, except for microcosms for which the salinity was adjusted to 15 ‰, in which case, both culturable and total cell counts increased (Figure 2). At salinities of 5, 25 and 35‰, an initial decrease in number of culturable cells was noted, which continued in 5‰ and 35‰ microcosms. At 25‰ salinity, however, after the second day of incubation, culturable counts gradually increased throughout the experiment.

Growth of *V. cholerae* at 20 C was influenced by salinity, indicated by a significant difference ($p \leq 0.05$) in culturable and total counts after incubation for two days with the salinity adjusted to 15‰ and no significant change ($p \leq 0.05$) in the inoculum size at salinities adjusted to 5‰, 25‰ and 35‰ (Figure 3). By the fifth day, however, populations of *V. cholerae* at all salinities demonstrated a significant increase ($p \leq 0.05$) above inoculum size. After incubation for 5 days, maximum culturable and total population counts were reached at 25‰ salinity.

Results obtained for microcosms incubated at 25 C were similar to those at 20 C, although no lag in growth of *V. cholerae* at any of the salinities tested were noted (Figure

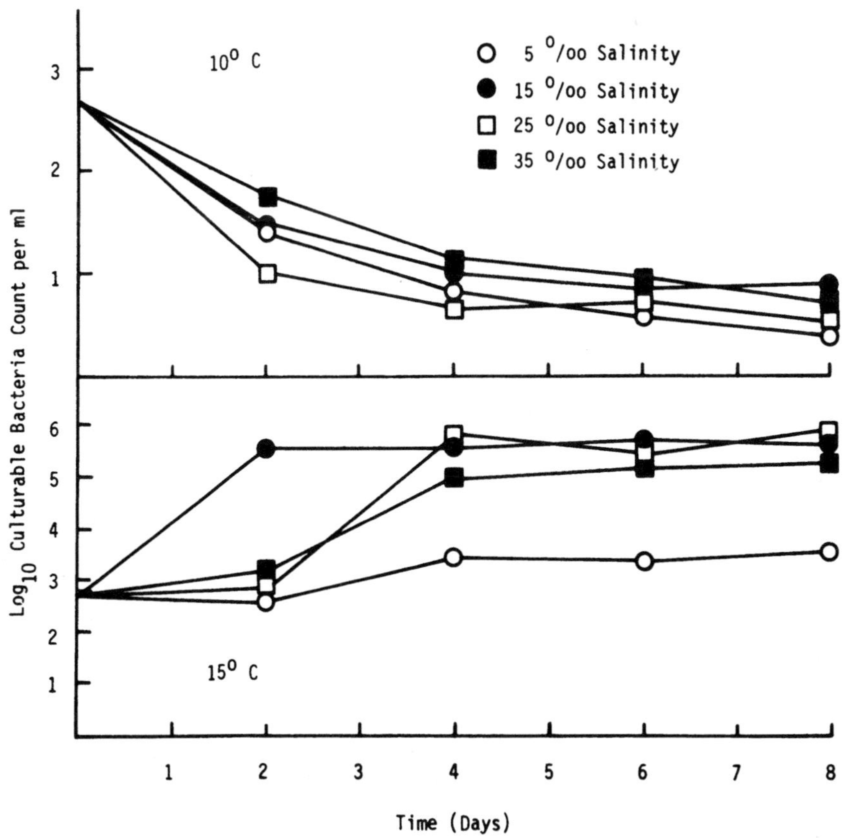

Fig. 2. Comparison of counts of *Vibrio cholerae* grown at 10°C and 15°C in a medium of various salinities.

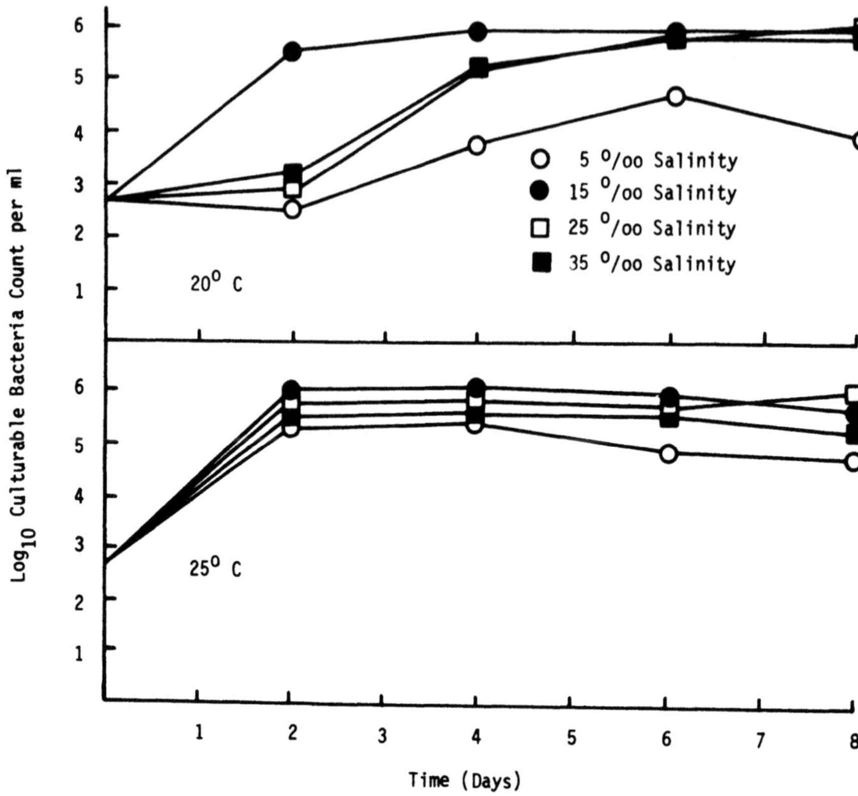

Fig. 3. Comparison of plate counts of *Vibrio cholerae* grown at 20°C and 25°C in a medium with the salinity adjusted to 5, 15, 25 and 35 parts per thousand ($^o/_{oo}$).

3). Both total and culturable counts increased to a maximum by the fourth day of incubation. During the last four days, although total counts remained stable at all salinities, with significant decreases ($p \leqslant 0.05$) in culturable counts were detected at 5 $^o/_{oo}$ and 35 $^o/_{oo}$ salinities.

After incubation for 8 days, samples were collected and inoculated into 25 ml of basal salts solution prepared to the same salinity as the microcosms. Fresh basal salts solution was amended with a ^{14}C-labelled amino acid mixture, incubated at the same temperature as the original microcosm, and heterotrophic activity of *V. cholerae* measured. At 25 C and 20 C, *V. cholerae,* from microcosms for which the salinity was adjusted to 25$^o/_{oo}$, utilized more amino acids than cultures grown at other salinities (Table 2). Lowest uptake values at 20 C and 25 C were obtained for populations in microcosms of 5$^o/_{oo}$ salinity.

Since the original microcosms contained different population sizes of *V. cholerae*, to obtain a more representative comparison of the influence of temperature and salinity on heterotrophic activity, uptake of ^{14}C–amino acid on a per culturable cell and per total cell number was calculated (Table 2). For the total population incubated at 25 C, largest uptake per cell was obtained at 25$^o/_{oo}$ salinity. Uptake of cells at all other salinities was approximately equivalent, but approximately 50% less than at 25 $^o/_{oo}$. This was

Table 2. Heterotrophic uptake of ^{14}C-labeled amino acids by *Vibrio cholerae* at selected salinities and temperatures.

Temperature (°C)	Salinity (°/oo)	Uptake rate[a] (μg/ℓ/hr x 10^{-2})	Uptake rate/ culturable cell[b] (μg/ℓ/hr)	Uptake/total cell number[c] (μg/ℓ/hr)
25	5	2.43	6.93 x 10^{-7}	1.08 x 10^{-7}
	15	4.78	1.16 x 10^{-7}	8.68 x 10^{-8}
	25	14.40	1.75 x 10^{-7}	1.81 x 10^{-7}
	35	2.74	3.38 x 10^{-7}	8.64 x 10^{-8}
20	5	2.95	6.82 x 10^{-6}	3.58 x 10^{-6}
	15	7.36	9.97 x 10^{-8}	1.13 x 10^{-7}
	25	12.9	1.33 x 10^{-7}	1.66 x 10^{-7}
	35	4.94	1.14 x 10^{-7}	1.71 x 10^{-7}
15	5	N.D.[d]	–	–
	15	3.36	4.94 x 10^{-8}	6.87 x 10^{-8}
	25	N.D.	–	–
	35	N.D.	–	–
10	5	N.D.	–	–
	15	0.54	–	–
	25	N.D.	–	–
	35	N.D.	–	–

[a] Mean of duplicate flasks per treatment.

[b] Obtained from mean culturable colony count.

[c] Obtained from acridine orange direct microscopic count (AODC) (8, 11, 14).

[d] None detected, when compared with killed controls.

not true, however, when uptake per culturable cell was compared, in which case more uptake occurred at 5°/oo and 35 °/oo. Similar results were obtained at 20 C, although greatest uptake per cell was at 5 °/oo.

To determine whether the observed effects of salinity on viability and survival of *V. cholerae* was due, in part, to a requirement for specific ion(s), a series of microcosms, each containing a basal salts solution prepared with no added Na^+ was used to determine whether *V. cholerae* requires Na^+ for growth. Also, to determine whether a Na^+ requirement, if any, could be satisfied by the presence of another monovalent cation, and to minimize changes in salinity, molar equivalents of LiCl or KCl were added as the NaCl concentration was decreased. When the NaCl concentration was decreased from 0.30 M to 0.10 M and the KCl concentration increased to 0.20 M, the *V. cholerae* population size increased, although not significantly, when analyzed by Duncan's multiple comparison (Table 3). As the NaCl concentration was decreased to 0.01 M, the *V. cholerae* population size decreased. When no NaCl was added, no culturable *V. cholerae* cells were detected. When LiCl was used to replace NaCl, no growth of *V. cholerae* occurred at any of the LiCl concentrations used.

Since no growth of *V. cholerae* occurred in microcosms containing Li^+, a washed-

Table 3. *Vibrio cholerae* population sizes in microcosms amended with selected concentrations of NaCl, KCl and LiCl.

NaCl (Molar)	KCl (Molar)	LiCl (Molar)	Mean Log_{10} Culturable count/ml	Mean Log_{10} Total cell count/ml
0.30	0	0	5.550 ± 0.045[a]	5.821 ± 0.030
0.15	0.15	0	5.584 ± 0.028	5.947 ± 0.005
0.10	0.20	0	5.778 ± 0.035	6.000 ± 0.029
0.05	0.25	0	5.640 ± 0.041	5.808 ± 0.028
0.01	0.29	0	5.480 ± 0.056	5.687 ± 0.149
0	0.30	0	N.D.[b]	N.D.
0.15	0	0.15	N.D.	N.D.
0.10	0	0.20	N.D.	N.D.
0.05	0	0.75	N.D.	N.D.
0.01	0	0.29	N.D.	N.D.
0	0	0.30	N.D.	N.D.

[a] Mean ± standard error.

[b] None detected.

cell suspension of *V. cholerae* was used to evaluate the influence of Na^+, K^+, and Li^+ on heterotrophic activity (Table 4). Uptake of ^{14}C-amino acids increased with decreasing Na^+ concentration and increasing Li^+ concentration to 0.20 M NaCl and 0.10 M LiCl. Similar results were obtained when KCl was added to compensate for decreasing NaCl concentration. However, maximum uptake occurred in the presence of 0.01 M NaCl and 0.29 M KCl. Lowest uptake of amino acids occurred in the absence of NaCl.

To determine if, indeed, Na^+ was required for growth of *V. cholerae*, culture tubes containing basal salts solution amended with different substrates and salt concentrations were inoculated with a washed-cell suspension of *V. cholerae*. From the growth patterns obtained, it was evident that Na^+ is required for growth of *V. cholerae* (Table 5). In the

Table 4. Effect of Na^+, Li^+ and K^+ on uptake of ^{14}C-amino acids by *Vibrio cholerae*.

Molar quantity added			Mean uptake rate	Respiration:
NaCl	LiCl	KCl	($\mu g \ell^{-1}$ hr^{-1} x 10^{-1})	incorporation
0.30	–	–	4.18	1:1.2
0.295	0.005	–	5.80	1:1.3
0.25	0.05	–	8.83	1:1.2
0.20	0.10	–	9.18	1:1.2
0.15	0.15	–	8.20	1:1.2
0	0.30	–	2.36	1:0.3
0.15	–	0.15	3.76	1:1.0
0.05	–	0.25	3.29	1:0.86
0.01	–	0.29	3.92	1:0.42
0.005	–	0.295	2.34	1:0.34
0.0005	–	0.2995	1.51	1:0.16
0	–	0.30	1.40	1:0.14

Table 5. Growth of *Vibrio cholerae* in basal salts solution amended with selected substrates and concentrations of NaCl, KCl and LiCl.

	Incubation time (days) before growth					
Added salt(s) concentration (Molar)	1	2	4	8	10	14
NaCl:						
0.30	+					
0.20	+					
0.10	+					
0.075	+					
0.05	+					
0.025	+					
0.01	–	+				
0	–	–	–	–	–	–
NaCl + KCl:						
0.30 + 0	+					
0.20 + 0.10	+					
0.10 + 0.20	+					
0.075 + 0.225	+					
0.05 + 0.25	+					
0.025 + 0.275	–	+				
0.01 + 0.29	–	–	–	–	–	–
0 + 0.30	–	–	–	–	–	–
NaCl + LiCl:						
0.30 + 0	+					
0.20 + 0.10	+					
0.10 + 0.20	+					
0.075 + 0.225	+					
0.05 + 0.25	+					
0.025 + 0.275	+					
0.01 + 0.29	–	+[a]	+			
0 + 0.30	–	–	–	–	–	–

[a] slight growth.

presence of 1% (w/v) tryptone, growth of *V. cholerae* occurred in the presence or absence of added NaCl, whereas, basal salts solution amended with either 0.05% (w/v) yeast extract or 1% (w/v) glucose yielded no growth of *V. cholerae*. A combination of 0.05% (w/v) yeast extract and 1% glucose indicated a requirement of Na^+ by *V. cholerae* (Table 5). At lower NaCl concentrations, an extended lag period occurred before growth took place. Results obtained also demonstrated that neither K^+ nor Li^+ can satisfy the Na^+ requirement.

The hypothesis of Colwell *et al.* (7) which considers *V. cholerae* to be a member of the autochthonous bacterial community of brackish water and estuarine systems, offers a new perspective on the ecology of this organism. Results reported herein support the hypothesis of *V. cholerae* as an autochthonous organism of estuarine and brackish water systems and emphasizes the need for an ecological approach in studying the role of *V. cholerae* in nature and in human disease.

Under simulated environmental conditions, all strains of *V. cholerae* tested, both 01 and non-01 serovars, grew to approximately the same population size (Table 1). For example, a clinical isolate from a patient who developed cholera, following ingestion of improperly prepared seafood, *V. cholerae* strain LA 4808 grew to approximately the same population size as type strain *V. cholerae* CA 401 and an 01 serovar, V-69, from Chesapeake Bay.

West (28) employed *in situ* growth chambers to evaluate survival of *V. cholerae* in aquatic systems in Great Britain and found that the growth pattern of *V. cholerae* was similar to that obtained in microcosms reported herein. Based on these results, as well as those previously reported (6, 7, 27), it is concluded that under a proper regime of nutrient, temperature, and salinity, *V. cholerae* is clearly capable of growth in the natural environment.

Also supporting the hypothesis that *V. cholerae* is a brackish water and estuarine denizen is its requirement for Na^+ for growth (Table 5). A requirement for Na^+ reported for many marine bacteria has been firmly established by MacLeod and co-workers (12, 19-21). An obligate requirement for Na^+ is considered by some investigators to be a characteristic useful in differentiating marine and estuarine bacteria from those of freshwater habitats (19).

In the turbidimetric assay employed in this study, the requirement of *V. cholerae* for Na^+ was demonstrated. However, when 1% (w/v) glucose and 0.05% (w/v) yeast extract were both added to the salts solution, growth of *V. cholerae* occurred both in the presence and absence of Na^+ if 1% tryptone was present. These seemingly contradictory results can be explained as follows. From quantitative analyses of tryptone (1) it has been established that tryptone contains Na^+ to approximately 2.7%, by weight. A 1% tryptone solution, thus, contains *ca.* 0.0012 M Na^+, enough to support the growth of *V. cholerae.*

Growth patterns of *V. cholerae* under conditions simulating various estuarine and marine habitats indicate a preference of the organism for moderate salinity, i.e., 15‰-25‰ (Figure 1). Also, uptake of ^{14}C-amino acids by *V. cholerae*, in microcosms of different salinities and within a given temperature range, demonstrated a significant influence of salinity on the metabolic state of the cells (Table 2). When uptake per culturable cell at 25 C or 20 C was compared, greater uptake occurred at 5‰ salinity. Since uptake per culturable cell was greater than at other salinities tested, i.e., 15 ‰, 25 ‰, or 35 ‰, a need for the cells to metabolize rapidly to maintain viability because of environmental stress is suggested, i.e., physiologically stressed cells, strongly indicated by the respiration to incorporation ratios. Stressed cells are those with a ratio greater than 1.0 (D. Kushner, personal communication).

If *V. cholerae* is, in fact, an indigenous member of the bacterial community of estuarine systems, possessing the ability to survive for extended periods under adverse conditions, many of the limited outbreaks of cholera in regions of no known, or apparent, source of the agent can be explained. Recent outbreaks of cholera in Louisiana (3) and Texas (5) have been associated with consumption of shellfish. An environmental reservoir of *V. cholerae*, such as shellfish or planktonic crustaceans, can serve as a source of cholera, either via a non-specific association or, as has been hypothesized (7), by interaction of *V. cholerae* in a commensal relationship with organisms of higher trophic levels. *V. cholerae* enterotoxin may, quite possibly, fill a role in the salt tolerance and/or osmoregulation of crustaceans.

Another potential ecological role of *V. cholerae* enterotoxin may be to sequester Na^+ for growth of the organism itself. When *V. cholerae* adheres to and colonizes the small intestine, cholera toxin binds to mucosal cell receptors and stimulates intestinal adenylate cyclase activity. The resulting cyclic AMP then inhibits NaCl uptake by the villi and stimulates active Cl^- secretion by the crypt cells. This causes osmotic loss of water, producting the symptoms associated with cholera in humans (10, 15, 17, 25, 26). Should cholera toxin affect epithelial cells of crustaceans similarly, *V. cholerae*, when in association with, or attached to, these organisms, would thus have a means of obtaining sufficient Na^+ from its host for survival and growth when the concentration of Na^+ in the environment falls below that required to sustain *V. cholerae.*

Based on results reported herein, *V. cholerae* is concluded to be, as hypothesized by Colwell *et al.* (7), an indigenous member of the bacterial community of estuarine systems, evident not only from its requirement for Na^+ for growth, but also by its obvious preference for a salinity regime typical of brackish water areas and estuaries. It is important to note that the distribution of *V. cholerae* would not be limited to estuaries, since the requirement for Na^+ can be spared if a sufficiently high nutrient concentration is present (27). Results of this study demonstrate the usefulness of combined laboratory and field studies in gaining an understanding of the role(s) and function(s) of *V. cholerae* in the natural environment.

REFERENCES

1. Anon. 1972. *Difco Manual of Dehydrated Culture Media and Reagents for Microbiological and Clinical Laboratory Procedures,* 9th Ed., Difco Laboratories, Inc., Detroit, MI.
2. Bashford, D. J., T. J. Donovan, A. L. Furniss, and J. V. Lee. 1979. *Vibrio cholerae* in Kent. Lancet **ii**:436-437.
3. Blake, P. A., D. T. Allegra, J. D. Snyder, T. J. Barrett, L. MacFarland, C. T. Caraway, J. C. Feeley, J. P. Craig, J. V. Lee, N. D. Puhr, and R. A. Feldman. 1980. Cholera - a possible endemic foucus in the United States. N. Engl. J. Med. **302**:305-309.
4. Blake, P. A., M. L. Rosenberg, J. Bandeira Costa, P. Soares Ferreira, C. Levy Guimaraes, and E. J. Gangarosa. 1977. Cholera in Portugal, 1974. I. Modes of transmission. Am. J. Epidemiol. **105**: 337-343.
5. Centers for Disease Control. Cholera-Texas. Morbidity and Mortality Weekly Report. August 21, 1981, **30**(32):389-390.
6. Colwell, R. R., J. Kaper, and S. W. Joseph. 1977. *Vibrio cholerae, Vibrio parahaemolyticus*, and other Vibrios: occurrence and distribution in Chesapeake Bay. Science **198**:394-396.
7. Colwell, R. R., R. J. Seidler, J. Kaper, S. W. Joseph, S. Garges, H. Lockman, D. Maneval, H. Bradford, N. Roberts, E. Remmers, I. Huq, and A. Huq. 1981. Occurrence of *Vibrio cholerae* serotype 01 in Maryland and Louisiana estuaries. Appl. Environ. Microbiol. **41**:555-558.
8. Daley, R. J., and J. E. Hobbie. 1975. Direct counts of aquatic bacteria by modified epifluores-cence technique. Limnol. Oceanogr. **20**:875-882.
9. Dutt. A. K., S. Alwi, and T. Velauthan. 1971. A shellfish-borne cholera outbreak in Malaysia. Trans. R. Soc. Trop. Med. Hyg. **65**:815-818.
10. Finkelstein, R. A. 1973. Cholera. Crit. Rev. Microbiol. **2**:553-623.
11. Francisco, D. E., R. A. Mah, and A. C. Rabin. 1973. Acridine orange epifluorescence technique for counting bacteria in natural waters. Trans. Amer. Microscop. Soc. **92**:416-421.
12. Gow, J. A., R. A. MacLeod, M. Goodbody, D. Frank, and L. DeVoe. 1981. Growth characteristics at low Na^+ concentration and the stability of the Na^+ requirement of a marine bacterium. Can. J. Microbiol. **27**:350-357.
13. Hobbie, J. E., and C. C. Crawford. 1969. Corrections for bacterial uptake of dissolved organic compounds in natural water. Limnol. Oceanogr. **14**:528-532.

14. Hobbie, J. E., R. J. Daley, and S. Jasper. 1977. Use of nuclepore filters for counting bacteria by fluorescence microscopy. Appl. Environ. Microbiol. **33**:1225-1228.
15. Holmgren, J. 1981. Actions of cholera toxin and the prevention and treatment of cholera. Nature **292**:413-416.
16. Kaper, J. B., H. Lockman, R. R. Colwell, and S. W. Joseph. 1979. Ecology, serology, and enterotoxin production of *Vibrio cholerae* in Chesapeake Bay. Appl. Environ. Microbiol. **37**:91-103.
17. King, C. A., and W. E. van Heyningen. 1975. Evidence for the complex nature of the ganglioside receptor for cholera toxin. J. Infect. Dis. **131**:643-648.
18. Kosinski, R. J., F. L. Singleton, and B. G. Foster. 1979. Sampling culturable heterotrophs from microcosms: a statistical analysis. Appl. Environ. Microbiol. **38**:906-910.
19. MacLeod, R. A. 1965. The question of the existence of specific marine bacteria. Bacteriol. Rev. **29**:9-23.
20. MacLeod, R. A., and E. Onofrey. 1957. Nutrition and metabolism of marine bacteria. III. The relation of Na^+ and K^+ to growth. J. Cell. Comp. Physiol. **50**:389-401.
21. MacLeod, R. A., and E. Onofrey. 1963. Studies on the stability of the Na^+ requirement of marine bacteria. *In* Symposium on Marine Microbiology. C. H. Oppenheimer (ed.). Charles C. Thomas Publisher, Springfield, IL. pp. 481-489.
22. Merson, M. H., W. T. Martin, J. P. Craig, G. K. Morris, P. A. Blake, G. F. Croun, J. C. Feeley, J. C. Camacho, and E. J. Gangarosa. 1977. Cholera on Guam, 1974. Epidemiological findings and isolation of non-toxinogenic strains. Am. J. Epidemiol. **105**:349-361.
23. Muller, H. E. 1978. Occurrence and ecology of NAG vibrios in surface water. Zentralbl. Bacteriol. Parasitenkd. Infektionskr. Hyg. Reihe B. **167**:272-284.
24. Ott, L. 1977. *An Introduction to Statistical Methods and Data Analysis.* Wadsworth Publishing Co., Inc., Belmont, CA.
25. Pierce, N. F., W. B. Greenough, III, and C. C. J. Carpenter, Jr. 1971. *Vibrio cholerae* enterotoxin and its mode of action. Bacteriol. Rev. **35**:1-13.
26. Sahyoun, N. and P. Cuatrecasas. 1975. Mechanism of activation of adenylate cyclase by cholera toxin. Proc. Natl. Acad. Sci. USA **72**:3438-3442.
27. Singleton, F. L., R. W. Attwell, M. S. Jangi, and R. R. Colwell. 1982. Influence of salinity and nutrient concentration on survival and growth of *Vibrio cholerae* in aquatic microcosms. Appl. Environ. Microbiol. **43**:1080-1085.
28. West, P. A. 1980. Ecology and taxonomy of the genus *Vibrio*. Ph. D. Thesis. University of Kent at Canterbury, England.

Advances in Research on Cholera and Related Diarrheas, eds., S. Kuwahara, N. F. Pierce, 113–120.

LYSOGENICITY OF *VIBRIO CHOLERAE*

Makoto Ohashi, Takeshi Terayama, Hiroshi Ushioda, Yasuo Kudoh, Masaaki Tsuno, Shigeru Matsushita, Kenji Ohta, Senzo Sakai and Orasa Suthienkul*

Department of Microbiology, Tokyo Metropolitan Research Laboratory of Public Health, Tokyo 160, Japan
**Department of Microbiology, Faculty of Public Health, Mahidol University, Bangkok 4, Thailand*

In 1963, Takeya and Shimodori described a certain temperate phage infecting a majority of strains of *Vibrio cholerae* biotype *eltor* isolated in the western Pacific region and named it as kappa type phage(1). Then, on the basis of the individual strains' lysogenicity by, and their sensitivity to, this phage, they classified the eltor type vibrio into three types, namely (i) Celebes type, which is lysogenic, (ii) cured type, non-lysogenic and sensitive, and (iii) classical-Ubon type, non-lysogenic and insensitive(2).

Furthermore, they advocated the kappa phage detection system as an efficient method for early detection of carriers of this organism(3, 4). We applied this method for analyzing the cause of the cholera outbreak occurring in Japan in 1978, and confirmed its efficiency in practical field(5).

By using this system, we noticed recently that the frequency of finding strains lysogenized by kappa phage was decreasing among isolates of the eltor type vibrio. Then, we have collected and examined these organisms isolated in many different parts of the world to see the presence of kappa phage. As a result, the recently isolated strains revealed a frequency of lysogenic strains as low as 34 per cent(6), in contrast to the level of 95 per cent reported by Takeya and his colleagues among strains examined from 1959 through 1963(2). Moreover the frequency varied from one country to another and also from year to year. This paper describes these findings.

During the course of this study, we have encountered some strains of biotype *cholerae* carrying kappa phage, which was originally described by Takeya as being highly specific to the eltor type vibrio. We also learned that some strains were doubly lysogenized by other phages in addition to kappa phage. This paper will also discuss these findings as well as the relation between the lysogenicity and enterotoxin production of *Vibrio cholerae*.

Strains of *Vibrio cholerae* biotype *cholerae* were kindly provided by T. Naito, the Institute for Tropical Medicine, Nagasaki University, and M. Nagao, Tokyo Quarantine Station.

Naito's strains had been isolated in 1946 at Nagasaki mainly from patients among post-war repatriates from China, their contacts and secondary infection cases, and Nagao's strains in East Pakistan from 1968 to 1970. Strain NIH 41 and several other old stock cultures were also submitted to the study.

Strains of biotype *eltor* were isolated in Japan, Gilbert and Ellice Islands, Malaysia, Nigeria, the Philippines and Thailand from 1977 to 1981. Non-0-group 1 strains were isolated in our laboratory from travellers' diarrheal cases and sea foods.

Lysogenicity was tested by the method described previously employing H218 SM^r and TSI 4 strains as indicators[6].

The former kindly provided by Y. Zinnaka is the indicator which is used by Takeya's group, and the latter is the gift of C. Yamada, National Institute of Health, Tokyo and is a phage- and vibriocin-production negative mutant obtained by nitrosoguanidine treatment of a laboratory stock of the Institute. Phage-sensitivity was tested by the spot method described by Takeya. Temperate phage of *Vibrio cholerae* biotype *eltor*, strain P6973 or strain CH 25 propagated on strain TSI 4, was employed as the reference preparation of kappa phage.

First of all, the frequency of lysogenic strains among *V. cholerae* biotypes *cholerae* and *eltor* and non-0-group 1 isolates was studied. As shown in Table 1, 31 strains or 63 per cent were found lysogenic out of 49 strains of biotype *cholerae*, whereas 284 or 36 per cent out of 792 strains studied were found lysogenic for biotype *eltor*. On the other hand, none of 58 strains of non-0-group 1 were lysogenic in so far as they were examined with these indicators.

During the course of these lysogenicity tests, we realized that there existed some strains of biotype *cholerae* producing temperate phages whose plaques on strain H218 SM^r were uniform while showing on TSI 4 two different kinds of morphology. Strains NIH 41 and CV 3 were most typical among those strains. When the lysogenicity of strain NIH 41 was examined on TSI 4, turbid and large plaques similar to those produced by the reference kappa phage were observed in addition to less turbid and smaller ones. However, the very same sample, when examined on H218 SM^r, has shown only the former type plaques without the latter. On the other hand, CV 3 strain formed only plaques with less turbidity on both indicators. However, the plaques formed on TSI 4 showed a larger variation in size.

The variability in plaque formation on different indicator strains was observed also in terms of the number of plaques formed. As shown in Table 2, the number of plaques formed on TSI 4 was consistently larger than those on H218 SM^r in both cases of strains NIH 41 and CV 3.

On the basis of these results, we have speculated the presence of two different temperate phages lysogenizing the respective strains. The temperate phage of strain NIH 41 producing turbid plaques was tentatively named ϕNIH 41-t and the other ϕNIH 41-c,

Table 1. Prevalence of lysogenic strains in *Vibrio cholerae* 0-group 1, biotypes *cholerae* and *eltor*, and non-0-group 1.

0-group and biotype	Number of strains tested	Number of lysogenic strains(%)
0 1, *cholerae*	49	31(63.3)
eltor	792	284(35.9)
Non-0 1	58	–

Table 2. Results of titration of temperate phages induced from strains NIH 41 and CV 3 on two different indicator strains.

Culture filtrate tested	PFU/ml counted on indicator strain:	
	TSI 4	H218 SM^r
NIH 41	7.8×10^7	1.0×10^7
CV 3	4.2×10^5	1.6×10^5

and CV 3 strain's phages producing large-size and small-size plaques on TSI 4 were named ϕCV 3-1 and ϕCV 3-s, respectively.

Next, the host range of these isolated phages, which were propagated on strain TSI 4 was studied. The results are summarized in Table 3. Phage ϕNIH 41-t, similar to the reference kappa phage preparation, lysed TSI 4, H218 SM^r and CV 3, whereas ϕNIH 41-c lysed strain TSI 4 only. ϕCV 3-1 demonstrated a lytic range identical to ϕNIH 41-c, whereas ϕCV 3-s phage lysed strains TSI 4, H218 SM^r and NIH 41. These results suggest that ϕNIH 41-t is kappa phage and ϕNIH 41-c is identical to ϕCV 3-1, although it is not kappa phage, and that ϕCV 3-s is different from kappa phage, ϕNIH 41-c or ϕCV 3-1.

The results of the host range experiment also support the idea that NIH 41 and CV 3 strains are doubly lysogenized by kappa phage plus ϕNIH 41-c and by ϕCV 3-1 plus ϕCV 3-s, respectively.

In order to confirm this idea, TSI 4 strain or H218 SM^r strain was experimentally lysogenized by each phage and thus cross immunity test was performed.

For isolation of experimentally lysogenized clones, 0.02 milliliter of a phage preparation in 10 routine test dilutions was placed on the alkaline agar plate overlaid with soft agar containing an overnight culture of the indicator strain, TSI 4 or H218 SM^r, and after an overnight incubation at 37°C, the cells surviving in the lytic zone were spread on other alkaline agar plates. Several tens of colonies thus isolated were then examined as to their sensitivity to the phage concerned. Then the inducibility of the infected temperate

Table 3. Host range of temperate phages derived from strains NIH 41 and CV 3.

Strain	Lysis by phage preparation*:				
	Reference kappa**	ϕNIH 41-t (kappa)	ϕNIH 41-c (tau 1)	ϕCV 3-1 (tau 1)	ϕCV 3-s (tau 2)
TSI 4	+	+	+	+	+
H218 SM^r	+	+	–	–	+
NIH 41	–	–	–	–	+
CV 3	+	+	–	–	–
P 6973	–	–	–	–	–

* Phage preparation of 10^6 – 10^7 PFU/ml was used.

** Reference kappa phage was derived from strain P 6973.

Table 4. Lytic pattern of experimentally lysogenized clones of strain TSI 4 and H218 SM^r.

Lysogenized clone: Strain(temperate phage)	Lysis by phage preparation*: Reference kappa	ϕNIH 41-t (Kappa)	ϕNIH41-c (tau 1)	ϕCV 3-1 (tau 1)	ϕCV 3-s (tau 2)
TSI 4(kappa)	–	–	+	+	+
〃 (ϕNIH 41-t)	–	–	+	+	+
〃 (ϕNIH 41-c)	+	+	–	–	+
〃 (ϕCV 3-1)	+	+	–	–	+
〃 (ϕCV 3-s)	+	+	+	+	–
〃 (ϕNIH 41-t, ϕNIH 41-c)	–	–	–	–	+
〃 (ϕNIH 41-t, ϕCV 3-1)	–	–	–	–	+
〃 (kappa, ϕNIH 41-c)	–	–	–	–	+
〃 (kappa, ϕCV 3-1)	–	–	–	–	+
H218 SM^r(kappa)	–	–	–	–	+
〃 (ϕCV 3-s)	+	+	–	–	–
(kappa, ϕCV 3-s)	–	–	–	–	–
Control: TSI 4	+	+	+	+	+
H218 SM^r	+	+	–	–	+

* Phage preparation of $10^6 - 10^7$ PFU/ml was used.

phage was studied as the final indication of lysogenicity, in the clones thus established as insensitive.

As clearly shown on Table 4, clone of strain TSI 4, which was lysogenized doubly by ϕNIH 41-t and ϕNIH 41-c acquired immunity not only to the homologous phages but also to the reference kappa phage and ϕCV 3-1, and reproduced the lytic pattern of strain NIH 41. Similarly, TSI 4 strains lysogenized by both ϕNIH 41-t and ϕCV 3-1 reproduced the lytic pattern identical to that of the clone mentioned above. The results did not change, when ϕNIH 41-t was replaced by the reference kappa phage. In other words, double lysogenicity of NIH 41 strain was thus established and one of the temperate phages carried was identified as kappa phage by these evidences. Furthermore, ϕNIH 41-t was neutralized by anti-kappa phage serum and *vice versa*, and ϕCV 3-1 was neutralized by immune serum against ϕNIH 41-c and *vice versa.*

The indicator strain, H218 SM^r, which was employed by Takeya's group for kappa phage detection, was found to be sensitive to ϕCV 3-s but insensitive to ϕNIH 41-c or ϕCV 3-1. However, as far as TSI 4 was used as the indicator strain, it was impossible to induce any temperate phage from this strain. The lytic pattern demonstrated by clone of strain H218 SM^r resembled very much that of NIH 41, when this strain was experimentally lysogenized by kappa phage or ϕNIH 41-t, and it resembled that of strain CV 3 when the strain was lysogenized by ϕCV 3-s, suggesting the possibility of H218 SM^r being a defective lysogenic strain by ϕNIH 41-c or ϕCV 3-1, although there is no evidence, so far, to prove the absence of surface exclusion mechanism to these phages. Clones insensitive to any of the phages, kappa, ϕNIH 41-t, ϕNIH 41-c, ϕCV 3-1 and ϕCV 3-s were successfully obtained from strain H218 SM^r as a result of double lysogenization by kappa and ϕCV 3-s phages.

Table 5. Lysogenicity and kappa-, tau 1- and tau 2-sensitivity in *V. cholerae* biotype *cholerae.*

Lysogenicity determined on TSI 4	Sensitivity to phage: Kappa	Tau 1	Tau 2	Number of strains	
+	–	–	–	18	31
	+	–	–	12	
	–	–	+	1	
–	–	–	–	7	18
	–	–	+	11	
Total					49

The group of phages represented by ϕNIH 41-c and ϕCV 3-1 will be referred to as tau 1 phage and the other represented by ϕCV 3-s as tau 2 phage.

Next, the sensitivity of isolates of *Vibrio cholerae* to these phages, kappa, tau 1 and tau 2, was studied. The results on biotype *cholerae* are summarized in Table 5. The lysogenic strains which were sensitive to kappa but not sensitive to tau 1 and tau 2, as represented by strain CV 3, were encountered in 12 out of 31. The lysogenic strain sensitive to tau 2 but not to kappa and tau 1 was only one, strain NIH 41.

On the other hand, a wide variety of lytic patterns were encountered among biotype *eltor* strains. As shown in Table 6, strains sensitive to tau 1 or 2 or to both were encountered among lysogenic strains which may correspond to the Celebes type of Takeya's typing schema. The strains with the same lytic pattern were also found in the cured type which were non-lysogenic and kappa-sensitive. All the 9 strains of Takeya's

Table 6. Lysogenicity and kappa-, tau 1- and tau-2 sensitivity in *V. cholerae* biotype *eltor.*

Lysogenicity determined on TSI 4	Sensitivity to phage: Kappa	Tau 1	Tau 2	Number of strains		Possible correspondence to Takeya's type
+	–	–	–	190	243	Celebes
	–	+	–	47		
	–	–	+	1		
	–	+	+	5		
–	+	–	–	305	453	Cured
	+	+	–	145		
	+	–	+	1		
	+	+	+	2		
–	–	–	–		9	Classical-Ubon
Total					705	

Table 7. Lysogenicity, phage-sensitivity and enterotoxin production in *V. cholerae* biotype *cholerae*.

Lysogenicity determined on TSI 4	Sensitivity to phage: Kappa	Tau 1	Tau 2	Number of strains tested	Enterotoxin production* (–)	1 – 4	8 – 32	64 –
+	–	–	–	18	1	4	12	1
	+	–	–	12	–	2	10	–
	–	–	+	1	–	–	1	–
–	–	–	–	7	–	4	1	2
	–	–	+	11	3	2	3	3
Total				49	4	12	27	6

* ng/ml determined by the reversed passive hemagglutination test

classical-Ubon type, which were non-lysogenic and kappa-insensitive, were insensitive to tau 1 and tau 2, at the same time.

Enterotoxin production was studied in 49 strains of biotype *cholerae* and 130 of biotype *eltor.* Toxin production was quantitated by the reversed passive hemagglutination test which was developed in our laboratory and reported in the 14th Joint Cholera Conference held at Karatsu, 1978, by Kudoh *et al.*[7] The results obtained on biotype *cholerae* isolates are shown in Table 7. No relation between the enterotoxin production and the phage-sensitivity was observed. As shown in Table 8, no significant difference in the amount of enterotoxin produced among strains with different phage sensitivity patterns was observed, although all the 3 non-lysogenic and insensitive strains were found to produce no detectable amount of the toxin. No difference in the amount of enterotoxin produced was also observed between strain TSI 4 and its lysogenized clones (Table 9).

Table 8. Lysogenicity, phage-sensitivity and enterotoxin production in *V. cholerae* byitype *eltor.*

Lysogenicity determined on TSI 4	Sensitivity to phage: Kappa	Tau 1	Tau 2	Number of strains tested	Enterotoxin production* (–)	1 – 4	8 – 32	64 –
+	–	–	–	29	5	20	4	–
	–	+	–	8	3	3	2	–
–	+	–	–	63	10	41	11	1
	+	+	–	26	6	19	1	–
	+	–	+	1	–	1	–	–
–	–	–	–	3	3	–	–	–
Total				130	27	84	18	1

* ng/ml determined by the reversed passive hemagglutination test

Table 9. Enterotoxin production of experimentally lysogenized clones of TSI 4 strain.

Lysogenized clone: Strain(temperate phage)	Amount of exterotoxin produced (ng/ml)
TSI 4 (kappa*)	16
〃 (ϕNIH 41-t)	16
〃 (ϕNIH 41-c)	16
〃 (ϕNIH 41-t, ϕNIH 41-c)	16
〃 (kappa, ϕNIH 41-c)	16
〃 (ϕCV 3-1)	16
〃 (ϕCV 3-s)	16
〃 (kappa, ϕCV 3-s)	16
Control: TSI 4	16
CH 25	32
NIH 41	8
CV 3	32

* Kappa phage derived from strain CH 25 was used.

Contrary to the discussion of Takeya and his colleagues, who reported kappa phage as being a specific temperate phage to *Vibrio cholerae* biotype *eltor*, it was also found in biotype *cholerae* as result of this study. The different sources of test strains used may have been responsible for this discrepancy. However, the most important contribution was the choice of our indicator for temperate phage detection, strain TSI 4, phage- and vibriocin-production negative mutant. The use of this indicator strain enabled us to discover double lysogenicity of certain strains of biotype *cholerae* by two different phages. As has been clearly demonstrated in the present investigation, the use of several different strains experimentally lysogenized by kappa and tau phages is very useful for identification of temperate phages. However, it is not easy to identify all temperate phages carried by many lysogenic strains and to determine if they were kappa, tau 1, tau 2 or the others for individual strains. Therefore we decided to look at sensitivities to those phages in this investigation. And by doing so, we realized that this system was capable of classifying the vibrio more precisely than did Takeya. The findings obtained in this study may also help us give a more logical endorsement to the phage typing system of the organism.

In *Corynebacterium diphtheriae* and other organisms, certain temperate phages are known to control their toxigenicity. However, Gerdes and Romig reported that they could not discover such a temperate phage in *Vibrio cholerae*[8]. The present investigation also confirmed their conclusion, although the classical-Ubon type, neither lysogenic nor sensitive to kappa phage, was considered very weakly toxigenic if any at all. Therefore, the relationship between the lysogenicity and enteropathogenicity of the organism will remain as an interesting subject for future studies.

REFERENCES

1. Takeya, K., and S. Shimodori(1963): Prophage-typing of El Tor vibrios. J. Bacteriol., **85**: 957-958.
2. Takeya, K., Y. Zinnaka, S. Shimodori, Y. Nakayama, K. Amako, and K. Iida(1965): Lysogeny in

El Tor vibrio. pp. 24-29. *In* Proceedings of the cholera research symposium, 1965, Honolulu Hawaii, US Government Printing Office, Wahsington, D. C.

3. Takeya, K., S. Shimodori, and Y. Zinnaka(1963): New method for early diagnosis of Celebes type El Tor vibrio carriers. J. Bacteriol., **90**: 824-825.
4. Takeya, K., S. Shimodori, and Y. Zinnaka(1967): Studies of kappa-type phage. pp. 61-66. *In* Proceedings of the symposium on cholera, 1967, Palo Alto, National Institutes of Health, Bethesda.
5. Ohashi, M. (1980): Laboratory aspects on the cause of the cholera outbreak in Japan, originating from a public wedding hall, in 1978. pp. 334-345. *In* Proceedings of the 15th Joint Conference on cholera, US-Japan Cooperative Medical Science Program, Bethesda, 1979(NIH Publication No. 80-2003), National Institutes of Health, Bethesda.
6. Ohashi, M., T. Terayama, H. Ushioda, Y. Kudoh, M. Tsuno, and S. Sakai(1981): Lysogenicity of the strains of *Vibrio cholerae*, biotype *eltor* recently isolated in various countries. Microbiol. Immunol., **25**: 613-616.
7. Kudoh, Y., S. Yamada, S. Matsushita, K. Ohta, M. Tsuno, M. Ohashi, T. Muraoka, and N. Ohtomo(1979): Detection of heat-labile enterotoxin of *Escherichia coli* by reversed passive hemagglutination test with specific immunoglobulin against cholera toxin. pp. 266-273. *In* proceedings of the 14th Joint Conference, US-Japan Cooperative Medical Science Program, 1978, Karatsu, Toho University, Tokyo.
8. Gerdes, J. C., and W. R. Romig(1975): Genetic Basis of toxin production and pathogenesis in *Vibrio cholerae*: Evidence against phage conversion. Infect. Immun. **11**: 445-452.

Advances in Research on Cholera and Related Diarrheas, eds., S. Kuwahara, N. F. Pierce, 121–125.

HEMAGGLUTININS (COLONIZATION FACTORS?) PRODUCED BY *VIBRIO CHOLERAE*

Richard A. Finkelstein and Larry F. Hanne*

Department of Microbiology
University of Missouri School of Medicine
Columbia, Missouri 65212

Although cholera is the prototype of the enterotoxic enteropathies in which the etiologic agents (after passing the gastric barrier) adhere to and colonize the epithelial surface of the small bowel (and there liberate their enterotoxin), relatively little is known about the mechanism(s) of attachment. Suggestive evidence that *Vibrio cholerae* have fimbriae (pili) was presented in 1968 (21), but this isolated report has not been substantiated by subsequent investigations. Observations in our laboratory (6, 16, 17) provided no support for the participation of surface organelles in adherence; rather, the evidence suggested that adherence was the result of a more direct interaction between the surface coat of the vibrios and the tips of the microvilli of the host intestinal epithelial cells.

In 1961, Bales and Lankford (1) observed that cholera vibrios could directly agglutinate erythrocytes (RBC) and that broth cultures exhibited high titers of hemagglutinating activity. Finkelstein and Mukerjee (8) in 1963, reported that El Tor, but not classical, biotype vibrios, when grown on solid media, agglutinated chicken RBC. Since that time *V. cholerae* have been shown to produce a variety of hemagglutinins (HAs) which have been proposed as possible mediators of attachment (2, 4-6, 10-13). A partially purified "soluble" HA (called "cholera lectin"), isolated from culture supernatants of a classical biotype strain, inhibited attachment of an El Tor biotype strain to rabbit tissue and thus is a likely candidate as a relevant adhesive factor (6).

The present work examines the distribution of the various hemagglutinins among the cholera vibrios and describes the isolation and characterization of the "soluble" HA ("cholera lectin") which is produced by all strains examined.

Studies with ten strains, representing both Inaba and Ogawa serotypes and El Tor and classical biotype strains from different epidemics, confirmed that agar-grown El Tor vibrios were hemagglutinative for chicken RRC whereas classical biotypes were not. This cell-associated HA was inhibited by D-mannose (and D-fructose).

Supernatants of late log phase tryptic soy broth (TSB) cultures of both biotypes

*Present address: Department of Microbiology and Immunology, University of Oregon, Portland, Oregon 97201. This work constitutes a portion of the dissertation of Larry F. Hanne, submitted in partial fulfillment of the requirements for the Ph.D. degree, University of Texas Health Sciences Center at Dallas, of which the majority was performed *in absentia* at the University of Missouri-Columbia.

(and serotypes) were hemagglutinative. This "soluble" HA was active on only a proportion (10/18) of RBCs tested, from different chickens, and it required Ca^{++} for maximal activity. "Non-responder" chicken RBC could be converted to "responder" RBC by treatment with mixed glycosidase (Miles Laboratories, Inc.). The soluble HA was not inhibited by any sugar tested (D-mannose, L-fucose, D-galactose, D-mannitol, D-glucosamine, D-fructose, D-ribose, D-glucose, N-acetyl-galactosamine, dextran) or by mixed gangliosides, phosphatidyl choline, or dithiothreitol.

A third HA activity, which was cell-associated and was inhibited by L-fucose, was found in early log phase broth-grown cells of some strains of the classical biotype and in spontaneous mutants of the El Tor biotype which lacked the mannose-sensitive hemagglutinin ($MSHA^-$) and which had been selected following co-sedimentation of the $MSHA^+$ parents with responder chicken RBC.

Interestingly, cells of a classical *V. cholerae* strain (which do not ordinarily express a cell-associated HA *in vitro*), harvested from the intestinal fluids of infected infant rabbits, were found to agglutinate responder, but not non-responder RBC. This observation suggests that the soluble HA may be expressed *in vivo* in a cell-associated form.

Because of the previous evidence suggestive of its potential role as a colonization factor (6) and its ubiquity among cholera vibrios, the soluble HA (cholera lectin) was purified to apparent homogeneity, from fermentor-grown TSB culture supernatants, by a sequence of procedures including concentration by membrane ultrafiltration, $(NH_4)_2SO_4$ precipitation, Sephadex gel filtration and preparative isoelectric focusing in a Sephadex gel matric (Ultradex, LKB). Three pH isotypes, with pIs of pH 6.3, 5.3, and 4.7, respectively, were isolated. Of these, the predominant pI 6.3 form was homogeneous in disc gel electrophoresis in sodium dodecyl sulfate (SDS-PAGE) whereas the other products still contained small amounts of contaminating proteins. SDS-PAGE, with and without boiling in SDS prior to electrophoresis, revealed that each of the preparations consisted of noncovalently associated oligomers of identically sized (32,000 m.w.) protein subunits. Reduction, with 2-mercapteothanol, had no effect indicating that there were no interchain disulfide bonds.

The HA activity was heat-labile: it was totally destroyed by heating for less than 1 hour at 60 C; it lost all activity on incubation for 24 hours at 37 C and by one week at 25C; but it was relatively stable at 4 C. Although only fractions with HA activity were pooled for further purification during the isolation procedure, recovery of activity during purification was poor (0.2 %) and the specific activity (HA units/mg protein) did not increase during purification. This was despite the fact that the inactive protein which was discarded constituted the vast majority of the starting material. These observations suggested the possibility that the HA activity was diminishing through effects of protease(s).

Consequently, the purified material was examined and found to have protease activity on azoalbumin (Sigma) and dimethyl casein. Further, when purified HA was subjected to disc electrophoresis, the protease activity co-migrated with the HA activity, which corresponded, in position, with the single band observed in a gel run in parallel which was stained for protein.

Protease activity was monitored, in parallel with HA activity, during the purification. As did the HA, the protease also isoelectrically focused at pHs of 6.3 and 5.3

to 4.7. If the protease and the HA are a single molecule, it would be expected that their specific activities should fluctuate in parallel at each step in purification. However, this was not the case: the most purified HA preparation had a lower ratio of HA/protease activity than the starting material.

Transmission electron microscopy, using uranyl acetate stain, revealed that the purified HA appeared as long filaments. It was further observed that whereas the HA was fully active at 4 C, the protease activity was maximal at 37 C and barely detectable when the assays were performed in the cold.

From the above information, we are led to the tentative operational hypothesis that the HA and protease activity reside on the same molecule and that the spontaneous self-aggregation into filaments may have a more marked effect on the HA activity than on the protease.

Further evidence that the HA molecule has both activities was provided by immunologic studies. Antisera were prepared in rabbits immunized with the different pH isotypes of the HA. These antisera gave reactions of identity in Ouchterlony tests with the different preparations. Thus, they are all immunologically identical. Further, antiserum against the pI 6.3 material gave only a single precipitin band (with a reaction of identity to the purified material) with concentrated crude culture supernatants of the parent strain and with all the other strains tested. This antiserum was used, in parallel with pre-immune serum from the same rabbit, in the following experiment.

Purified pI 6.3 material was subjected to disc electrophoresis in duplicate. One gel was stained for protein with Coomassie Brilliant Blue R (Sigma) and, as had been observed previously, only one protein stained band was obtained. The other gel was embedded in skim milk agar (20) to detect and localize protease activity. Two troughs were cut in the skim milk agar, parallel to and equidistant from the disc gel. Immune serum was placed in one trough and pre-immune serum in the other. After overnight incubation at 25 C, zones of proteolysis were observed on both sides of the embedded gel corresponding to the position of the protein band in the stained gel. However, the zone of proteolysis was markedly inhibited by the immune serum.

Fab fragments prepared from this serum significantly ($p<0.025$) inhibited in vitro attachment of ^{14}C-labelled vibrios to tissue discs of infant rabbit ileum in comparison with Fab fragments from the pre-immune control serum.

It should also be mentioned that antiserum against a partially purified *V. cholerae* protease, isolated independently by Schneider and Parker (18, 19), gave a precipitin reaction of identity with the purified soluble HA and our anti-HA serum.

It should be emphasized that although this HA has been isolated from culture supernatants and has therefore been called a "soluble HA," production and release of such a soluble adhesin would be disadvantageous to the vibrios unless its purpose was to promote *detachment* of the vibrios from host intestinal epithelial membrane receptors. The fact that it was isolated from culture supernatants may be an artifact of *in vitro* growth. The "soluble HA" may, in fact, be cell-associated in vivo as indicated by the finding that in vivo grown vibrios directly agglutinated responder but not non-responder RBC and by inhibition of binding studies. It may be found in the supernatants of late log phase cultures *in vitro* because of the vibrios' tendency to release outer membrane fragments by "blebbing." It is also worthy of further consideration that the soluble HA could serve both to facilitate attachment and to promote detachment (16) through its protease function.

From the present results and those of others, we propose that adherence by *V. cholerae* is a multi-factorial process which may involve motility of the vibrios, chemotactic events and trapping in the mucus gel (see Freter et al, 9); the "soluble HA-protease-cholera lectin" described here; and perhaps the mannose- and fucose-sensitive cell-associated HAs in certain circumstances. Different factors may be more important in some experimental models than in others and it remains to be determined which is/are most important in the natural host, man. It would of interest to ascertain whether active (passive) immunization with the purified HA (of the present work) is protective in animal models and whether antibody to this HA contributes to the immunity which has been observed in man following convalescence from the disease (14) and following oral immunization with the Texas Star-SR A^-B^+ attenuated mutant candidate vaccine strain (3, 15). Additional details of the experimental results summarized here are presented elsewhere (7, 11).

This study was supported, in part, by Public Health Service Grants AI-08877 and AI-17312 under the U.S.-Japan Cooperative Medical Science Program, from the National Institute of Allergy and Infectious Diseases.

Note added in proof:

The activity of the protease on fibronectin, mucin, lactoferrin, and other proteins, has been reprinted (6a).

REFERENCES

1. Bales, G. L., and C. E. Lankford. 1961. An adherence factor of *Vibrio cholerae*, p. 118. In Bacteriological Proceedings 1961; American Society for Microbiology, Washington, D. C.
2. Bhattacharjee, J. W., and B. S. Srivastava. 1978. Mannose-sensitive haemagglutinins in adherence of *Vibrio cholerae* El Tor to intestine. J. Gen. Microbiol. **107**:407-410.
3. Boesman-Finkelstein, M., and R. A. Finkelstein 1982. Protection in rabbits induced by the Texas Star-SR attenuated A^-B^+ mutant candidate live oral cholera vaccine. Infect. Immun., **36**:221-226.
4. Chaicumpa, W., and N. Atthasishtha. 1977. Study of intestinal immunity against *V. cholerae*: Role of antibody to *V. cholerae* haemagglutinin in intestinal immunity. Southeast Asian J. Trop. Med. Pub. Health **8**:13-18.
5. Chaicumpa, W., and N. Atthasishtha. 1979. Study of intestinal immunity against *V. cholerae* El Tor haemagglutinin and the protective role of its antibody in experimental cholera. Southeast Asian J. Trop. Med. Pub. Health **10**:73-80.
6. Finkelstein, R. A., M. Arita, J. D. Clements, and E. T. Nelson. 1978. Isolation and purification of an adhesive factor ("cholera lectin") from *Vibrio cholerae*, pp. 137-151. In Proceedings of the 13th Joint Conference on Cholera, U. S.-Japan Cooperative Medical Science Program, Atlanta, GA, 19-21 September 1977 (DHEW Pub. No. 78-1590). National Institutes of Health, Bethesda, MD.

6a. Finkelstein, R A., M B.-Finkelstein and P. Holt. 1983. *Vibrio cholerae* hemagglutinin/lectin/protease hydrolyzes fibronectin and ovomucin : F. M. Burnet revisited. Proc. Natl. Acad. Sci. USA. **80**:1092-1095.

7. Finkelstein, R. A., and L. F. Hanne. 1982. Purification and characterization of the soluble hemagglutinin ("cholera lectin") produced by *Vibrio cholerae*. Infect. Immun.,**36**:1199-1208.
8. Finkelstein, R. A., and S. Mukerjee. 1963. Hemagglutination: A rapid method for differentiating *Vibrio cholerae* and El Tor vibrios. Proc. Soc. Exp. Biol. Med. **112**:355-359.
9. Freter, R., B. Allweiss, P. M. C. O'Brien, S. A. Halstead, and M. S. Macsai. 1981. Role of chemo-

taxis in the association of motile bacteria with intestinal mucosa: in vitro studies. Infect. Immun. **34**:241-249.

10. Freter, R., and G. W. Jones. 1976. Adhesive properties of *Vibrio cholerae*: Nature of the interaction with intact mucosal surfaces. Infect. Immun. **14**:246-256.
11. Hanne, L. F., and R. A. Finkelstein. 1982. Characterization and distribution of the hemagglutinins produced by *Vibrio cholerae*. Infect. Immun., **36**:209-214.
12. Jones, G. W., G. D. Abrams, and R. Freter. 1976. Adhesive properties of *Vibrio cholerae*: Adhesion to isolated rabbit brush border membranes and hemagglutinating activity. Infect. Immun. **14**:232-239.
13. Jones, G. W., and R. Freter. 1976. Adhesive properties of *Vibrio cholerae*: Nature of the interaction with isolated rabbit brush border membranes and human erythrocytes. Infect. Immun. **14**: 240-245.
14. Levine, M. M., R. E. Black, M. L. Clements, L. Cisneros, D. R. Nalin, and C. R. Young. 1981. Duration of infection-derived immunity to cholera. J. Infect. Dis. **143**:818-820.
15. Levine, M. M., R. E. Black, M. L. Clements, C. R. Young, T. Honda, and R. A. Finkelstein. 1981. Texas Star-SR: Attenuated *Vibrio cholerae* oral vaccine candidate. In Proceedings of the 17th Joint Conference on Cholera, U.S.-Japan Cooperative Medical Science Program, Baltimore, MD, 25-28 October 1981, in press.
16. Nelson, E. T., J. D. Clements, and R. A. Finkelstein. 1976. *Vibrio cholerae* adherence and colonization in experimental cholera: electron microscopic studies. Infect. Immun. **14**:527-547.
17. Nelson, E. T., M. Hochli, C. R. Hackenbrock, and R. A. Finkelstein. 1977. Electron microscopic observations on intestinal colonization by *Vibrio cholerae*: Freeze-etching studies, pp. 81-86. In Symposium on Cholera: Sapporo 1976 (Proceedings of the 12th Joint Conference, U.S.-Japan Cooperative Medical Science Program, Cholera Panel; ed., H. Fukumi and Y. Zinnaka). National Institute of Health, Tokyo, Japan.
18. Schneider, D. R., and C. D. Parker. 1978. Isolation and characterization of protease-deficient mutants of *Vibrio cholerae*. J. Infect. Dis. **138**:143-151.
19. Schneider, D. R., and C. D. Parker. 1982. Purification and characterization of the mucinase of *Vibrio cholerae*. J. Infect. Dis., **145**:474-482.
20. Sokol, P. A., D. E. Ohman, and B. H. Iglewski. 1979. A more sensitive plate assay for detection of protease production by *Pseudomonas aeruginosa*. J. Clin. Microbiol. **9**:538-540.
21. Tweedy, J. M., and R. W. A. Park. 1968. Evidence for the presence of fimbriae (pili) on vibrio species. J. Gen. Microbiol. **51**:235-244.

Advances in Research on Cholera and Related Diarrheas, eds., S. Kuwahara, N. F. Pierce, 127–134.

EXPERIMENTAL CHOLERA IN GERM-FREE AND GNOTOBIOTIC PIGLETS

Eiji Tokunaga, Toyoharu Muraoka, Shunsuke Akiyama
Kazusuke Kudo and Nobuya Ohtomo

The Chemo-Sero-Therapeutic Research Institute,
Kumamoto 860, Japan

Introduction

We have previously reported that two to five weeks old germ-free piglets developed cholera-like watery diarrhea consistently after orogastric inoculation with cholera toxin or *Vibrio cholerae* Inaba 569B.[1] Because Inaba 569B is an extraordinarily hyper-toxigenic strain of *Vibrio cholerae*, we have further evaluated the germ-free piglet model by using strains with lower toxigenicity as the challenge organism. *Vibrio cholerae* El Tor Inaba P6973, El Tor Inaba T348 and Ogawa NIH41, which produce toxin at the same level as current isolates, were used as challenge strains.[2]

We have also expanded our piglet model to include gnotobiotic piglets. Germ-free piglets were inoculated with known nonpathogens and then challenged with *Vibrio cholerae* Inaba 569B or cholera toxin.

Materials and Methods

Piglets. (1) Germ-free piglets. They were produced in our laboratory according to Kashiwazaki *et al.*[3] A healthy pregnant sow was introduced one or two days before the expected delivery day, and under anesthesia its uterus was taken out and transferred aseptically into a sterile isolator. Piglets were delivered out of the incised uterus and transferred separately into other sterile isolators. They were then fed with SPF milk (Borden Chemical, Norfolk, Va.). (2) Gnotobiotic piglets. Germ-free piglets were fed with known nonpathogenic microorganisms to establish intestinal florae prior to challenge. The bacteria introduced were *Enterobacter cloacae, Staphylococcus epidermidis* and a strain of gram-positive anaerobe. Those nonpathogenic microorganisms were isolated from healthy specific pathogen free piglets in our laboratory.

Preparation of inocula. Viable cell inocula were prepared by serially diluting 18hrs heart infusion agar slant cultures of an appropriate strain in sterile 0.85% saline. Viable counts for colony-forming units (CFU) per milliliter were determined by the mix-culture method in nutrient agar plate. Serial dillutions of purified cholera toxin were made in phosphate buffered saline. The cholera toxin was prepared as described elsewhere.[4]

Orogastric challenge. Either germ-free or gnotobiotic piglets, two weeks old, were subjected to the experiment after they had been ketp in isolators. Prior to challenge, the piglets were fasted overnight. As previously reported, *Vibrio cholerae* or cholera toxin in 30 ml of a 6% sodium bicarbonate solution was introduced into the piglet's stomach through a 10 Fr., 33 cm silicon rubber catheter (Terumo Co., Tokyo).[1] Germ-free piglets were challenged with *Vibrio cholerae* El Tor Inaba P6973, El Tor Inaba T348 or Ogawa NIH41. Gnotobiotic piglets were challenge with *Vibrio cholerae* Inaba 569B or cholera toxin.

Examinations. After challenge, piglets were inspected 7 days for stool status. The stool of healthy piglets was of a moderate consistency with brown to darkbrown color. As stool consistency bacame liquid, there was a color change. In this work, we used four terms for characterizing the stool status: *normal stool* meant moderate consistency with brown to darkbrown color, *soft stool* loose consistency with yellowish color, *diarrhea* amorphous stool with yellowish color, and *watery diarrhea* literally watery flow but still yellowish. Rectal swabs were taken and streaked directly on TCBS agar or cultured for 6hrs in 1% alkaline peptone water at pH 9.0 before subculturing on TCBS agar. *Vibrio cholerae* were identified by colonial appearance and by an appropriate aggultination test.

Results

Diarrheal response in germ-free piglets. Nine germ-free piglets were divided into 2 groups: 6 challenge piglets and 3 control piglets, for which the challenge was done with approximately 10^8 CFU of *Vibrio cholerae.* This challenge dose generated cholera-like syndroms irrespective of the challenge strain. Every two germ-free piglets were infected with either *Vibrio cholerae* Inaba P6973, Inaba T348 or Ogawa NIH41. Three control piglets were given sterile bicarbonate solution only. As illustrated in Fig. 1, one of two piglets, inoculated with P6973, developed diarrhea at 9hrs followed by watery diarrhea at 12hrs. This piglet's stool gradually improved to soft consistency. The other piglet began to discharge watery diarrhea at 9hrs and died at 18hrs. Piglets, inoculated with T348, demonstrated diarrhea 9 and 15hrs after the challenge, respectively, with one of them developing watery diarrhea at 15hrs. Piglets, challenged with NIH41, developed diarrhea at 15hrs followed by watery diarrhea at 18 and 24hrs. Control piglets were asymptomatic.

Diarrheal response in gnotobiotic piglets. Eight germ-free piglets were divided into two groups. *Enterobacter cloacae* and *Staphylococcus epidermidis* were established as the specific flora in the first group of 5 piglets. The second group was infected with gram-positive anaerobes to establish the specific flora. The gnotobiotic piglet model was highly sensitive to orogastric challenge with *Vibrio cholerae* Inaba 569B or cholera toxin. Challenge results of gnotobiotic piglets, having defined flora of *Enterobacter cloacae* and *Staphylococcus epidermidis*, are shown in Fig. 2. Two piglets developed diarrhea 6hrs after receiving 10^8 CFU of Inaba 569B, with onset of watery diarrhea at 9hrs. The watery diarrhea continued until 45 and 51hrs postchallenge. Piglets, given 50 μg of purified cholera toxin, also showed watery diarrhea. However, the onset of watery diarrhea was delayed and its duration was short; beginning at 18hrs and lasting for 9 to 12hrs. The control piglet was asymptomatic. Fig. 3 shows the challenge results of gnotobiotic piglets with gram-positive anaerobes as the defind flora. Both piglets, given 10^8 CFU of *Vibrio cholerae* Inaba 569B, demonstrated diarrhea beginning at 12 and 18hrs. Watery diarrhea commensed at 15 and 27hrs, respectively.

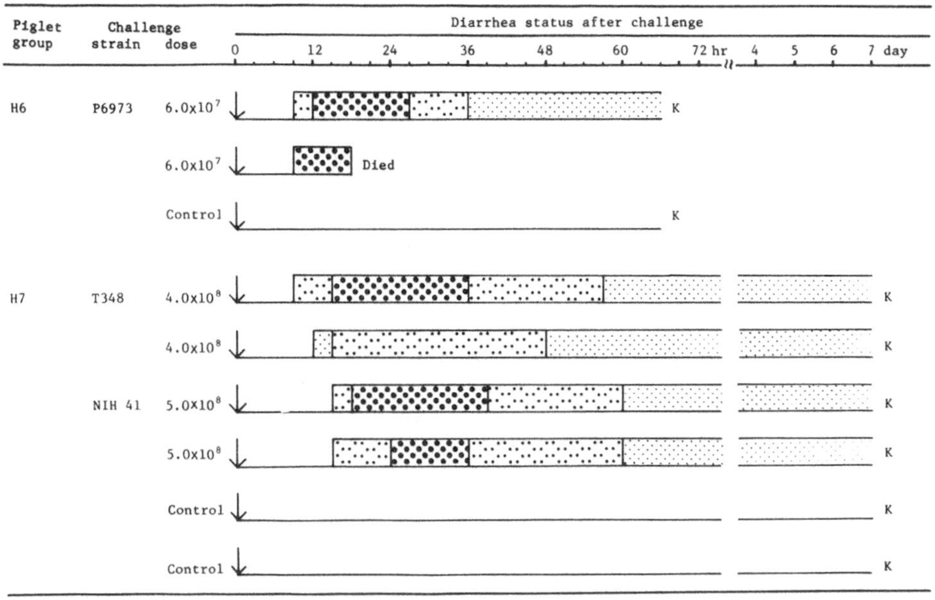

Fig. 1. Diarrhea in germ-free piglets after orogastric inoculation with *Vibrio cholerae*. Piglets were sacrificed for autopsy as indicated by K. Symbols: [soft stool symbol] soft stool, [diarrhea symbol] diarrhea, [watery diarrhea symbol] watery diarrhea.

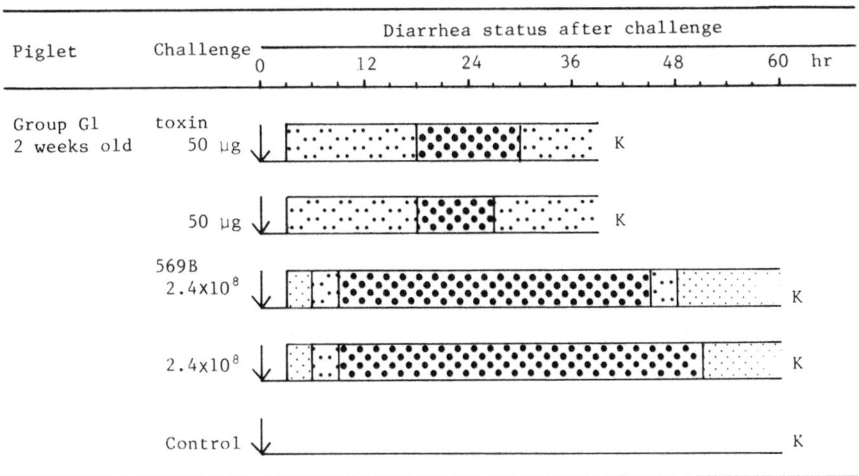

Fig. 2. Diarrhea in gnotobiotic piglets, previously given *Enterobacter cloacae* and *Staphylococcus epidermidis*, after orogastric inoculation with cholera toxin or *Vibrio cholerae* Inaba 569B. Piglets were sacrificed for autopsy as indicated by K. Symbols are the same as shown in Fig. 1.

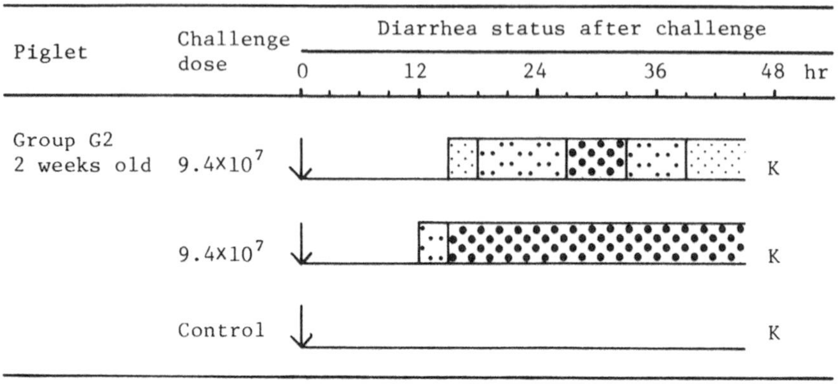

Fig. 3. Diarrhea in gnotobiotic piglets, previously given a strain of gram-positive anaerobe, after orogastric inoculation with *Vibrio cholerae* Inaba 569B. Piglets were sacrificed for autopsy as indicated by K. Symbols are the same as shown in Fig. 1.

Excretion of Vibrio cholerae in germ-free and gnotobiotic piglets. Results of rectal swab tests on germ-free piglets before and after challenge with *Vibrio cholerae* are shown in Table 1. *Vibrio cholerae* excretion began 3 to 12hrs after the challenge and continued throughout the observation period. Quantitative counts of vibrios in the stool of 3 germ-free piglets were also made throughout the observation period. Fig. 4 shows the results of two piglets infected with Inaba T348 and one piglet with Ogawa NIH41. The number of secreted vibrios decreased gradually from 10^{10} CFU/ml at 15hrs to 10^{8}-10^{9} CFU/ml on the sixth day. Table 2 shows the results of the rectal swab test on gnotobiotic piglets. Piglets began to excrete vibrios between 3 to 12hrs after challenge. Excretion continued 2 to 3 days until the piglets were sacrificed. Fig. 4 shows the quantitative counts of vibrios in the stool of the gnotobiotic piglets with gram-positive anaerobes as the defined flora. The number continued to increase and reached to a peak of about 10^{10} CFU/ml at 33hrs. after which they declined.

Table 1. Excretion of *V. cholerae*[1)] in germ-free piglets after orogastric challenge.

Piglet group	Challenge strain	dose	0	3	6	9	12	15	18	21	24hr	2	3	4	5	6	7days
H6	P6973	$6.0x10^{7}$		–	–		+++	+++	+++	+++	+++	+++	+++	K[2)]			
		$6.0x10^{7}$			+++	+++	+++	+++	+++	Died							
H7	T348	$4.0x10^{8}$		+++	+++	+++	+++	+++	+++	+++	+++	+++	+	+++	+	+++	+++ K
		$4.0x10^{8}$		+++	+++	+++	+++	+++	+++	+++	+++	+++	+++	+++	+++	+++	+++ K
	NIH 41	$5.0x10^{8}$		+	++	+++	+++	+++	+++	+++	+++	+++	+++	+++	+++	+++	+++ K
		$5.0x10^{8}$		+++	+++	+++	+++	+++	+++	+++	+++	+++	+++	+++	+++	+++	+++ K

1. Not quantitative. Symbols represent the grades of growth of stool culture.
2. Piglets were sacrificed for autopsy as indicated by K.

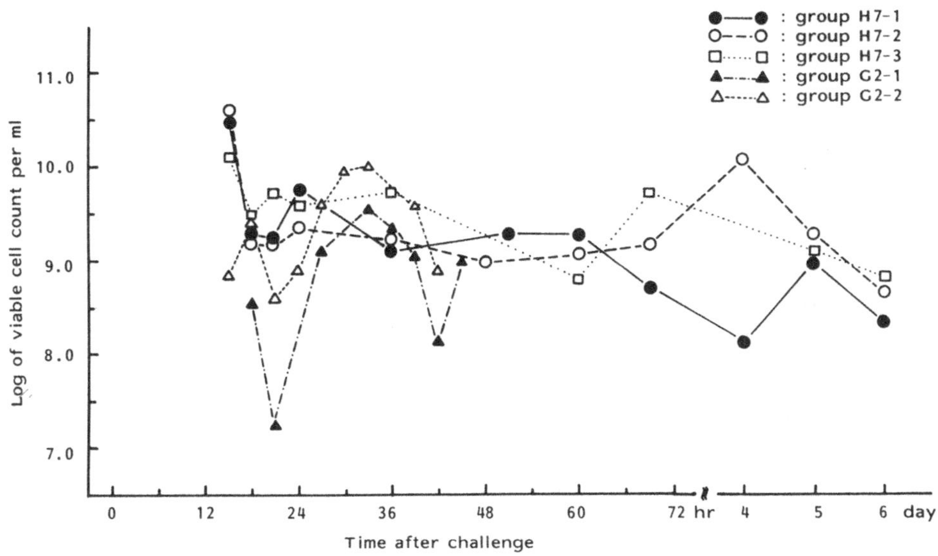

Fig. 4. Time course of vibrio excretion in HPCD piglets after orogastric challenge. Symbols: ●–● and ○–○ germ-free piglets challenged with T348, □···□ germ-free piglet challenged with NIH41, ▲-·-▲ and △–△ gnotobiotic piglets, previously given a strain of gram-positive anaerobe, challenged with 569B.

Virulence of piglet-passaged Vibrio cholerae. As described above, piglets challenged with 569B or other strains demonstrated watery diarrhea starting about 10 to 20hrs after the challenge and then gradually improved, but they still excreted vibrios throughout the observation period. Therefore, there was a possibility that *Vibrio cholerae* might lose the virulence through the piglet passage. The pathogenicities of stock strains and piglet-passaged strains were compared by the rabbit ileal loop test. As shown in Table 3, piglet-passaged strains demonstrated an obviously positive FA ratio just as did the stock strains and a statistical analysis revealed that there was no significant difference between the

Table 2. Excretion of *V. cholerae*[1)] strain 569B in gnotobiotic [2)] piglets after orogastric challenge.

Piglet group	Challenge dose	Time after challenge 0	3	6	9	12	15	18	21	24hr	2	3 days
G1	$2.4x10^8$		++	++	+		⧻	⧻			⧻	⧻ K[3)]
	$2.4x10^8$		++	++	⧻		⧻	⧻			⧻	⧻ K
G2	$9.4x10^7$		–	–	–	⧻	⧻	⧻	⧻	⧻	⧻	K
	$9.4x10^7$		–	+	–	+	⧻	⧻	⧻	⧻	⧻	K

1. Not quantitative. Symbols represent the grades of growth of stool culture.
2. Flora : group G1 ; *Enterobacter cloacae* and *Staphylococcus epidermidis*,
   group G2 ; a strain of gram-positive anaerobe.
3. Piglets were sacrificed for autopsy as indicated by K.

Table 3. Comparison of virulence of *V. cholerae* in the rabbit ileal loop test between the stock and piglet-passaged strains.

Challenge strain	dose[1)]	No. of animals	Fluid accumulation[2)] ml/cm
T348	$4.0x10^8$	3	1.48±0.32
T348 (H7–1)[3)]	$4.0x10^8$	3	2.04±0.34
T348 (H7–2)	$4.0x10^8$	3	2.08±0.53
NIH 41	$4.0x10^8$	4	1.89±0.33
NIH 41 (H7–3)	$4.0x10^8$	4	2.00±0.25
NIH 41 (H7–4)	$4.0x10^8$	4	1.44±0.24
569B	$4.0x10^8$	4	2.34±0.42
569B (G2–2)	$4.0x10^8$	4	2.08±0.36
Saline		4	0.01±0.01

1. Approximate number estimated by an optical absorbance method.
2. Ml per cm length of the loop, expressed as the mean.
3. *V. cholerae* with parenthesis means the piglet-passaged strain.

stock strains and piglet-passaged strains ($P<0.05$). From this result, it appears that fairly long excretion of *Vibrio cholerae* in piglets is not due to a loss of virulence.

Localization of Vibrio cholerae. The localization of vibrios in the gastrointestinal content of germ-free and gnotobiotic piglets was examined at autopsy. The results of germ-free piglets are shown in Table 4. *Vibrio cholerae* were detected predominantly in the colon with smaller numbers in the small intestine. Sometimes vibrios could not be detected in the duodenum. Similar trends were observed in the gnotobiotic piglets (Table 5).

Table 4. Detection of *V. cholerae* from organs of germ-free piglets at autopsy.

Piglet group	Challenge strain	dose	Organ Stomach	Gallbladder	Duodenum	Jejunum	Ileum	Colon
H6	P6973	$6.0x10^7$	–[1)]	(+)	(+)	+	+++	+++
		$6.0x10^7$	+++	–	+++	+++	+++	+++
H7	T348	$4.0x10^8$	–	+	++	+ $2.1x10^6$[2)]	+++ $5.1x10^8$	+++ $1.0x10^9$
		$4.0x10^8$	–	–	(+)	++ $1.8x10^7$	++ $1.1x10^7$	+++ $1.1x10^9$
	NIH 41	$5.0x10^8$	–	–	+	+	+++	+++ $2.4x10^9$
		$5.0x10^8$	–	–	+	++	+++ $2.0x10^9$	+++ $3.3x10^9$

1. Estimated on TCBS agar. Symbols represent the grades of growth of stool culture, that in parenthesis means the result by enrichment in peptone water.
2. The number means viable count per ml of the content of the organ estimated by means of mix-culture.

Table 5. Detection of *V. cholerae* strain 569B from organs of gnotobiotic[1)] piglets at autopsy.

Piglet	Challenge dose	Stomach	Gallbladder	Duodenum	Jejunum	Ileum	Colon
				Organ			
Group G2	$9.4x10^7$	–[2)]	–	(+)	(+)	++	+++
2 weeks old					$6.1x10^6$	$3.5x10^6$	$1.1x10^9$
	$9.4x10^7$	–	–	(+)	+	+	+++
					$1.2x10^7$	$4.9x10^7$	$4.3x10^7$

1. Flora : a strain of gram-positive anaerobes.
2. Estimated on TCBS agar. Symbols represent the grades of growth of stool culture, that in parenthesis means the result by enrichment in peptone water.
3. The number means the viable counts per ml of the content of the organ estimated by means of mix-culture.

Discussion

The present study confirms and extends the previous findings on the usefulness of germ-free piglets for experimental study of cholera. In a previous paper we reported that germ-free piglets consistently developed cholera-like watery diarrhea after orogastric inoculation with either *Vibrio cholerae* Inaba 569B or cholera toxin.[1)] However, Inaba 569B is an extraordinarily hypertoxigenic strain of *Vibrio cholerae.* Therefore, it seemed necessary to conduct the challenge experiment in germ-free piglets with other strains to evaluate its applicability. The three strains of *Vibrio cholerae* tested in this experiment produce toxin at the same level as do current isolates and are virulent in other animal models, such as the ligated ileal loop model of rabbits and guinea pigs, and the infant mouse oral challenge model.[2)] As described in the results, all germ-free piglets challenged with either of these strains developed diarrhea with watery flow. From the results reported in the previous and this paper, it is quite evident that germ-free piglet is sensitive enough to challenge with various strains of *Vibrio cholerae* and/or cholera toxin.

In addition to the germ-free piglets, we had an opportunity to conduct a challenge experiment in gnotobiotic piglets with either *Vibrio cholerae* Inaba 569B or cholera toxin. Gnotobiotic piglets responded quite sensitively and regularly to either *Vibrio cholerae* or cholera toxin. In consequence it is conceivable that either the germ-free or the gnotobiotic piglet is adoptable as a reliable animal model for cholera study.

As previously reported we performed pathogenicity tests of hypotoxinogenic mutant strains, *tox*-101TIN4 and *tox*-101TIN6, by the germ-free piglet model in addition to the rabbit ligated ileal loop model and infant mouse oral challenge model.[2,5,6)] These tests revealed that both strains were avirulent. It is likely that the germ-free and gnotobiotic piglet models will provide a reliable virulence test for any strain of *Vibrio cholerae.*

The sensitivity of the germ-free piglet model has been proved to be reliable as far as 5 weeks but no longer observation has been made as yet. If these piglets keep the sensitivity for a further period, the model will be able to be applied to immunological studies.

REFERENCES

1. Ohtomo, N., Muraoka, T., Tokunaga, E., Akiyama, S., Kudo, K. and Taneno, H. 1980. Experimental cholera in hysterectomy-produced colostrum-deprived (HPCD) piglets. *In* Proc. 16th US-Japan Joint Cholera Conference, Gifu, 266-275.
2. Ohtomo, N., Muraoka, T., Kudo, K., and Murphy, J. R. 1979. Toxigenicity and pathogenicity of a mutant strain *tox*-101TIN4 derived from *Vibrio cholerae* 569B Inaba. *In* Proc. 15th US-Japan Joint Cholera Conference, Bethesda, 345-361.
3. Kashiwazaki, M., Namioka, S., Umoto, K. and Shibata, S. 1967. Studies on the rearing of germ-free pigs. I. A germ-free rearing isolator apparatus and procurement of baby pigs. (In Japanese.) Experimental animals. **19**:85-92.
4. Ohtomo, N., Muraoka, T., Tashiro, A., Zinnaka, Y. and Amako, K. 1976. Size and structure of cholera toxin molecule and its subunits. J. Infect. Dis. **133**:suppl. S31-S40.
5. Nichols, J., Murphy, J. R., Robb, M., Echeverria, P. and Craig, J. P. 1978. Isolation and characterization of *Vibrio cholerae* mutant which produce defective cholera toxin. *In* Proc. 14th US-Japan Joint Cholera Conference, Karatsu, 192-199.
6. Tokunaga, E., Muraoka, T., Akiyama, S., Ohtomo, N., Nichols, J. C. and Murphy, J. R. 1981. Pathogenicity test in HPCD piglets of hypotoxinogenic mutant strain, *tox*-101TIN4 of *Vibrio cholerae*. *In* Proc. 16th US-Japan Joint Cholera Conference, Gifu, 276-281.

Advances in Research on Cholera and Related Diarrheas, eds., S. Kuwahara, N. F. Pierce, 135–143.

ISOLATION OF HYBRIDOMA CELL LINES PRODUCING ANTIBODY AGAINST CHOLERA ENTEROTOXIN

M. Robb, J.C. Nichols, and J.R. Murphy

Department of Microbiology and Molecular Genetics, Harvard Medical School, Boston, Massachusetts 02115

1. Introduction

We have previously reported the *in vitro* synthesis of cholera toxin-related polypeptides in *Escherichia coli* cell free translation mixtures. These polypeptides were immunologically detected following treatment of reaction mixtures with anti-subunit A or anti-cholera toxin sera (1). Addition of cholera toxin to reaction mixtures was shown to bolck immunoprecipitation. These experiments strongly suggested that *in vitro* synthesis of cholera toxin-related polypeptides was being detected. However, identification was dependent on the purity of antisera used for immunoprecipitation. Since there was a possibility that the sera used contained minor components which might precipitate proteins other than cholera toxin-related polypeptides, we decided to develop a collection of cell lines producing monoclonal antibodies against cholera toxin and its subunits. These antibodies would be important in the study of cholera toxin precursors and the secretion of cholera toxin from *Vibrio cholerae*.

Kohler and Milstein were the first to describe hybridoma methodology (2, 3). In this method, spleen cells from immunized mice are immortalized by fusion with cultured mouse myeloma cells. Some of the fused or hybrid cells produce antibody against the immunizing antigen. These cells can be selected and tissue culture then provides a continuous source of antibodies with a single, defined antigenic specificity. We have immunized mice with cholera toxin and have isolated cell lines which produce monoclonal antibody against each of the subunits of cholera toxin.

Materials and Methods

Purification of Cholera Toxin and its Subunits. A hypertoxinogenic mutant of *Vibrio cholera* 569B, Htx-D, was grown overnight in a 10 l fermentor as follows: cells from an 8 h, two liter shake culture were isolated by centrifugation, resuspended and used to inoculate 10 l of CYE (4) broth supplemented with 500 ml of 5X M63 buffer (5) and 100 ml 20% sucrose. The culture was incubated at 30°C and aerated vigorously with air and compressed oxygen. Toxin was purified from the supernatant fluid essentially as described by Mekalanos (4). The protein fraction of the supernatant was co-precipitated with sodium hexametaphosphate. The precipitate was redissolved in 0.1 M sodium phosphate, pH 8.3, equilibrated with 10 mM sodium phosphate, pH 7.0, and chromatographed on phosphocellulose; purified toxin was eluted with 0.2 M sodium phosphate, pH 8.3. Subunit $A_1 A_2$ was prepared from purified toxin which had been dialyzed against water and dissociated in 6 M urea at pH 2.7; after the pH was adjusted to 7.0, toxin was rechromatographed over phosphocellulose at pH 7.0 in 6 M urea. Subunit $A_1 A_2$ was recovered in the void volume and subunit B was eluted with 0.2 M sodium phosphate, pH 8.3. Subunit A preparations were equilibrated with 10 mM carbonate buffer, pH 8.8, as Subunit A deteriorates in phosphate buffer.

E. coli heat labile toxin was the generous gift of Dr. John C. Clements.

Immunization. Twenty-eight to thirty-five day old female BALB/c mice (Charles River Breeding Labs, Wilmington, M.A.) were immunized as follows (T. Springer, personal communication) : approximately 30 days prior to spenectomy (day -30), mice were injected intraperitoneally (IP) with 5 ng of toxin plus 50 μg of toxoid; on day -7 mice received an IP injection of 100 μg of subunit $A_1 A_2$; on days –3 and –1, 100 μg of subunit $A_1 A_2$ was injected intravenously; and on day –2 100 μg subunit $A_1 A_2$ was injected IP.

Media and Chemicals. Dulbecco's modified Eagle's medium without pyruvate (incomplete DMEM) was purchased from Grand Island Biochemicals, New York. Complete DMEM was made up as follows: Dulbecco's modification of Eagle's medium (with pyruvate) (Flow Laboratories, Rockville, M.D.) was supplemented with nonessential amino acids, penicillin-streptomicin, glutamine, and 20% bovine sera (10% fetal/10% newborn bovine sera). HT media (HT–DMEM) was prepared by adding 13.6 μ 13.6 μg/ml hypoxanthine and 3.88 μg/ml thymidine to complete DMEM; HAT–DMEM was prepared by adding 0.175 μg/ml aminopterin to HT–DMEM. Ten grams polyethylene glycol MW 1500 (PEG) (Aldrich Chemical Co., Milwaukee, W.I.) was autoclaved, cooled and added to 10 ml incomplete DMEM; the pH was adjusted to 7.6–7.8. Noble agar (Difco, Detroit, M.I.) in complete DMEM was used for soft agar cloning.

Mouse IgG, rabbit anti-mouse IgG, and peroxidase conjugated anti-mouse IgG were purchased from Cappell Laboratories, Cochranville, Pennsylvania. Mouse IgG typing sera was purchased from Miles Laboratories, Elkhart, Indiana. The nonionic detergent Brij-58 was purchased from Sigma Chemical, St. Louis, Missouri. 0-dianisidine 3,3'-dimethoxybenzidine dihydrochloride) was purchased from Aldrich Chemical Company, Metuchen, New Jersey. CoStar (Cambridge, M.A.) 96- and 24-well microtiter plates were used for tissue culture; untreated 96-well microtiter plates (Linbro, Division of Flow Laboratories, Hamden, C.T.) were used for Enzyme-Linked Immuno-Sorbent Assays (ELISA).

Hybridization. Cells were fused using a modification of the PEG fusion method of Nowinski, *et al.* (6). The myeloma cell line BALB/c P-3NS1/1AG4-1 (NS1) was kindly provided by Dr. S. Burstin.

Spleens were removed by blunt dissection and washed three times in ice cold incomplete DMEM. Spleen cells were isolated by perfusion and fused with NS1 cells in a 4:1 ratio with 50% PEG according to the following schedule:

Time (min)	Treatment
0–0.5	Add 1 ml 50% PEG dropwise while stirring with tip of 1 ml pipette
0.5–2.0	Allow to stand at 37°C with occasional stirring
2.0–5.0	Add 5 ml incomplete DMEM (37°C) slowly with stirring
5.0–6.0	Add 14 ml imcomplete DMEM (37°C)
6.0	Add 30 ml complete DMEM (37°C)

Following centrifugation, the supernatant was aspirated and cells were resuspended to 3×10^6 input spleen cells/ml and dispensed in 100 μl volumes into 96-well microtiter dishes. Cells were maintained for 29 days in HAT-DMEM; after day 30, cells were maintained in HT-DMEM medium for two weeks, and thereafter in complete DMEM.

After screening for the presence of antibody to cholera toxin, cells from positive wells were transferred into 20mm, 24-well tissue culture plates. After re-screening, cells from positive wells were cloned in soft agar (7). Clones were picked and grown in liquid media in 96-well microtiter plates and retested for antibody production in an ELISA; cells which remained positive were grown in 75 cm^2 tissue culture flasks and supernatnats were regularly collected.

Screening for Antibody to Cholera Toxin and Subunits. An Enzyme-Linked Immuno-Sorbent Assay was used to screen for anti-cholera toxin producing cells. Cholera toxin (10 μg/ml in phosphate buffered saline [PBS]) or subunit A (10 μg/ml in sodium carbonate, pH 8.8) was dispensed in 200 μl volumes into 96-well microtiter dishes which were incubated overnight at 4°C or for 2 hours at 37°C. Plates were washed three times and incubated for 2 h at 37°C with 200 μl aliquots of 1:4 dilutions of hybridoma culture fluids or supernatants. All washes and antibody dilutions were made in PBS containing Brij-58 at a final concentration of 0.05% to minimize nonspecific protein-protein interaction. After three more washes, 200 μl aliquots of a 1:5000-1:10000 dilution of peroxidase conjugated anti-mouse IgG were added to each well, plates were incubated for 2 h at 37°C, and again washed. To prepare the substrate solution, fresh hydrogen peroxide (30%) was diluted 1:100 in H_2O. This hydrogen peroxide solution was further diluted 1:100 in 0.1M sodium phosphate buffer, pH 6.0. Substrate-dye solution was prepared by adding 0.042 ml of o-dianisidine (1% in methanol) to 5.0 ml substrate solution. Peroxidase activity was detected colorimetrically following addition of 0.05 ml substrate-dye solution to each well.

SDS-Polyacrylamide Gel Elecrophoresis. 15% SDS-polyacrylamide gels were prepared according to the method of Laemmli (8). Samples were boiled in gel application buffer for 5 min and electrophoresed for 15 h at 40V. Molecular weight standards (Pharmacia Fine Chemicals, Piscataway, N.J.) were run on all gels.

Western Blotting (9). Electrophoretic transfer and immunologic detection of proteins on nitrocellulose was a modification of the technique described by Towbin *et al.* (10). After two washes in deionized water, unstained SDS gels were soaked for 60 min in three changes of Tris-glycine transfer buffer. A nitrocellulose-gel "sandwich" was assembled and inserted into an electrophoretic transfer apparatus with nitrocellulose paper (Schleicher and Schuell, Keene, N.H.) closest to the positive electrode; proteins were transferred from the SDS gel to the nitrocellulose paper for 16 h at 100V. After transfer, the nitrocellulose sheet closest to the gel was washed for 1 h in at least two changes of 10 mM Tris, 0.5 M NaCl, 0.1% Brij-58 (TNB) buffer and incubated for 2 h at room temperature with hybridoma supernatant fluids diluted in TNB buffer. The nitrocellulose was washed again for 60 minutes in at least three changes of TNB buffer, incubated for 1-2 h in 20 mls of a 1:5000 to 1:10000 dilution of peroxidase conjugated rabbit mouse IgG in TNB buffer, and washed in 2 changes of TNB buffer. Peroxidase activity was detected colorimetrically by addition of chromergen solution (0.05 ml o-dianisidine [1% in methanol] and 0.02 ml hydrogen peroxide were added to 100 ml of 10 mM Tris-0.5 M NaCl). If two sheets of nitrocellulose paper were used, the sheet distal to the gel was stained for total protein with amido black stain.

Neutralization Assays. The ability of monoclonal antibodies to neutralize cholera toxin activity was assessed in a S49 lymphosarcoma assay (11). Culture supernatant fluids from each cell line were serially diluted in DMEM and 100 μl aliquots were added to microtiter plates containing either 100 pg or 25 pg/well of cholera toxin. Plates were incubated for 60 min at 37°C; 100 μl of S49 cells (6-8 $\times$ 10^5 cells/ml) were then added. Controls included wells with toxin alone, supernatant dilutions alone, and dilutions of U.S. Standard Cholera Antitoxin (Bureau of Biologics, Bethesda, M.D.). The phosphodiesterase inhibitor Ro 20-1724/1 (Hoffman-LaRoche, N.Y.) was added to a final concentration of 5 $\times$ 10^{-5}M and gentamicin (Schering, Union, N.J.) was added to 50 μ g/ml. Toxicity assays were read after 96 hours of incubation. Rabbit skin permeability factor (PF) assays (12) were performed by Dr. Jack Craig at Downstate Medical Center, Brooklyn, New York.

Determination of Hybridoma IgG concentration. Radial immune diffusion was used to determine the hybridoma IgG concentration in tissue culture supernatant fluids. Rabbit antimouse IgG was diluted 1:100-1:1000 in 1% agarose tempered to 55°C. Standard concentrations of mouse IgG and aliquots of diluted and undiluted antibody preparations were added to wells in agarose. Samples were allowed to diffuse in a humid atmosphere at room temperature for 12-24 h; plates were then dried and stained in Coomassie blue. Hybriodama IgG concentration was determined by comparing the precipitin ring size of mouse IgG standards and samples.

IgG Typing. The initial screening assay selected for IgG producing clones; typing was therefore limited to the four sub-classes of IgG (IgG_1, IgG_{2a}, IgG_{2b}, IgG_3). Typing was determined by precipitin line formation with murine IgG typing sera.

Results

Detection of HYbrid Cell Lines Producing Monoclonal Antibody to Cholera Toxin. Twenty microtiter plates were seeded with mouse myeloma-spleen cell fusion mixture. After two weeks of growth, culture supernatant fluid from each well was tested in an ELISA for production of antibody to cholera toxin. Approximately 300 (15%) of the 2000 wells tested gave positive reactions. Three days later, wells were retested for production of antibodies to cholera toxin and subunit A; although approximately 30% of the wells were lost due to fungal contamination, all surviving wells which previously reacted with cholera toxin continued to do so. In addition, 40 new wells were detected which reacted with subunit A only. Ten days later, 120 surviving wells were again tested for anti-CT and anti-A activity and about 75% remained positive. Twenty of the positive

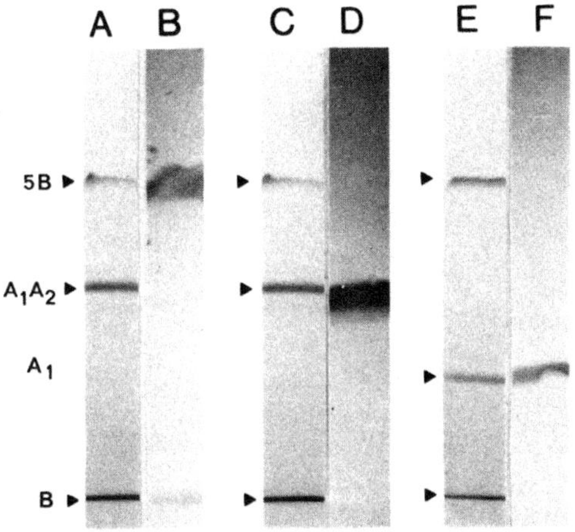

Figure 1. Western blots demonstrating cholera toxin subunit specificity of monoclonal antibodies. Lanes A, C, and E are stained SDS-polyacrylamide gel profiles. In Lanes B, D, and F gel proteins have been transferred to nitrocellulose, reacted with monoclonal antibody, and treated with peroxidase conjugated anti-mouse IgG. Lane B: treated with culture fluid of clone 9E2. Lanes D and F: treated with culture fluid of clone 14E11.

wells were cloned in soft agar; clones derived from 11 of these gave positive ELISA reactions.

Subunit Specificity of Antibody Producing Clones. Although the ELISA proved to be a useful screening technique, its utility in defining subunit specificity of clones was limited by the need for large quantities of highly purified subunits. Western blots provided a simple and specific way to clearly define subunit reactivity: subunits were cleanly separated on SDS gels; after transfer to nitrocellulose paper and reaction with hybridoma antibody, unambiguous results were obtained. This was not found to be the case with the ELISA since low levels of subunit contamination gave ambiguous results. Figure 1 demonstrates Western blots which have been exposed to anti-subunit A and anti-subunit B producing clones.

The left lane of each pair is a photograph of a Coomassie blue stained SDS gel. Lanes A and C are identical-both contain a mixture of heated and unheated cholera toxin. The three bands observed are pentameric subunit B (CT-5B), subunit A (CT-A_1A_2), and monomeric subunit B (CT-B). In lane E, the same mixture has been treated with reducing agent to produce subunit A_1(CT-A_1). The right hand column of each pair shows these same proteins which have been transferred to nitrocellulose, and treated with monoclonal antibody and peroxidase conjugated anti-mouse IgG. Using this technique, subunit specificity can clearly be assigned for each clone. For example, Clone 9E2 reacts with pentameric and monomeric subunit B. (Fig. 1, lane B). Reactions with monomeric subunit B are consistently less intense than those observed with pentameric subunit B. In lanes D and F, proteins were treated with clone 14E11 which reacts with the A_1 portion of subunit A.

Figure 2 shows the same sort of analysis with *E. coli* heat labile enterotoxin (LT) as

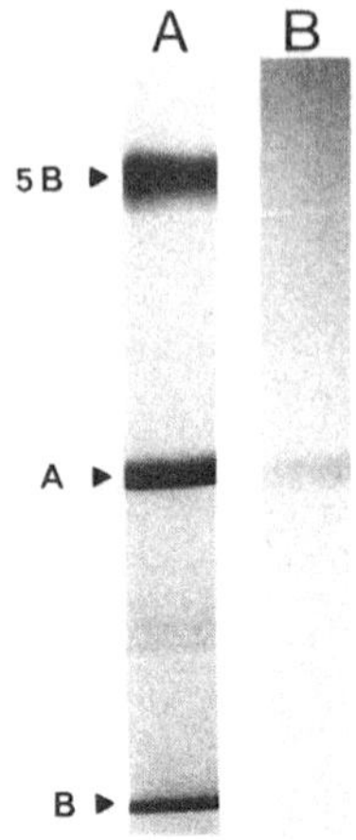

Figure 2. Determination of subunit specificity of monoclonal antibody for *E. coli* heat labile toxin by Western blot analysis. A: stained gel profile of LT. B: Western blot of LT reacted with clone 10E10.

antigen. The left hand column is again a Coomassie blue stained gel and the right hand column is a Western blot of the same polypeptides. There are three protein species present on the gel (lane A) : LT pentameric B (LT-5B), subunit A (LT-A) and monomeric subunit B (LT-B). In this case, clone 14E11 reacts only with LT-A (lane B).

Western blot data for all clones is summarized in Table 1. Five clones (6E3, 9E1, 10B6, 10E10, 14E11) react with subunit A of cholera toxin. This specificity can be further assigned to the A_1 portion of subunit A. All five clones also react with LT subunit A. Clone 14E11 consistently reacts less intensely with LT-A than CT-A. Two clones (9E2 and 9H4) react with CT-5B and CT-B, although less well with monomeric than with pentameric subunit B. Clones 9E2 and 9H4 do not react with pentameric or monomeric

Table 1. Monoclonal antibody specificity for cholera toxin and *Escherichia coli* heat labile enterotoxin subunits.

monoclonal cell line	Cholera toxin				LT		
	A1A2	A1	5B	B	A1A2	5B	B
6E3/1	++	++	–	–	++	–	–
9E1/1	++	++	–	–	++	–	–
10B6/3	+++	+++	–	–	+++	–	–
10E10/1	++	++	–	–	++	–	–
14E11/1	++	++	–	–	++	–	–
9E2/1	–	–	+++	+	–	–	–
9H4/1	–	–	+++	+	–	–	–
14F12/1	++	++	++	+	++	–	–

subunit B of LT. Since proteins are transferred to nitrocellulose after exposure to SDS, it was possible that a reactive site on LT subunit B might be more sensitive to SDS denaturation than CT-B. However, neither anti-CT-B clone reacts with LT in a non-denaturing system (data not shown). One clone (14F12) appears to react with both subunit A and subunit B of cholera toxin (Table 1 and Figure 3, lanes B and D). 14F12 is currently being recloned to determine if there are two cell lines with different specificities, or if there is a single monoclonal cell line producing antibody(s) which reacts with both subunits.

Neutralization of Toxic Activity. Monoclonal antibodies were tested for the ability to neutralize cholera toxin activity. Anti-toxic activity was measured in the S-49 tissue culture assay for cholera toxin activity and in the rabbit skin permeability factor assay. The two anti-CT-B clones (9E2 and 9H4) were clearly the best neutralizing antibodies in both assays (Table 2). Anti-subunit A clones have less antitoxic activity, consistent with data on polyclonal antibody (13); clone 10B6 demonstrated the greatest antitoxic activity in both assays and clone 10E10 demonstrated the least activity. With the exception of 14F12 (subclass IgG_{2a}), typing has shown that all clones belong to the IgG_1 subclass; this is not surprising since IgG_1 is the most frequent class of IgG in mouse sera.

Discussion

In 1975, Kohler and Milstein demonstrated that permanent cultures of antibody producing hybrid cell lines could be created by fusing mouse myeloma cells with spleen cells from immunized mice. By varying the selection process, hybrid cells can be isolated which produce monoclonal antibody to specific components of an immunoge. Using hybridoma technology, we have isolated and characterized a family of monoclonal antibody producing cell lines directed against cholera toxin. The monoclonal antibodies

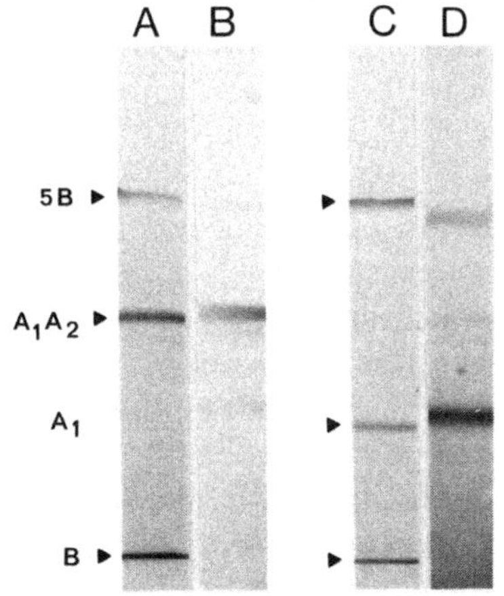

Figure 3. Cholera toxin subunit specificity of clone 14F12. A and C: stained gel profiles of CT. B&D: Western blot of 14F12.

Table 2. Antitoxin activity of monoclonal antibodies against cholera toxin.

monoclonal cell line	μg IgG/ml	S49 ASSAY Antitoxin Units*/ml	PF ASSAY Antitoxin Units*/ml	Antitoxin Units*/ng IgG
6E3/1	210	0.25	0.84	4
9E1/1	170	0.025	1.25	7
10B6/3	100	1.25	2.6	26
10E10/1	<25	0	<0.43	0
14E11/1	130	0.12	0.91	7
9E2/1	55	25	93	1860
9H4/1	235	250	160	680
14F12/1	<25	0.12	2.5	>100

*One unit neutralized 40 ng of cholera toxin.

isolated fall into two major subclasses: those which react with determinants on subunit B of cholera toxin and those which react with antigenic determinants on subunit A. Hybridoma antibody directed against the B subunit is effective in neutralization of cholera toxin activity in an *in vitro* and *in vivo* assay for cholera toxin biological activity. In contrast, monoclonal antibodies directed against the A subunit are weakly neutralizing or ineffective in neutralizing toxic activity.

One clone, 14F12, appears to produce antibody which reacts with both the A and B subunits of cholera toxin. This could be the result of cross reactivity between the two subunits, or it is possible that one cell line produces antibody with two specificities (14).

The *E. coli* heat labile enterotoxin, LT, is structurally and functionally very similar to cholera toxin (15, 16, 17); immunological cross reactivity has been demonstrated (18). Monoclonal antibodies directed against the B subunit of cholera toxin do not react with the B subunit of LT; however, all monoclonal antibodies which react with the A subunit of cholera toxin also react with the A subunit of LT.

Isolation of monoclonal antibodies to subunit A as our predominant class clearly demonstrates some advantages of this technique for producing antibodies. Subunit A is a notoriously poor immunogen and is difficult to purify free from subunit B contamination. Since hybridoma technology precludes the need for purified antigen, it is now possible to obtain anti-subunit A sera with relative ease.

We anticipate that monoclonal antibodies directed against cholera toxin will prove to be useful functional probes. A set of antibodies directed against various antigenic sites on the cholera toxin molecule should allow us to map those domains on the cholera toxin polypeptide which are involved in binding, enzymic activity, and those which function as major immunogenic sites. In addition, we should be able to identify those functional sites which may differ between cholera toxin and *E. coli* heat labile toxin.

REFERENCES

1. Nichols, J. C., P. C. Tai, and J. R. Murphy. 1980. Cholera toxin is synthesized in precursor form on free polysomes in *Vibrio cholerae* 569B. J. Bacteriol. **144**:518.
2. Kohler, G., and C. Milstein. 1975. Continuous cultures of fused cells secreting antibody of predetermined specificity. Nature (London). **256**:495.
3. Kohler, G., and C. Milstein. 1976. Derivation of specfic antibody-producing tissue culture and tumor lines by cell fusion. Eur. J. Immunol. **6**:511.
4. Mekalanos, J. J., R. J. Collier, and W. R. Romig. 1978. Purification of cholera toxin and its subunits: New methods of preparation and the use of hypertoxinogenic mutants. Infect. Immun. **20**: 552.
5. Miller, J. H. 1974. Experiments in Molecular Genetics. Cold Spring Harbor Press. Cold Spring Harbor, N. Y. p. 431.
6. Nowinski, R. C., M. E. Lostrom, M. R. Tam, M. R. Stone, and W. N. Burnette. 1979. The isolation of hybrid cell lines producing monoclonal antibodies against the p 15(E) protein of ecotopic murine leukemia viruses. Virol. **111**:126.
7. Cotton, R. G. H., D. S. Secher, and C. Milstein. 1973. Somatic mutation and the origin of antibody diversity. Clonal variability of the immunoglobulin produced by MOPC 21 cells. Eur. J. Immunol. **3**:135.
8. Laemmli, U. K. 1970. Cleavage of structural proteins during assembly of the head of bacteriophage T4. Nature (London). **227**:680.
9. Burnette, W. N. 1981. "Western Blotting": Electrophoretic transfer of proteins from sodium dodecyl sulfate-polyacrylamide gels to unmodified nitrocellulose and radio-graphic detection with antibody and radioiodinated Protein A. Anal. Biochem. **112**:195.
10. Towbin, H., T. Staehelin, and J. Gordon. 1979. Electrophoretic transfer of proteins from polyacrylamide gels to nitrocellulose sheets: procedure and some applications. Proc. Natl. Acad. Sci. USA **76**:4350.
11. Ruch, F. E., J. R. Murphy, L. H. Graf, and M. Field. 1978. Isolation of nontoxinogenic mutants of *Vibrio cholerae* in a colorimetric assay for cholera toxin using the S49 mouse lymphosarcoma cell line. J. Inf. Dis. **137**:747.
12. Craig. J. P. 1966. Preparation of vascular permeability factor of *Vibrio cholerae*. J. Bact. **92**:793.
13. Ohtomo, N., T. Muraoka, and K. Kudo. 1978. Consideration to the role of anti-cholera toxin subunit A, anti-SA, in cholera. Proceedings of the 14th Joint U.S.-Japan Conference on Cholera. p. 108.
14. Kubota, E., H. I. Ishikawa, and K. Saito. 1981. Evidence for a cloned hybridoma (HO-13-4-9) producing 2 kinds of antibody molecules different in specificity, one directed to THY 1.2 gene products and the other to antigen on a subpopulation of THY 1.1 thymocytes. J. Immunol. **127**: 1498.
15. Clements, J. D., and R. A. Finkelstein. 1979. Isolation and characterization of homogeneous heat-labile enterotoxins with high specific activity from *Escherichia coli* cultures. Infect. Immun. **24**:760.
16. Dallas, W. S., and S. Falkow. 1980. Amino acid sequence homology between cholera toxin and *Escherichia coli* heat-labile toxin. Nature (London). **288**:499.
17. Gill, D. M., and S. H. Richardson. 1980. Adenosine diphosphate-ribosylation of adneylate cyclase catalysed by heat-labile enterotoxin of *Escherichia coli* comparison with cholera toxin. J. Inf. Dis. **141**:64.
18. Clements, J. D., and R. A. Finkelstein. 1978. Immunological cross-reactivity between a heat-labile enterotoxin(s) of *Escherichia coli* and subunits of *Vibrio cholerae* enterotoxin. Infect. Immun. **21**:1036.

CLINICAL STUDIES

Advances in Research on Cholera and Related Diarrheas, eds., S. Kuwahara, N. F. Pierce, 147–149.

EFFICACY OF BICOZAMYCIN IN TREATMENT OF ACUTE DIARRHEA CAUSED BY ENTEROTOXIGENIC *ESCHERICHIA COLI*

Charles D. Ericsson, Herbert L. DuPont, Peggy Sullivan, Emma Galindo, Dolores G. Evans, Jean Hinlicky, Jorge Olarte, Doyle J. Evans Jr.

University of Texas Medical School at Houston, Texas and
Hospital Infantil de Mexico, Mexico, D.F.

Bicozamycin is a new antibiotic first reported by Miyoshi, *et al.*, in 1972.[1] Bicozamycin is poorly absorbed from the gastrointestinal tract. Its spectrum of activity includes many enteropathogens including *Escherichia coli* in which bicozamycin appears to interfer with biosynthesis of lipoprotein and its incorporation into peptidoglycan in the cell wall.[2] Bicozamycin has no apparent activity against gram-positive, anaerobic organisms, Proteus or Pseudomonas. Finally, plasmid-mediated resistance has been looked for, but only chromosomal resistance to bicozamycin has so far been demonstrated. In view of these features of bicozamycin, a prospective, randomized, double-blind, placebo controlled study of bicozamycin in the empiric treatment of acute diarrhea in a population of U.S. adults newly arrived in Guadalajara, Mexico, was conducted.

All subjects had acute diarrhea of less than 48 hours duration. Diarrhea was defined as passage of ≥4 unformed stool/24 hours plus ≥1 associated symptom of enteric disease like cramps, nausea, vomiting or temperature elevation. Subjects submitted an unformed stool sample prior to enrollment and this stool was cultured for Salmonella and Shigella, and 5 representative *E. coli* colonies were picked, placed on stabs and transported to Houston for assay for enterotoxin production. LT-toxin was assessed using a standard Y-1 adrenal cell assay. ST-toxin was assessed using a standard suckling mouse assay.

Subjects were treated with bicozamycin (500 mg orally four times a day) or placebo for 3 days. All subjects were treated as outpatients and took fluids ad lib.

Of the 140 subjects whose experience could be analyzed the number of patients with enterotoxigenic *E. coli* is listed in Table 1.

Table 1. Number of patients with Enterotoxigenic *E. coli* Disease.

ETEC Category	Bicozamycin Group (n=72)	Placebo Group (n=68)
ST/LT	18	12
ST-only	9	3
LT-only	4	3

There were no significant differences in pretreatment severity of diarrhea between the bicozamycin and placebo groups in either of the ETEC subgroups. Efficacy of bicozamycin was assessed by analyzing time to last unformed stool, mean number of stools per 24 hours, degree of cramps and degree of overall illness. Also, some subjects had illness which worsened within or persisted beyond the 5-day period of observation and these subjects were analyzed as "treatment failures". Unless stated otherwise data were analyzed by the Wilcoxon Rank Sum Test. The following Tables show the results of these analyses.

Table 2. Comparison of number of subjects who continue to pass unformed stools after 1 day of therapy with bicozamycin or placebo.

	Bicozamycin	Placebo	Significance
ALL ETEC	14/31 (45%)	14/18 (78%)	P = 0.05 (Chi-square test)

Table 3. Comparison of total treatment failures occurring in the bicozamycin and placebo groups.

	Bicozamycin	Placebo	Significance
ALL ETEC	2/31 (6%)	6/18 (33%)	P = 0.02 (Fisher exact test)

Table 4. Comparison of number of subjects who continue to pass unformed stools in ETEC subgroups by day of study when significant differences first occur.

Etiology	Day of Treatment	Bicozamycin	Placebo	Significance
ST/LT	2	2/18(11%)	8/12(67%)	p=0.003
ST-only	3	0/9(0%)	2/3(67%)	p=0.05
LT-only	-	-	-	N.S.

Table 5. Comparison of mean number of stools/24 hours in ETEC subgroups by day of study when significant differences first occur.

Etiology	Day of Treatment	Bicozamycin	Placebo	Significance
ST/LT	1	3.1	6.3	p=0.03
ST-only	2	1.6	5.0	p=0.05
LT-only	-	-	-	N.S.

Table 6. Comparison of mean index for cramps in ETEC subgroups by day of study when significant differences first occur, where mild (tolerable)=1, moderate (distressing) = 2 and severe (incapacitating) = 3.

Etiology	Day of Treatment	Bicozamycin	Placebo	Significance
ST/LT	2	0.6	1.4	p=0.01
ST-only	3	0.0	1.3	p=0.01
LT-only	-	-	-	N.S.

Table 7. Comparison of mean index for overall diarrheal illness in ETEC subgroups by day of study when significant differences first occur. Cramps, nausea or vomiting are ranked 1, 2 or 3 as in Table 6. Diarrhea is ranked 1, 2, 3, 4 or 5 for 2-3, 4-5, 6-7, 8-9 or ⩾10 uniformed stools/24 hours, respectively.

Etiology	Day of Treatment	Bicozamycin	Placebo	Significance
ST/LT	2	1.2	3.2	p=0.01
ST-only	2	0.9	3.7	p=0.01
LT-only	-	-	-	N.S.

Table 8. Comparison of duration of diarrhea (mean hours) in ETEC subgroups.

Etiology	Bicozamycin	Placebo	Significance
ST/LT	30	70	p=0.03
ST-only	25	92	p=0.05
LT-only	-	-	N.S.

These data show that bicozamycin was effective therapy for ST/LT and ST-only disease. Therapy with bicozamycin significantly shortened the course of diarrhea and relieved cramps compared to placebo. Since enterotoxigenic *E. coli* account for a large proportion of diarrhea in travelers to developing countries, these data may form the cornerstone of an empiric approach to therapy of travelers' diarrhea. Particularly for longer term travelers and until effective immunologic interventions become available, this empiric approach may be more reasonable than use of currently available agents like prophylactic antibiotics or bismuth subsalicylate.

REFERENCES

1. Miyoshi T., Miyairi N., Aoko H., *et al.*: Bicyclomycin, a new antibiotic. The J. Antib. **25**:569-575, 1972.
2. Tanaka, N.: Mechanism of action of bicozamycin. The J. Antib. **29**:155-168, 1976.

Advances in Research on Cholera and Related Diarrheas, eds., S. Kuwahara, N. F. Pierce, 151–157.

ENDOSCOPY OF THE SMALL INTESTINE IN ETEC AND NAG VIBRIO DIARRHEA

Tetsuo Morishita, Rafiqul Islam, Pradip K. Bardhan, Yoshio Munakata, Toshifumi Hibi, Hitoshi Asakura, and Masaharu Tsuchiya

Department of Internal Medicine, School of Medicine, Keio University, Tokyo, International Centre for Diarrhoeal Disease Research, Bangladesh, Dacca

The authors have already reported the endoscopic[1], microscopic[2] and electron microscopic findings[3] of the small intestine in human cholera. In order to investigate the diarrheal mechanism further, endoscopy and simultaneous biopsy of the small intestine were done in patients with enterotoxicogenic Escherichia coli (ETEC) or Non-O Group 1 Vibrio cholerae or Nonagglutinating (NAG) vibrio diarrhea.

Subjects and Methods

The endoscopy was performed in 4 patients with ETEC, 6 patients with NAG vibrio diarrhea who were admitted to the International Centre for Diarrhoeal Disease Research, Bangladesh (ICDDR,B), former Cholera Research Laboratory, during 1980, and in 9 control subjects.

The clinical findings and laboratory data pertaining to the patients are summarized in Table 1. Clinical diagnosis was confirmed bacteriologically in each case. All strains

Table 1. Clinical and laboratory data in 10 patients with ETEC or NAG vibrio diarrhea.

Patients	No	Age	Sex	Stool(L/24h)	Dehydration	Hct	Toxin
ETEC	1	22	M	3.82 liquid	+~++	35	ST·LT
	2	23	M	3.42 watery	+~++	39	ST·LT
	3	23	M	2.27 watery	++	45	ST·LT
	4	26	M	0.10 watery	++	42	ST·LT
NAG	1	30	M	3.00 watery	++	43	
	2	28	M	0.99 loose	+	37	
	3	20	M	1.61 watery	++	44	
	4	23	M	2.37 watery	++	46	
	5	43	M	0.85 loose	+	43	
	6	20	M		+	39	

from the ETEC patients yielded both heat stable (ST) and heat labile toxins (LT). The endoscopes used were a small intestinal fiberscope, Olympus SIF type B[1] and a magnifying endoscope, Olympus GIF-HM[4]. The mucosa of the gastrointestinal tract was observed endoscopically to points 10 to 20 cm beyond the ligament of Treitz in the jejunum (Figure 1).

Endoscopy was performed in the patients within 24 hours of admission, and control subjects fasted overnight. Mucosal biopsy was done simultaneously under direct vision.

Results

In the control subjects, peristaltic movement ceased after 40 mg of butylscopolamine bromide was injected intramuscularly. The smooth mucosal surface of the small intestine was unblemished by reddening, erosion or ulceration.

In contrast, the small intestinal mucosa in the ETEC or NAG vibrio diarrhea patients was edematous. Hyperperistalsis was seen in all ETEC and NAG vibrio diarrhea cases (100%) despite the intramuscular injection of 40 to 80 mg of butylscopolamine bromide (Figure 2). Prominent hypersecretion was also seen in all cases (100%) (Figure 3). In some patients secreted fluid was in bubbles or foams. Mucosal reddening, spotted or zonal, was noted in all cases (100%) (Figure 4). Changes of erosion were observed in 2 cases with ETEC (50%) and 2 cases with NAG vibrio diarrhea (33%) (Figure 5). The biopsy specimen from the erosion revealed staining abnormality, capillary congestion, mononuclear cell infiltration in the lamina propria, loss of definition of brush border. And desquamation of epithelial cells with fibrin deposition was observed (Figure 6). The endoscopic findings are summarized in Table 2.

A comparison between the endoscopic findings and clinical data of the patients was

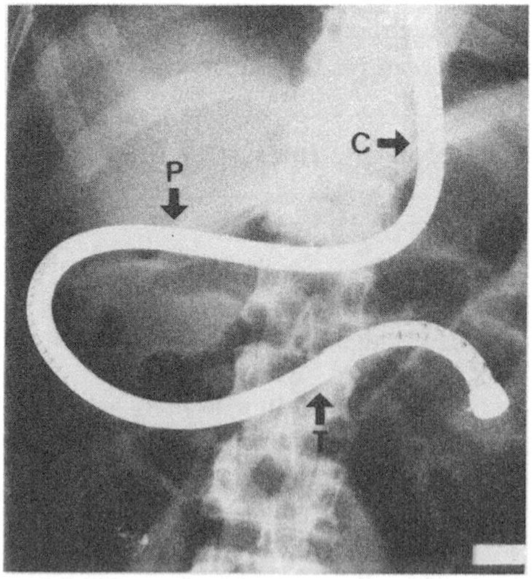

Fig. 1. Small intestinal endoscope inserted through the duodenum into the jejunum (C-cardia, P-pylorus, T-ligament of Treitz).

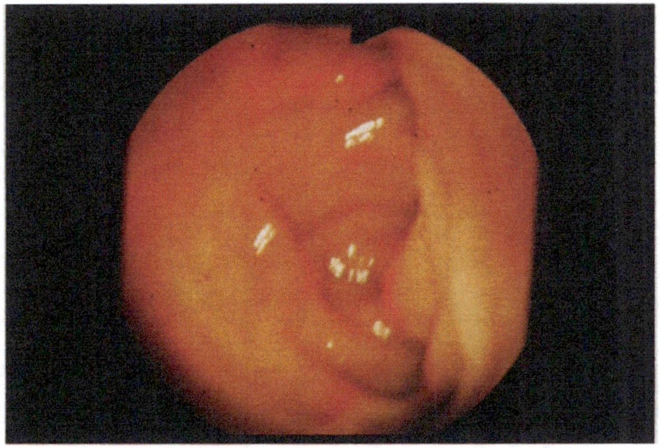

Fig. 2. Hyperperistalsis of the small intestinal tract. Reddened spots are also seen. (NAG vibrio diarrhea case)

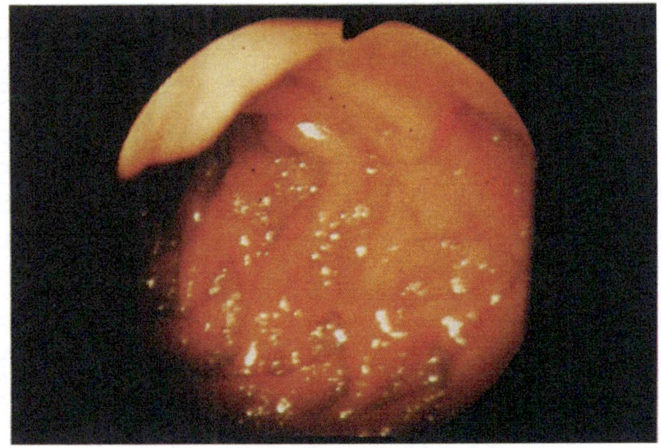

Fig. 3. Prominent hypersecretion. (ETEC diarrhea case)

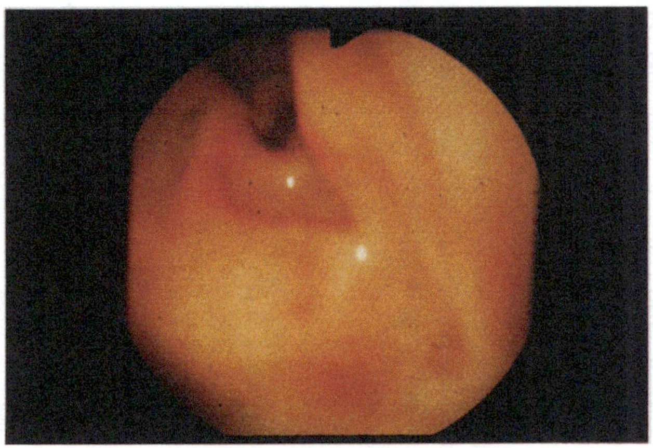

Fig. 4. Spotted or zonal reddening of the mucosa. (NAG vibrio diarrhea case)

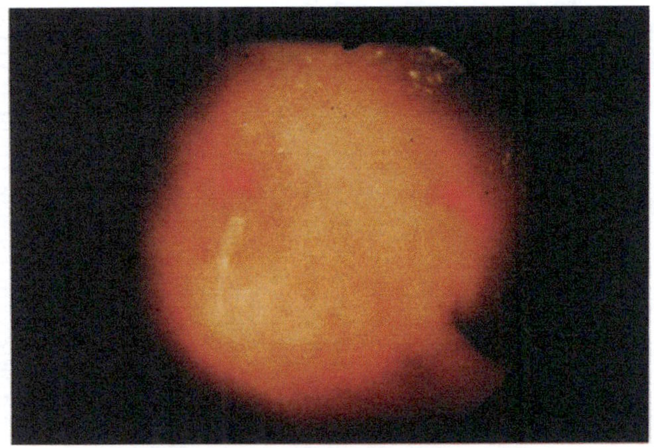

Fig. 5. Mucosal erosions. (NAG vibrio diarrhea case)

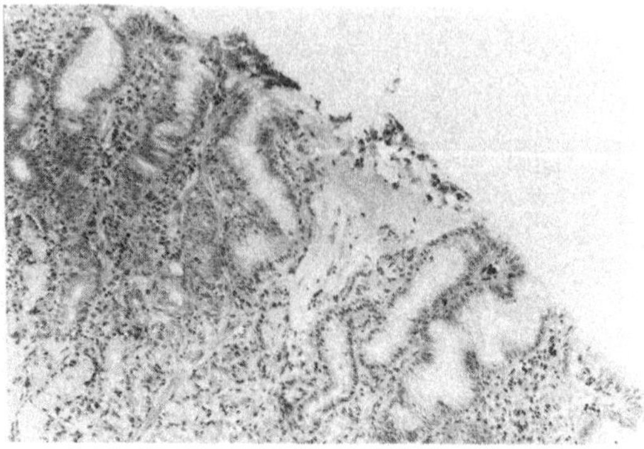

Fig. 6. Biopsy specimen from the erosive lesion. Staining abnormality, capillary congestion, mononuclear cell infiltration in the lamina propria, loss of definition of brush border, desquamation of epithelial cells with fibrin deposition are seen (HE x200).

made. Hematocrit ratio is a quotient of the hematocrit on admission divided by the one on discharge. A higher hematocrit ratio means a severer grade of diarrhea and dehydrated condition in the patient. In the ETEC diarrhea cases, there was a tendency that the more prominent mucosal edema or hyperperistalsis the higher hematocri ratio. Concerning the mucosal erosion, a significant difference of the hematocrit ratio could be seen between the patients with erosion (1.49±0.11) and those without erosion (1.18±0.04) ($P<0.05$) (Table 3). In NAG vibrio diarrhea cases, patients with mucosal edema or hypersecretion showed a greater stool volume in 24 hours after admission. A significant difference in the hematocrit ratio could be found between the group with erosion (1.37±0.06) and that without erosion (1.08±0.12) ($P<0.05$) (Table 4).

Discussion

Since the denudation concept of the intestinal lesion in asiatic cholera by Virchow [5] in 1879, there have been controversies as to whether there are pathological changes of the small intestinal mucosa in human cholera. The denudation concept was denied by Gangarosa and Fresh[6], who did the intestinal biopsies using a biopsy instrument of Crosby, which were blind biopsies.

Table 2. Endoscopic features of the small intestinal mucosa in 10 patients with ETEC or NAG vibrio diarrhea.

Patients / Features	ETEC				NAG					
	1	2	3	4	1	2	3	4	5	6
Erosions	–	–	+	+	–	–	+	+	–	–
Reddening	++	+	+	++	++	+	++	+	++	+
Edema	++	+	++	+	++	+	++	++	+	+
Reticular pattern	±	±	±	±	±	±	±	±	±	±
Hypersecretion	++	+	++	+	++	+	++	++	+	++
Hyperperistalsis	++	+	++	++	+	++	++	++	+	+

Table 3. Relationship between endoscopic features and clinical data in 4 patients with ETEC diarrhea.

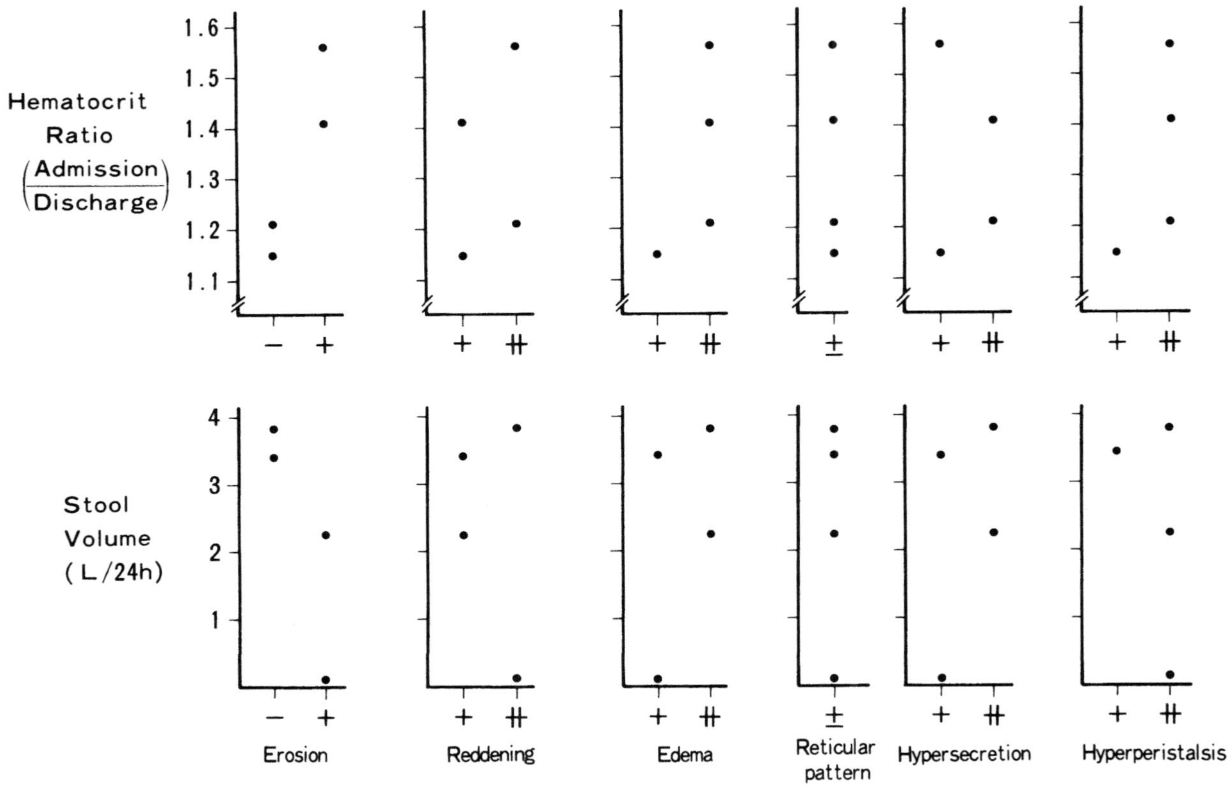

Table 4. Relationship between endoscopic features and clinical data in 6 patients with NAG vibrio diarrhea.

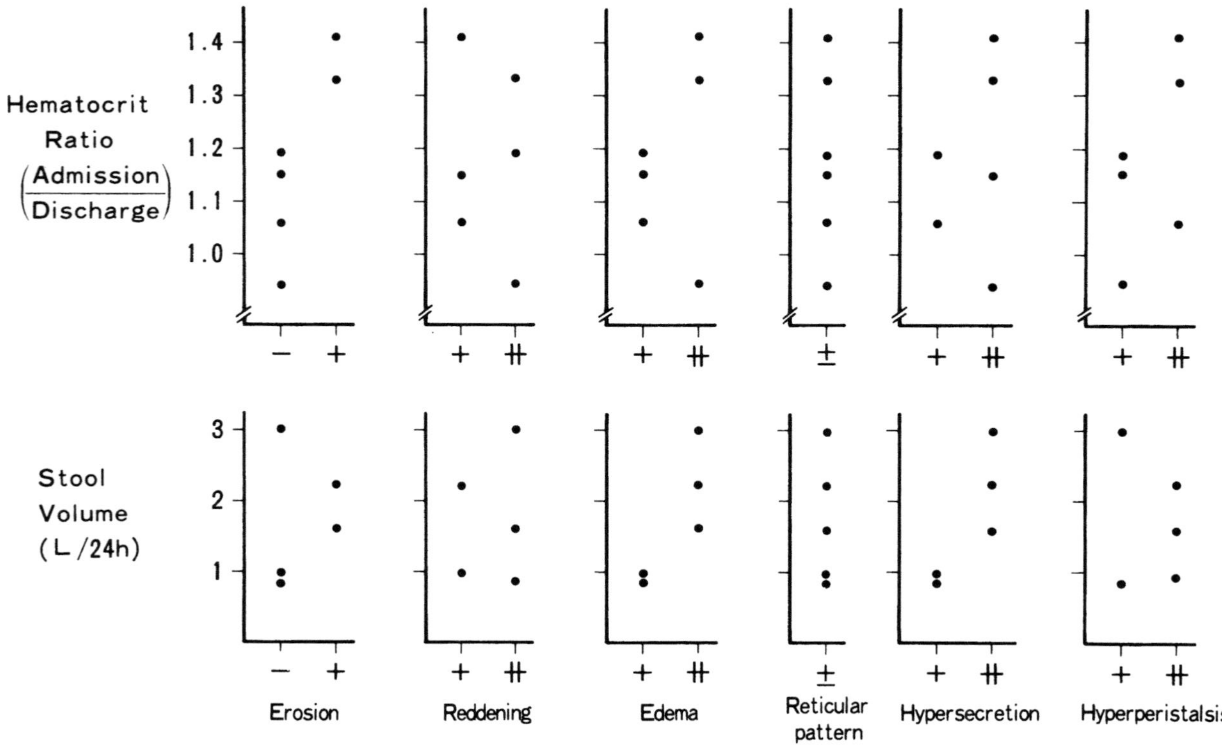

However, the endoscopic study performed by us revealed the mucosal erosions, multiple patchy and scattered, in the jejunum of cholera patients[1].

This study showed the mucosal erosions of the small intestine in 2 cases with ETEC (50%) and 2 cases with NAG vibrio diarrhea (33%). Mucosal reddening, edema, hypersecretion and hyperperistalsis were seen in all cases (100%).

The patients with erosions showed the significantly higher hematocrit ratio ($P<0.05$), that is, they had suffered from the severer diarrhea and dehydration.

There seem to be a few possibilities concerning the significance of mucosal erosions.

Some strains of ETEC and NAG vibrio may cause erosions and be biologically similar to Vibrio cholera as regards the formation of erosions.

In turn it is possible that erosions may not be the result of infection but a factor which facilitate the susceptibility to infections, accelerating the colonization and growth of bacteria in the intestinal tract. The change of erosions may boost the fluid loss caused by ETEC and NAG vibrio infection.

Haglund *et al.*[7] reported denuded villi and ulceration of the lamina propria of the small intestine of 4 patients in shock and in 3 patients with local intestinal hypotension. The similar mucosal changes in ETEC and NAG vibrio diarrhea might be due to hypovolemia.

What roles the pathologic changes including erosions may play in disturbed fluid transport and in ETEC and NAG vibrio infection remains to be elucidated.

REFERENCES

1) Morishita, T., Hibi, T., Asakura, H., Tsuchiya, M., Pescante, M. and Uylangco, C.: Endoscopy of the jejunal mucosa in human cholera. Gastrointestinal Endoscopy, **24**:284-285, 1978.
2) Asakura, H., Morita, A., Morishita, T., Tsuchiya, M., Fukumi, H., Ohashi, M., Uylangco, C. and Castro, A.: Pathological findings from intestinal biopsy specimens in human cholera. Am J Dig Dis, **18**:271-278, 1973.
3) Asakura, H., Tsuchiya, M., Watanabe, Y., Enomoto, Y., Morita, A., Morishita, T., Fukumi, H., Ohashi, M. and Castro, A.: Electron microscopic study on the jejucal mucosa in human cholera. Gut, **15**:531-544, 1974.
4) Morishita, T., Asakura, H., Miura, S., Kamiya, T. and Tsuchiya, M.: Magnifying endoscopic findings of the duodenum in a case of intestinal lymphangiectasia. Gastroenterological Endoscopy, **23**:133-141, 1981.
5) Virchow, R.: Gesammelte Abhandlungen auf dem Gebiete der öffentlichen Medizin: **1**:151-184, Hirschwald; Berlin, 1879.
6) Gangarosa, E. J., Beiser, W. R., Benyajati, C., Sprinz, H. and Piyaratn, P.: The nature of the gastrointestinal lesion in Asiatic cholera and its relation to pathogenesis: A biopsy study. Amer J Trop Med, **9**:125-135, 1960.
7) Haglund, U., Hultén, L., Åhren, C., Lundgren, O.: Mucosal lesions in the human small intestine in shock. Gut, **16**:979-984, 1975.

Advances in Research on Cholera and Related Diarrheas, eds., S. Kuwahara, N. F. Pierce, 159–167.

HISTOLOGIC AND BACTERIOLOGIC FINDINGS IN INFANTS WITH ENTEROPATHOGENIC *E. COLI* INFECTION

Robert J. Rothbaum, A. James McAdams, Ralph A. Giannella,
D.B. Shah, Pamela Smith, and John C. Partin

Children's Hospital Research Foundation and
University of Cincinnati College of Medicine, Cincinnati, Ohio

Escherichia coli infection causes diarrhea by a variety of mechanisms. These include elaboration of heat-labile or heat stable enterotoxins or cytopathic toxin and invasion of the intestinal mucosa. Enteropathogenic strains have been implicated as the cause of diarrhea outbreaks in infants but the nature and pathogenesis of EPEC diarrhea have remained obscure. In this report, we describe studies of infants evaluated between October, 1979 and March, 1981 who presented with protracted diarrhea apparently due to an enterocyte adherent strain of the classical enteropathogenic *E. coli* 0119:B14.

Patient Population

These fifteen infants presented with a syndrome of watery diarrhea and poor growth and were evaluated at Children's Hospital Medical Center, Cincinnati, Ohio. With discontinuation of oral feedings, watery green stools persisted with volumes often reaching 100 gm/Kg/day. Multiple attempts at enteral feedings were unsuccessful because of worsening of diarrhea and continued weight loss.

Methods

Routine clinical investigation included blood studies for assessment of hematologic, renal and hepatic function, measurement of serum albumin and immunoglobulins, sweat chloride determination and urine culture. At least three stool cultures from each infant were examined for Salmonella, Shigella, Yersinia and campylobacter using Standard American Society of Microbiology techniques (1). Three to five colonies of *E. coli* were randomly selected to be serotyped using commercially available polyvalent and specific 0119:B14 typing sera (Difco Labs) (2). Stools were also examined directly for ova and parasites and for rotavirus by ELISA.

After obtaining informed consent, peroral small intestinal biopsy was performed with the 1.8 mm twin port Crosby-Kugler capsule passed to the proximal jejunum. Five patients had rectal mucosal biopsy performed with a 1.8 mm portsize Quinton multipurpose suction biopsy instrument. Biopsy specimens were proccessed for light and electron microscopy (3). In all patients, jejunal fluid was analyzed for tryptic activity and lipase (4,5) and cultured by pour plate in trypticase-soy agar at 37°C and on sheep's blood agar with and without kanamycin and vancomycin at 37°C in 10% CO_2, 5% hydrogen and 85% nitrogen and in pre-reduced thioglycolate broth. All isolates were speciated and *E. coli* were serotyped in 0119:B14 antisera (1).

Trypticase-soy broth cultures of *E. coli* 0119:B14 isolates were negatively stained with 1% phosphotungstinic acid and examined with a Phillips 400 transmission electron microscope. Hemagglutination testing of isolates was performed in guinea pig, bovine and Human Type A erthyrocyte by the method of Evans *et al.* (6). Heat-labile enterotoxin was sought from 15 jejunal and 22 stool isolates (7) heat-stable enterotoxin from 14 jejunal and 6 stool isolates (8), and cytopathic toxin from 16 isolates (9). In addition, whole trypticase soy broth cultures of 8 jejunal isolates were examined for fluid secretion in the 18 hour ligated rabbit ileal loop model (10).

Results

These fifteen infants ranged from 3 weeks to seven months of age. There were 6 males, nine females. All lived within a 25 mile radius of Cincinnati. Most (10/15) had gained weight poorly prior to this admission; nine had been hospitalized previously, 5 at Children's Hospital Medical Center, usually with short-lived diarrheal illness. At the time of isolation of *E. coli* 0119:B14, all infants had profuse diarrhea with dehydration and metabolic acidosis necessitating intravenous rehydration. Six infants appeared sufficiently ill to suspect septicemia and begin parenteral ampicillin and gentamicin. No patient had, however, documented bacteremia.

Laboratory evaluation revealed anemia in eight and hypoalbuminemia in nine of the 15 infants. Five patients had mildly and transiently elevated transaminases. No patient had pancreatic insufficiency, elevated sweat chloride concentration or significant immunoglobulin deficiency. Salmonella, Shigella, Yersinia, or Campylobacter were not isolated from any patient. Three infants had rotavirus, one grew cytomegalovirus from stool and jejunal fluid.

Because enteral feedings led to worsening of diarrhea and continued fluid and electroyte depletion, all infants required central venous alimentation through the infant Broviac catheter for nutritional support. Each received 100-110 cal/Kg/day as 20% dextrose and 10% or 20% Intralipid with 1.5-2.0 gm/Kg/day of protein as Aminosyn R. The average duration of total parenteral nutrition was 32 days (range 9-111 days).

Culture Results:

Multiple stool samples from all patients grew *E. coli* 0119:B14. Jejunal fluid from all fifteen also yielded the identical *E. coli* serotype at concentrations exceeding 50,000 CFU/ml (Table 1). Although small numbers of other enterobactereacae were present in 3 patients and anaerobes in one patient, *E. coli* 0119:B14 was the only organism recovered from the jejunum of 11 patients and the predominant organism in the other four.

Jejunal and Rectal Morphology

To elucidate the etiology of this severe diarrhea, all patients underwent jejunal and/or rectal biopsy. Table 1 details the timing of biopsies and histological findings. Hematoxylin and eosin-stained light microscopic sections of jejunum revealed moderate to severe atropy of villi, generally associated with a reduction in the total thickness of the mucosa. Commonly, there was atrophy of the surface epithelium with a disordered arrangement of enterocytes. Adherent bacteria often lined the luminal surface. The crypt epithelium usually demonstrated a distinctive subnuclear vacuolization. The lamina propria was populated by increased numbers of lymphocytes, plasma cells and eosinophils but there was never evidence of an acute enteritis. Paneth cells were often increased. Lipid stains (Sudan black, Nile blue, Sudan IV, Oil red 0) of sections snap-frozen in liquid nitrogen revealed no increase in mucosal lipid content.

Table 1. Time of biopsy, culture results and light microscopic findings in 15 patients

Pt. No.	Time to Biopsy From Admission (wk)	Jejunal Fluid Culture	Jejunal Biopsy	Rectal Biopsy
1	5	E. coli[a]	Moderate shortening of villi	
	7	None	Normal villi	
2	2-1/2			Mild inflammation
	4	E. coli	Severe shortening of villi	
3	2	E. coli, few Klebsiella[b]	Absence of villi	
4	1-1/2	E. coli	Severe shortening of villi	
	3-1/2	Staph. epidermidis, cytomegalovirus	height of villi	
5	2-1/2	E. coli, few Enterobacter	Severe shortening of villi	
6	3	E. coli	Severe shortening of villi	
7	1	Few E. coli[c]	Mild jejunitis	
	3			Atrophic epithelium
	4	E. coli	Absence of villi	
	5			Normal mucosa
8	2	E. coli, few Klebsiella	Moderate shortening of villi	Acute proctitis
9	2-1/2	E. coli, Viellonella alcalescens	Severe shortening of villi	Atrophic epithelium
10	2	E. coli, few Staph. aureus	Moderate shortening of villi	
11	1/2	E. coli	Moderate shortening of villi	
12	1	E. coli	Severe shortening of villi	
	3-1/2	Few E. coli[c], few Klebsiella	Mild jejunitis	
13	1	E. coli	Moderate shortening of villi	
14	1-1/2	E. coli	Severe shortening of villi	
	4	Few E. coli[c]	N.D.	
15	1-1/2	E. coli	N.D.	Atrophic epithelium
	6	N.D.	N.D.	Normal mucosa

[a] E. coli = ≥ 50,000 CFU/cc of E. coli 0119:B14. [b] "few" = ≤ 10^3 CFU/cc. [c] "few" E. coli ≤ 10^3 CFU/cc, not E. coli 0119:B14.

Light microscopic examination of thick sections (1–2μ) of plastic-embedded jejunum demonstrated adherent clusters of bacteria in all 15 patients. Microcolonies dotted the mucosal surface along the tips and sides of shortened villi (Figure 1). In electron microscopic examination of thin sections (40–60A), enterocytes had stubby microvilli that were decreased in number and possessed a sparse glycocalyx. In areas of bacterial adherence, there was dissolution of the glycocalyx and flattening or loss of microvilli (Figures 2 and 3). The actin filamentous backbone of microvilli and part of the terminal web had disappeared. At actual points of contact, the plasma membrane of the enterocytes was cupped along the adherent bacterium. Bacteria were never found within the substance of enterocytes or in the lamina propria. Intracellular organelles appeared relatively normal except in cells heavily coated with bacteria. Damaged enterocytes had numerous large lysosomes and distended smooth endoplasmic reticulum near the luminal surface. Often, mitochondria were severly deformed in watery, swollen cytoplasm. Some bacteria-laden cells sloughed into the lumen. Bacteria did not adhere to the microvilli of crypt cells nor to the surfaces of goblet, Paneth or argentaffin cells. The granules of Paneth cells were large with irregular contours and dense inclusions. In the lamina pro-

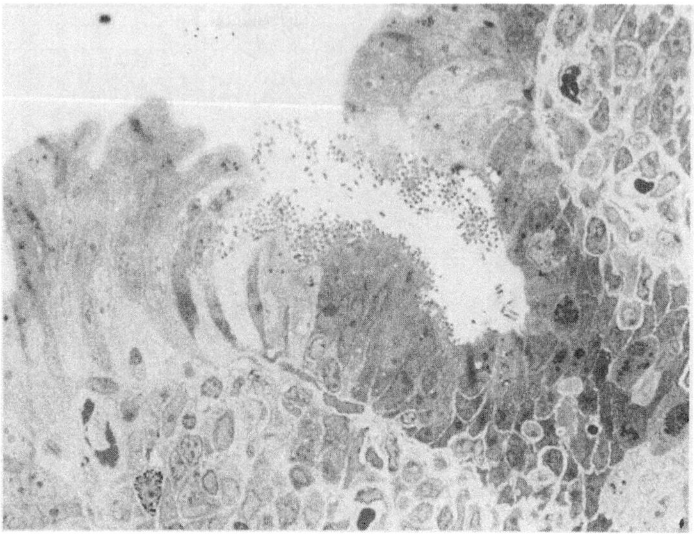

Figure 1: Thick Epon section shows myriad bacilli adherent to the surface epithelium. The microvillus border disappears in the area of bacterial attachment. (x 920)

pria, plasma cells possessed very distended rough endoplasmic reticulum.

Rectal mucosal biopsy revealed histological changes that were remarkably similar to those of the jejunum: The surface epithelium was atrophic and disorganized; the glandular epithelium showed subnuclear vacuolization. The lamina propria was edematous with a moderate lymphocyte and plasma cell infiltration. Also, as in the jejunum, electron microscopic examination revealed obliteration of microvilli at the areas of bacterial adherence with cupping of the enterocyte plasma membrane along the adherent organisms.

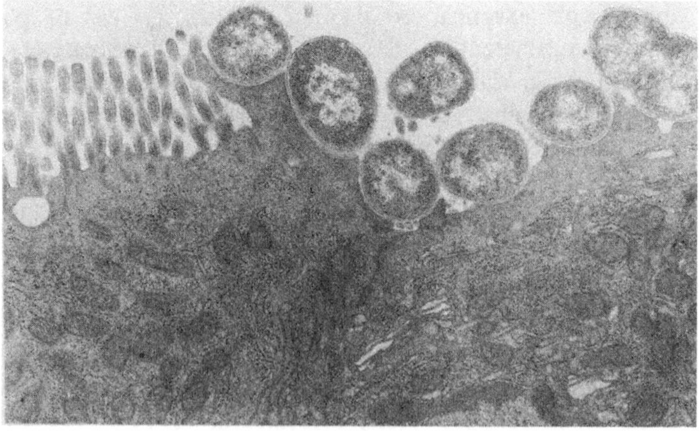

Figure 2: A bacterial microcolony adheres to neighboring enterocytes, obliterating glycocalyx and microvilli. The remaining microvilli and intracellular organelles appear relatively undisturbed. (x 25,000)

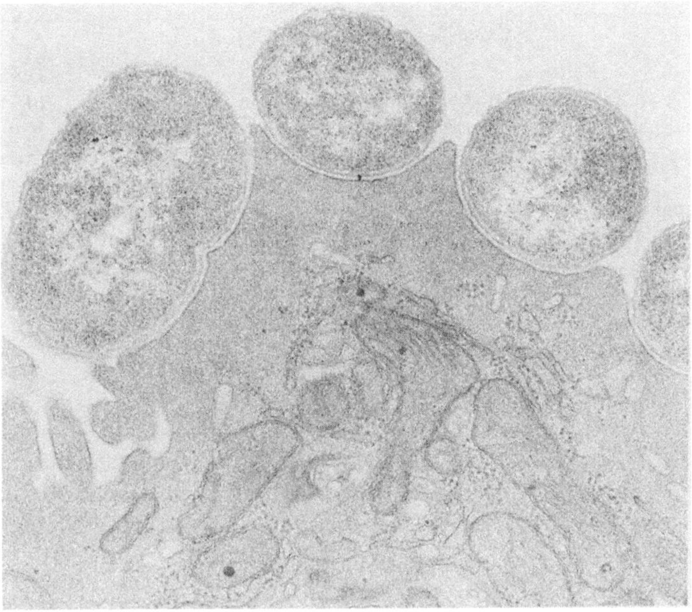

Figure 3: At areas of bacterial contact, the simplified enterocyte plasma membrane remains intact and cups the adherent organisms. The actin filaments of microvilli and cellular terminal web have disappeared. (x 55,000).

Hospital Course and Treatment

With documentation of *E. coli* 0119:B14 jejunal overgrowth, neomycin at a dose of 100 mg/Kg/day was administered orally for 5-7 days. Within three to five days of starting neomycin, *E. coli* 0119:B14 and most other aerobic flora disappeared from stool cultures. Repeat quantitative jejunal bacteriology was performed in patients 1,4,12 and 14 after 14 to 18 days. Jejunal fluid contained less than 10^3 CFU/ml, none of which were *E. coli* 0119:B14. In patients 11, 12, and 15, the return of normal enteric flora in stool cultures was accompanied by intermittent isolation of the pathogenic *E. coli* serotype. However, significant diarrhea did not recur. Histologic improvement with restoration of normal architecture of villi was documented by repeat jejunal biopsy in patients 1,4 and 12. Repeat rectal biopsy in patients 7 and 15 demonstrated disappearance of adherent bacteria and return of normal mucosal structure. Overall, neomycin therapy in conjunction with parenteral nutrition resulted in a marked decrease in diarrhea and substantial weight gain.

Table 2 outlines the major events of each infant's hospitalization: Time to initial isolation of *E. coli* 0119:B14 from stool, time to treatment with neomycin, duration of central alimentation and length of hospitalization.

The first eight patients were diagnosed by intestinal biopsy or by serotyping of stools when the diagnosis was suspected and patients 9 through 15 after serotying of stool cultures for *E. coli* 0119:B14 was instituted on a routine basis for infants with diarrhea who were less than six months of age. This change in surveillance led to more rapid diagnosis and earlier therapy with neomycin Decreases in duration of central alimentation

Table 2. Hospital course and treatment

Patients	Time to First Recognition of *E. coli* 0119:B14*	Time to Neomycin Therapy (After Hospitalization)*	Duration of Central TPN*	Duration of Hospitalization*
1 through 8	17	24	45	67
9 through 15	5	10	17	32

*All values represent mean in days

required and in the length of hospitalization then followed.

All infants, except patient 1 who died with *E. coli* (not 0119:B14) sepsis, gradually resumed enteral feedings with Pregestimil and progressed to a regular diet for age without diarrhea. None of the surviving infants has persistent intestinal or immunological disease.

Epidemiology

Twelve of these 15 infants were admitted with severe diarrhea and had *E. coli* 0119:B14 isolated from early stool cultures. Three patients (1,7, and 10) had nosocomial acquisition of *E. coli* 0119:B14 infection. Patient 1 was initially hospitalized for vomiting and poor weight gain, and 7 days after admission, developed severe diarrhea. Patients 7 and 10 were admitted with mild diarrhea, had initially negative stool cultures, and 7-10 days later, had marked worsening of diarrhea, with isolation of *E.coli* 0119:B14. In addition, patients 8 and 15 had been hospitalized previously at Children's Hospital Medical Center. Ten patients had received antibiotics (ampicillin and/or gentamicin) prior to or during this hospitalization.

From January, 1980 until June 1981, the Children's Hospital Medical Center Microbiology Laboratory has serotyped *E.coli* isolates from stool culture of all infants less than 6 months of age who were admitted with or subsequently developed diarrhea. In this survey of 900 patients, 4% had *E.coli* 0119:B14; half of these had severe illness that required intravenous alimentation and intensive investigation.

Further Studies In Other Infants With E.coli 0119:B14 in Stool and/or Jejunal Overgrowth

As the clinical syndrome and histologic findings of infants with *E.coli* 0119:B14 infection became clear, two important questions arose: (1) Did all infants with *E.coli* 0119:B14 in the stool have jejunal overgrowth and/or mucosal damage from this organism? (2) Did infants with jejunal overgrowth with other enteric organisms have adherent bacteria on jejunal biopsy and the same type of clinical illness? To answer these questions, two other groups of infants were studied: (1) Infants with *E.coli* 0119:B14 in stool only, and (2) infants with jejunal overgrowth with other enteric organisms. Table 3 summarizes the clinical illnesses, cultures and biopsy findings in these two groups and compares these 2 groups with the initial fifteen patients. All of these patients were hospitalized during the same period.

Infants with the pathogenic *E.coli* in both jejunal and stool had severe diarrhea, marked mucosal damage with bacteria adherent to jejunum and/or colon, required central

Table 3. Comparison of disease severity with site of isolation of *E. coli* 0119:B14

	Stool and Jejunum	Stool only	Jejunal Coliform Overgrowth
Number of Patients	15	6	6
Age (weeks)	3 – 28	4 – 16	1 – 40
Diarrhea	severe	moderate	mild to moderate
Mucosal Damage	severe	mild	mild to none
Central TPN	15	2	1
Length of Hospitalization (Mean in Days)	51	31	24

venous alimentation and were hospitalized for a mean of 51 days. Infants with *E.coli* 0119 in stool only, had less severe diarrhea, mild histological abnormalities in the colon or jejunum and did not have bacteria adherent to either mucosal surface. They usually tolerated feedings with elemental formula for nutritional support and were hospitalized for an average of one month. Infants with jejunal coliform overgrowth but no *E.coli* 0119 also had a less severe clinical illness and minimal jejunal mucosal changes without adherent bacteria. Only one infant required central alimentation and the average hospitalization was relatively short.

Characteristics of E.coli 0119:B14

To explore further the pathogenesis of diarrhea with *E.coli* 0119:B14, several studies of bacterial morphology and properties were performed. Negative staining revealed large numbers of pili and a capsule. Hemagglutination testing did not show a pattern consistent with colonization factor antigen I or II (9). *In vivo* and *in vitro* tests for heat-labile, heat-stable and vero cell toxins were negative for all duodenal and fecal isolates examined. *E.coli* 0119:B14 isolates were susceptible by disc diffusion to the aminoglycosides kanamycin, gentamicin and neomycin, but resistant to ampicillin and carbenicillin. Analysis of bacterial plasmids by DNA agarose gel electrophoresis revealed consistent carriage of 4 plasmids in *E.coli* 0119:B14 isolates from all 15 patients (11).

Discussion

Escherichia coli 0119 is a well-recognized enteropathogenic serotype. As illustrated by our 15 infants, the infection can be severe with protracted diarrhea that precludes enteral feedings and requires central venous alimentation and prolonged hospitalization. A striking feature of the illness caused by the present *E.coli* 0119:B14 was the ability of this organism to adhere to the jejunal and colonic mucosa and to colonize the small intestine. The specific properties responsible for adherence to intestinal mucosa were not identified.

These 15 infants may have been unusually susceptible to this pathogenic organism and to severe diarrheal illness. First, most were in a poor nutritional state that may alter the structure and function of enterocytes. Second, mucosal injury by prior enteric infection may have predisposed to later severe damage. Patients 7, 11, and 13 had documented rotavirus infection; patient 4 had cytomegelovirus. Third, since a consistent marker of *E.coli* 0119:B14 was ampicillin-resistance, prior treatment with ampicillin may have rendered ten of the 15 infants susceptible to this enteropathogen. Finally, three infants most likely acquired the organism in the hospital and two others had been exposed during previous CHMC admissions.

The exact mechanisms by which *E.coli* 0119:B14 and the other classical enteropathogenic *E.coli* produce diarrhea is unclear. For *E.coli* 0119:B14, production of heat labile, heat-stable or vero cell toxins seems to be excluded. We are currently investigating fractions from *E.coli* 0119:B14 lysates and filtrates for enterotoxin activity. *E.coli* 0119:B14 apparently does not have the ability to invade jejunal or colonic mucosa as this was not found by light or electron microscopic examination. An important part of the mechanism may be the damage to the glycocalyx, microvillus border and terminal web of enterocytes that occurs at the areas of bacterial adherence. Heavily conlonized enterocytes show damaged organelles, cell swelling and, presumably, eventual cell death. Atrophy of villi and disorganization of the remaining epthelium then follow. Similar changes at both the light and electron microscopic levels occur in the colonic mucosa.

Several findings support the conclusion that *E.coli* 0119:B14 is the cause of this enterocyte and mucosal damage, leading to severe diarrhea. First, patient 7 initially had mild diarrhea and poor weight gain with mild jejunal mucosal damage secondary to rotavirus. With the onset of *E.coli* 0119:B14 infection, he rapidly developed massive watery diarrhea, jejunal overgrowth with the pathogenic *E.coli* and marked injury to both jejunal and rectal mucosa with adherent bacteria in both locations. Secondly, eradication of the pathogenic *E.coli* from stool cultures and/or jejunum of these patients led to a marked reduction in diarrhea and resolution of the mucosal abnormalities. Nutritional support via intravenous alimentation also appeared important to allow repair of the damaged intestinal and colonic mucosa and to restore the normal mucosal functions of digestion, absorption and defense. Third, the 15 infants with *E.coli* 0119:B14 in both jejunum and stool had the most severe clinical disease and the most marked damage to epithelial cells of the jejunum and colon. Patients with the pathogenic serotype in stool only (Table 3) had mild diarrhea and did not have bacteria adherent to mucosal cells. Furthermore, jejunal overgrowth with other enteric organisms was associated with less severe diarrhea, less damage to vili and an absence of adherent bacteria on enterocytes (Table 3).

The exact conditions, mucosal and bacterial, that allow bacterial adherence and result in mucosal damage remain unclear. Adherence assays and toxin studies are being performed to define further the pathophysiology of this bacterial cause of diarrhea.

This work was supported in part by the True Order of Sisters of Ruth, Post #18, and CRC Grant #RR-00123.

REFERENCES

1. Lennette, E. (ed.) Manual of Clinical Microbiology (Third Edition) American Society of Microbiology, Wahsington, DC, 1980.
2. Orskov, I, Orskov, F, Jann, B and Jann K: Serology, chemistry, and genetics of 0 and K antigens of Escherichia Coli. Bact. Rev. **41**(3):667-710, 1977.
3. Partin, JC, Schubert, WK, and Partin, JS: Mitochondrial ultrastructure in Reye's Syndrome. N. Engl. J. Med. **285**:1339-1343, 1971.
4. Wiggins, HS: Simple method for estimating trypsin. Gut. **8**:415-416, 1967.
5. Erlansow, C and Bergstrom, B: Tributyrine as a substrate for determination of lipase activity of pancreatic juice and small intestinal content. Scan J. Gastroenterol. **5**:293-295, 1970.

6. Evans, D, Evans, D and DuPont, H: Hemegglutination patterns of enterotoxigenic and enteropathogenic *E. coli*. Infect. Immun. **23**:336-346, 1979.
7. Sack, D and Sack, BR: Test for enterotoxigenic *E. coli* using Y-1 adrenal cells in miniculture. Infect. Immuno. **11**(2):334-336, 1975.
8. Giannella, RA: Suckling mouse model for detection of heat-stable *E. coli* enterotoxin: characteristics of the model. Infect. Immun. **14**(1):995-99, 1976.
9. Konowalchuk, J, Spears, J and Stavric, S: Vero response to a cytotoxin of *E. coli*. Infect. Immun. **18**(3):775-779, 1977.
10. Giannella, RA, Formal, SB, Damimin, GJ and Collins, H: Pathogenesis of Salmonellosis: Studies of fluid secretion, mucosal invasion and morphologic reaction in the rabbit ileum. J. Clin. Invest. **52**:441-453, 1973.
11. Dey, RR, Loper, JC, Kurzepa, H and Rothbaum, RJ: Local isolates of human enteropathogenic *E. coli*: Plasmids and *in vitro* adherence. Presented to American Society of Microbiology, 1980.

GENETICS

Advances in Research on Cholera and Related Diarrheas, eds., S. Kuwahara, N. F. Pierce, 171–182.

PROPERTIES OF THE RELATED TRANSPOSABLE PHAGE VcA1 AND DEFECTIVE PROPHAGE dVcA1 IN EL TOR AND CLASSICAL BIOTYPES OF *VIBRIO CHOLERAE*

S.R. Johnson[1], B.C.S. Liu[2], D. Schreiber[2], and W.R. Romig[2]

[1]*Centers for Disease Control, Atlanta, Ga., and*
[2]*Department of Microbiology, University of California*
Los Angeles, California

Parker *et al.* (13) demonstrated that most classical strains of *Vibrio cholerae* produced defective phage structures after induction with mitomycin C, whereas pathogenic El Tor strains produced morphologically intact phage. Morphologically intact phage were also produced by an exceptional classical strain, NIH 41, which was subsequently shown by C. Parker to produce two different phages, both of which could infect or lysogenize the El Tor indicator strain, RJ1. These two phages, called VcA1 and VcA2, were heteroimmune, and VcA2 has been shown (4) to belong to the "Kappa type" phage group described by Takeya (18). Several biological properties of phage VcA1 have been described (21).

Later studies (4,5) revealed that classical strains such as 569B produced two kinds of defective phage tails that were morphologically and serologically related to phage VcA1 and VcA2, respectively. All 36 classical strains tested were immune to phage VcA1 and all but 8 of them were immune to phage VcA2. Defective prophage dVcA2 was eliminated from strain 569B, but defective prophage dVcA1 could not be eliminated from this, or other classical strains. No evidence for the involvement of either prophage in toxin production or in other aspects of pathogenicity of *V. cholerae* was detected.

Phages VcA1 and VcA2 have not been demonstrated to mediate generalized transduction, nor have the defective prophage attachment sites in classical strains been determined. However, phage VcA1 was presumed to chromosomally integrate in El Tor strain RJ1, because plasmids were not detected in DNA extracted from VcA1 lysogens of this strain (S. Johnson, unpublished). DNA extracted from mature VcA1 particles was a linear, double stranded molecule of approximately 22 megadaltons (R. Hudson, Ph. D. thesis, UCLA, 1977). Other biological properties of phage VcA1, including its similarities to coliphage Mu (3,19), were revealed by studies (10) on a unique conjugative plasmid, pSJ15, which are summarized below.

Conjugative plasmid pSJ15 apparently arose spontaneously in a derivative of classical mating strains 162 (1,15) that contained the hybrid P::Tn*1* plasmid, pSJ5 (7,8). Previous results showed that plasmid pSJ5 was formed by transposing the ampicillin resistance transposon Tn*1* (8) to the *V. cholerae* P factor (1,14). Plasmid pSJ5 retained normal P factor activities, including derepressed self-transfer at high frequency, lacunae formation (1,14), and low frequency, non-oriented chromosomal transfer.

It was unexpected, therefore, when a bacterial recombinant, that on the basis of its ampicillin resistance was presumed to contain plasmid pSJ5, was found to preferentially transfer the *his trp* region of the strain 162 chromosome. Further investigations revealed that the unique donor properties of this recombinant were plasmid determined. As described below, our results indicated that plasmid pSJ15 is a composite plasmid that was formed by transposing defective prophage dVcA1 from the *V. cholerae* strain 162 chromosome to conjugative plasmid, pSJ5.

Interactions of plasmid pSJ15 with the $VcA1^{+}$ prophage in several independently isolated lysogens of strains RJ1 strongly suggested that phage VcA1, like coliphage Mu, inserts promiscuously in El Tor strains that it lysogenizes. The genetic and physical evidence supported this interpretation and indicated that phage VcA1 resembles phage Mu in other properties. The results also suggest that all classical strains may contain the VcA1 prophage and that none of the El Tor strains are naturally lysogenic for this bacteriophage. Preliminary results indicate that the VcA1 prophage may be located at the same site and in the same orientation in all classical strains.

MATERIALS AND METHODS

Bacterial strains and plasmids. The El Tor and classical strains used for colony hybridizations included those described by Parker *et al.* (13) and by Gerdes and Romig (4,5); El Tor strains provided by J. Ogg, Colorado State University; and a group of classical strains provided by Betty Davis, CDC, Atlanta, Ga. Bacterial strains used for genetic studies and for other purposes are listed in Table 1. Bacteriophage VcA2 from classical strain NIH 41 were maintained as lysogens of strains RJ1.

Media. Meat extract agar (MEA) and brain heart infusion (Difco) were used as complete media for mating experiments and for routine bacteriological procedures (14). Synthetic media were minimal medium A (12) supplemented at previously reported (7) levels. Enriched minimal agar (19) was medium A supplemented with 200 μg/ml of Difco nutrient broth powder. Antibiotics were used at previously reported levels (7,10). TYC media (4) were used for preparing and assaying phages and for other manipulations involving phage VcA1.

Mating procedures. Quantitative matings for gene transfer and linkage analysis were performed in liquid medium as previously described, and donors were counterselected with antibiotics (7,14). Transconjugants that received P::Tn*1* plasmids were selected with ampicillin (8).

Bacteriophages. Phage were prepared, concentrated and assayed as described (4,5). Bacteria were lysogenized by placing drops of concentrated phage suspensions onto the surface of bacterial lawns in soft agar. Survivors were purified by repeated single colony isolation and tested for immunity by cross-streaking against concentrated phage suspensions. The ability to produce phage was determined by stabbing cells into indicator lawns of sensitive bacteria. VcA1-resistant strains were obtained by the same procedures except that resistant cultures which failed to produce phage and did not adsorb phage VcA1 were retained.

Restriction analyses and hybridizations. Phage VcA1 DNA was purified by phenol extraction and ethanol precipitation (12) and was stored in TE buffer at 4°C. Bacterial DNA was purified by the methods of Brenner et al. (2). Restriction endonucleases were

Table 1. V. cholerae strains and plasmids

162 derivatives	plasmid content and relevant properties[1]	Source
RV34(pSJ5)	pSJ5, Ap^r/ leu-1 pur 1	(10)
RV34(pSJ15)	pSJ15, Ap^r, $VcA1^{imm}$/leu-1 pur-1	This Paper
RV106(pSJ5)	pSJ5, Ap^r/ arg-1 his-1 ilv-1 Nal^r	(10)
RV129	none/leu-1 pur-1 lys-2 Str^r	(15)
RV169	none/arg-1 his-1 ilv-1 trp-1 met-2 Str^r	(15)
RV177	none/arg-1 his-1 ilv-1 trp-1 met-2 Spc^r	(15)
RV800(pSJ15)	PSJ15, Ap^r, $VcA1^{imm}$/leu-1 pur-1 Str^r	This Paper
RV94	none/arg-1 his-1 ilv-1 trp-1 Str^r	(15)
RJ1 derivatives		
RJ1	none/ prototrophic, VcA1 sensitive, plasmid-free	(7)
RJ1(pSJ5)	PSJ5, Ap^r/RJ1	(7,10)
RJ1(pSJ15)	pSJ15, Ap^r, $VcA1^{imm}$/RJ1	This Paper
RJ1($VcA1^+$)	none/RJ1, $VcA1^{imm}$	This Paper
RJ39	none/arg-7 ilv-5 thr-1 Rif^r Str^r	(7,9)
RJ44	none/arg-7 ilv-5 his-2 Rif^r Str^r	(7,9)
RJ47	none/arg-7 ilv-5 trp-2 Rif^r Str^r	(7,9)
RJ57	none/arg-7 ilv-5 met-4 thy-3 Rif^r Str^r	(7,9)
Plasmids		
P	naturally occurring *V. cholerae* conjugative plasmid 48 Mdal	(1,14)
pSJ5	P::Tn*1* conjugative plasmid, Ap^r, 52 Mdal	(7,8)
pSJ15	pSJ15::dVcA1, Ap^r, $VcA1^{imm}$, about 70 Mdal	This Paper
pSJ44	pSJ5::$VcA1^+$, Ap^r, $VcA1^+$, recombinant 70Mdal	This Paper

1. Conjugative plasmids and their properties appear before the slash line /; bacterial properties appear after the slash line /. Designations correspond to those of Parker *et al.* (14) and Johnson and Romig (7,10) for *V. cholerae.*

obtained from Bethesda Research Laboratories, Bethesda, MD., and used as recommended by the supplier. Electrophoresis in agarose gels was performed as previously described (10). Restriction fragments were blotted and hybridized by the Southern (17) procedure and ^{32}P-labeled DNA was prepared by the nick-translation procedures of Rigby *et al.* (16).

Colony hybridization. Colony hybridizations were performed by the procedure of Grunstein and Hogness (6) using nick-translated VcA1 DNA. Various levels of stringency were attained by hybridizing the filters in solutions containing 20%, 30%, or 50% formamide at 37°C for 16 hr, after which they were washed at 54°C, 60°C or 70°C, respectively for 1 hr. Essentially identical results were obtained at all levels of stringency.

Electron microscopy. Heteroduplexes of purified phage VcA1 DNA were prepared and spread for electron microscopy by our previously described procedures (8).

RESULTS

Donor RV106(pSJ5) was mated to strain RV129, a P^- derivative of strain 162, and Str^r *lys*$^+$ recombinants were selected. One such recombinant, strain RV800, that on the basis of its ampicillin resistance was presumed to contain conjugative plasmid pSJ5, was subsequently mated to another strain 162 derivative, RV177. As shown in Table 2, cross 1, strain RV800 transferred the *his* and *trp* genes at higher frequencies than other selected markers. Other strain 162 derivatives, such as strain RV34, that acquired ampicillin resistance from strain RV800 also gained the ability to transfer the *his* and *trp* genes at high frequency, indicating that the enhanced transfer ability was plasmid determined (Table 2, cross 2). Ampicillin resistant transconjugants of strain RV34 that acquired plasmid pSJ5 from donors other than RV800, transferred all chromosomal markers at about the same low frequencies (Table 2, cross 3).

These results suggested that strain RV800 contained a mutant plasmid, which we designated pSJ15, that mediated polarized chromosomal transfer from an origin near the *his* gene. Interrupted mating experiments and linkage analyses supported this conclusion, but did not directly reveal the nature of the mutation responsible for polarized transfer. It seemed possible that plasmid pSJ15 was a P-prime which had acquired the chromosomal *his* and *trp* markers. To test this possibility, it was introduced into strain RJ1, where its transfer properties were determined.

Unlike strain 162 transconjugants, ampicillin resistant transconjugants of El Tor strain RJ1 that received plasmid pSJ15 did not transfer the *his* and *trp* genes or other selected markers at enhanced frequencies. Moreover, further characterization of strain RJ1 transconjugants revealed that they had all (102/102) acquired immunity to phage VcA1, and that they efficiently co-transferred ampicillin resistance and VcA1 immunity to other strain RJ1 recipients. The latter observations were explained by assuming that plasmid pSJ15 contained all or part of defective prophage dVcA1, which was presumably trasnsposed from the strain 162 chromosome to conjugative plasmid pSJ5.

This hypothesis predicted (i) that potential strain RJ1 transconjugants that received plasmid pSJ15 should be zygotically induced and produce defective phage tails; (ii) that surviving ampicillin resistant transconjugants should be UV inducible; and (iii) that plasmid pSJ15 should be as much as one VcA1 genome larger (22 megadaltons) than plasmid pSJ5. Consistent with these predictions, more than 90% of the potential transconjugants of strain RJ1 were killed by mating them with RJ1 (pSJ15) donors, and large numbers of phage tails were visible in the supernatant fluids of the mating mixtures. Surviving ampicillin resistant transconjugants produced defective phage structures after UV induction, and plasmids extracted from these transconjugants or from strain RV800

Table 2. Transfer of selected markers by classical strain 162 donors that contain plasmid pSJ15.

		Transfer frequency of selected marker[1]				
Donor	Recipient	his-1	trp-1	met-2	ilv-1	arg-1
1. RV 800	RV177	350	250	6	5	1
2. RV34(pSJ15)	RV177	220	240	–	–	–
3. RV34(pSJ5)	RV169	6	5	–	3	4

[1] Frequencies are expressed as recombinants per 10^5 input donors. The order of markers corresponds to their order on the classical strain 162 genetic map (15).

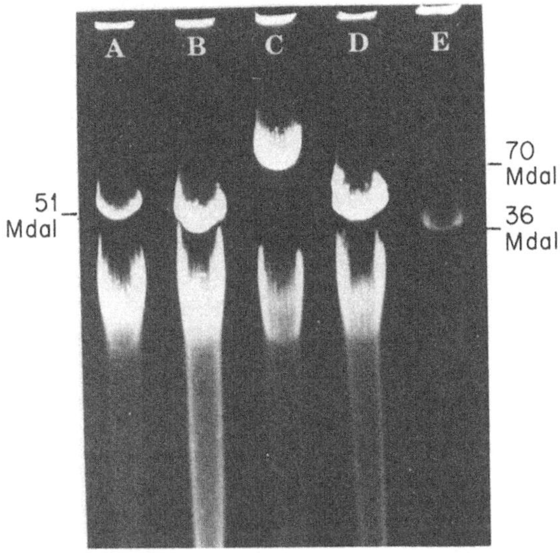

Fig. 1. Agarose gel electrophoresis of *V. cholerae* plasmids. Lane A, 52 Mdal pSJ5; Lanes B and D, plasmid deletion mutants derived from plasmid pSJ15 VcA1$^+$ recombinant plasmids; Lane C, 70 Mdal plasmid pSJ15; Lane E, plasmid RP4 control.

were about 70 megadaltons in size, which is about one VcA1 genome larger than the 52 megadalton parental pSJ5 plasmid (Fig. 1).

By transferring plasmid pSJ15 into strains of RJ1 that had previously been lysogenized with wild type VcA1, conjugative plasmids that co-transferred ampicillin resistance and the ability to produce wild type VcA1 phage were obtained. This class of plasmid appeared to arise by generalized recombination between the wild type prophage in VcA1$^+$ lysogens and the defective dVcA1 prophage in plasmid pSJ15. The recombinant plasmids were the same size as pSJ15, they were relatively stable, and were indefinitely transferrable from cultures that contained them. Two mutant plasmids that had lost transfer abilities and no longer produced infectious phages arose spontaneously in cells that received VcA1$^+$ recombinant plasmids. These were shown to be severely deleted plasmids that had simultaneously lost prophage and transfer sequences (Fig. 1).

The preceding results supported the contention that conjugative plasmid pSJ15 contained defective prophage dVcA1. It seemed likely therefore, that plasmid pSJ15 mediated the preferential transfer of the *his* region of classical strain 162 by integrating into its chromosome through the homologous prophage sequences near this region. Because the dVcA1 prophage has not been mapped, the latter interpretation was based on analogies between transfer properties of pSJ15-mediated donors and other Hfr-like donors whose transfer properties depend on similar "portable regions of homology" (11).

To more directly test the above hypothesis, several independently isolated VcA1$^+$ lysogens of strain RJ1 were converted into donors with plasmid pSJ15 and were separately crossed to a multiply auxotrophic recipient that had been lysogenized with phage VcA1 to prevent zygotic induction. The resulting donors expressed Hfr transfer abilities, but based on their transfer frequencies for selected markers, at least three different kinds

Table 3. Different Hfr transfer properties of strain RJ1(VcA1$^+$) lysogens that contain plasmid pSJ15.

RJ1(VcA1$^+$) (pSJ15) donor	Transfer frequency of selected marker[1] his–2	ilv–7	arg–5
RJ176	200	20	4
RJ178	5	8,000	800
RJ179	80	4,000	7

[1] Frequencies are presented as recombinants per 10^5 input donors.

of Hfr donors were detected (Table 3). Assuming the correctness of our model for Hfr formation, this implied that like coliphage Mu, VcA1 could integrate at multiple sites in cells that it lysogenizes.

The hallmark feature (3,19) of bacteriophage Mu is its ability to induce a range of different auxotrophic mutations in the bacteria that it lysogenizes. It was of interest, therefore, to determine if phage VcA1 likewise generated auxotrophic mutations by inserting into genes of *V. cholerae*. In the first experiments to test this, one auxotrophic mutant was identified among the 250 independently isolated VcA1 lysogens that were tested. Using the more efficient procedures of Taylor (19), a wide variety of auxotrophic mutants was isolated, and the frequency of their occurrence approached the 2-3% frequency reported for phage Mu (3,19). Auxotrophic mutations induced by phage VcA1 in strain RJ1 and other El Tor strains were generally non-leaky and with two exceptions, reverted at an undetectably low frequency, resembling in these respects, the mutations induced by wild type phage Mu (3).

According to our model for enchanced gene transfer, by acquiring the pSJ15 conjugative plasmid, VcA1-induced auxotrophic mutants should be converted into Hfr donors whose transfer origins originate within the mutated gene. As shown in Table 4, the transfer properties of these donors correspond with these expectations.

Previous results showed that most classical strains appeared to contain defective

Table 4. Hfr-like properties of VcA1-induced auxotrophs that contain plasmid pSJ15.

Donor[1]	Recipient[2]	Transfer frequency for selected marker[3] ilv-5	arg-7	thr-1	his-2	trp-2	met-4
ilv-21::VcA1	RJ39, RJ44	1400	1400	950	400	–	–
his-7::VcA1	RJ47, RJ44	30	14	–	170	2500	–
trp-5::VcA1	RJ57, RJ44	50	70	–	11	–	300
RJ1 wild type	RJ44	12	8	–	7	–	–

[1]Donors all contained plasmid pSJ15 and were counterselected with Str.

[2]Recipients were lysogenized with VcA1; see Table 1 for markers in each.

[3]Transfer frequencies as for Table 3.

prophages which were closely related to temperate phage VcA1. These findings prompted us to re-examine the distribution of VcA1 prophages in *V. cholerae* biotypes by a different technique. For this purpose, nick-translated ^{32}P-labeled VcA1 DNA was used to detect hybridizable sequences in classical and El Tor strains, using the colony hybridization procedures of Grunstein and Hogness (6). Representative results are presented in Fig. 2, which showed that all 51 classical strains tested, irrespective of their geographical origin or time of isolation, contained VcA1 sequences. None of the 16 El Tor strains were naturally lysogenic for phage VcA1, nor was any genetic relatedness between VcA1 or phage Mu revealed by these techniques.

These experiments confirmed that all classical strains contained VcA1 prophages, and that none of the El Tor strains were naturally lysogenic for phage VcA1. This finding, together with the finding that phage VcA1 can integrate at multiple sites in El Tor strains, raised the question of whether phage VcA1 was also integrated at many sites in the naturally lysogenic classical strains. Accordingly several classical strains were converted into donors with plasmid pSJ15 and were crossed to appropriate recipients. All of the

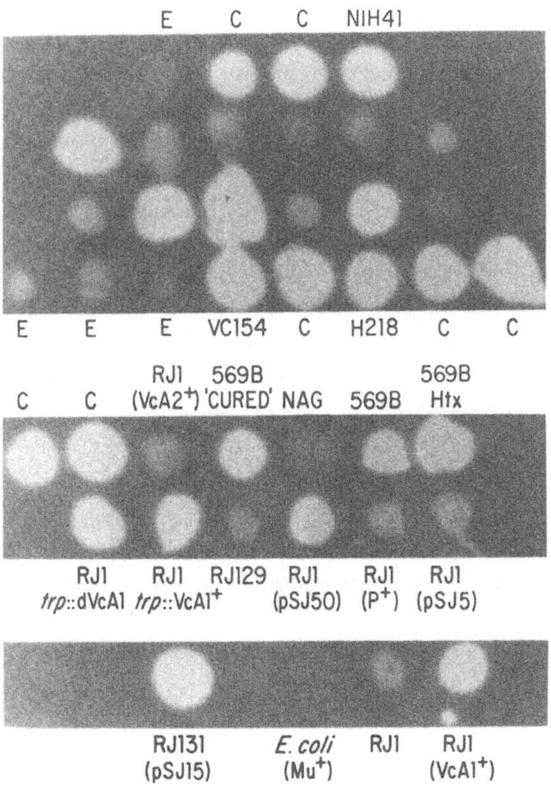

Fig. 2. Colony hybridizations of classical and El Tor strains using ^{32}P-labeled VcA1 DNA. "E" represents El Tor and "C" classical strains. Some strains are identified by strain numbers. 569 B 'cured' was cured of prophage dVcA2, but still contains dVcA1. Hybridization was at the 30% formamide stringency level. All classical strains, and no El Tor strains were naturally lysogenic for phage VcA1 by this procedure.

classical donors transferred the *his* and *trp* markers at enhanced frequencies (Table 5). By analogy with strain 162, these results indicated that the dVcA1 prophage was located in the same region and in the same orientation in all of them.

We also attempted to locate the VcA1 prophage in classical and El Tor strains by comparing restriction patterns of DNA extracted from mature phage and from various lysogenic hosts. After digestion with restriction endonucleases and electrophoresis through agarose gels (17), the DNA fragments were transferred to nitrocellulose filters and hybridized with ^{32}P-labeled VcA1 DNA (16). If phage VcA1 was integrated at the same site and in the same orientation in all strains, the sizes and positions of the prophage restriction fragments might well be identical; if it was integrated at different sites, the sizes and positions of fragments containing the prophage ends should vary from lysogen to lysogen.

Assuming that like phage Mu, phage VcA1 integrates linearly (3), we expected the number of VcA1-hybridizable fragments in the mature phage and prophage DNA preparations to be identical. However, the sizes, and hence the positions, of the fragments containing the end sections of the phage were expected to differ in the two kinds of preparations. This is because the sizes of the fragments that contain the prophage ends are determined by the amount of DNA between the restriction sites nearest either end of the phage DNA and the first restriction sites in the bacterial DNA sequences that flank the integrated prophages. Accordingly, the "fuzzy" restriction band in mature phage VcA1 DNA that corresponds to the "S" end of phage Mu DNA (3), was expected to be replaced by a discrete band of higher molecular weight in DNA preparations that contained the prophage.

Restriction patterns obtained after *Hind* III digestion of phage VcA1 DNA and of DNA extracted from VcA1-induced auxotrophic lysogens of strain RJ1 are presented in Fig. 3. Most of the VcA1-hybridizable bands appeared at the same positions in the two kinds of preparations and were presumed to correspond to internal fragments common to prophage and mature phage DNA. The broad band in VcA1 DNA corresponding to its S end has been replaced by discrete bands of different sizes in the *trp*::VcA1 and the *cys*::VcA1 lysogens; the mutation in the *cys*$^+$::dVcA1 lysogen did not alter the prophage restriction pattern. These results thus support the previous conclusion that the prophages in different VcA1-induced auxotrophs of strain RJ1 are inserted at different chromosomal sites.

Table 5. Transfer frequencies of various classical donors that contain conjugative plasmid pSJ15.

Donor[1]	Selected Marker[2]			
	ilv–1	arg–1	his–1	trp–1
NIH 41	1	2	180	74
569 B	14	17	4000	3000
Vc12	4	3	740	400
RV34	2	2	220	240

[1]Donors all contained conjugative plasmid pSJ15.

[2]Transfer frequencies as in Table 3.

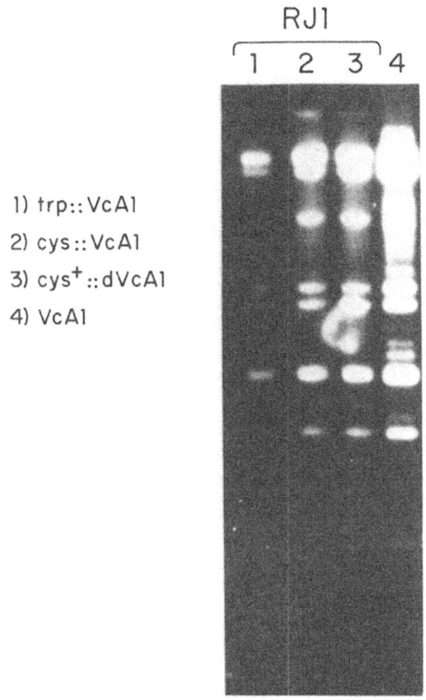

Fig. 3. Southern hybridizations of various VcA1-induced auxotrophs of strain RJ1. The *cys*$^+$::dVcA1 strain is a revertant of the *cys*::VcA1$^+$ auxotroph and fails to produce infectious phage. Lane 4 is DNA from mature phage. All DNAs were digested with *Hind* III and hybridized with ^{32}P-labeled VcA1 DNA.

DNA extracted from naturally lysogenic classical strains was similarly analyzed (Fig. 4). The VcA1-hybridizable bands that correspond to internal fragments were found at essentially the same positions in DNA prepared from classical strains as they were in DNA from the El Tor lysogens. Unexpectedly, however, there were more high molecular weight bands in the classical strain preparations that hybridized with VcA1 DNA than were predicted from the linear insertion model. To explain the discrepancy, our current working hypothesis is that classical strains contain two closely juxtaposed copies of the VcA1 prophage, although this possibility has not been established.

Regardless of the ultimate explanation for the band complexity observed in classical strain DNA preparations, it is apparent that the pattern of prophage restriction fragments is the same in all classical strains. This observation, together with the gene transfer data discussed above, indicate that the VcA1 prophage may be inserted at the same site in all classical strains.

DISCUSSION

Our results have shown that *V. cholerae* phage VcA1 is similar in many respects to the apparently unrelated *Escherichia coli* phage Mu. Similarities between these phages include their ability to transpose to different DNA sites within a cell; their ability to

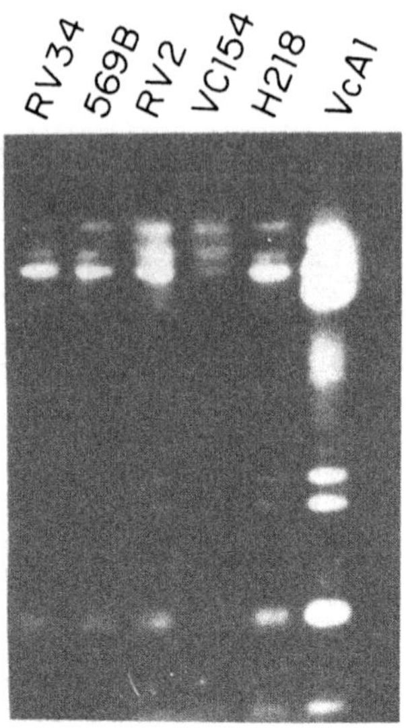

Fig. 4. Southern hybridizations of various classical strains. The last lane is DNA from phage VcA1. All DNAs were digested with *Hind* III and hybridized with ^{32}P-labeled VcA1 DNA.

induce a variety of auxotrophic mutations by integrating into the genes of bacteria that they lysogenize; and similarities in the structure and organization of their genomes.

That phage VcA1 might be functionally similar to phage Mu was first suggested by evidence indicating that plasmid pSJ15 was formed by transposing defective prophage dVcA1 to plasmid pSJ5. Since the ability to transpose is a distinguishing feature of phage Mu, this suggested that phage VcA1 might possess other properties in common with phage Mu. This possibility was supported by finding that about 2% of the El Tor strains lysogenized with phage VcA1 contained auxotrophic mutations that resulted from prophage insertions into the affected genes.

At the structural level, heterogeneous bacterial DNA was found at one, and possibly both, of the ends of the DNA from mature phage VcA1. This was revealed by an anomalously broad restriction band in *Hind* III and *Bam* H1 digested VcA1 DNA after electrophoresis through agarose gels. After transfer to nitrocellulose filters, this band, which was presumed to be analogous to the S end of phage Mu, hybridized strongly with ^{32}P-labeled chromosomal DNA. A much fainter band, which was presumed to correspond to the "C" end, was detected in some preparations. Heteroduplexes formed by denaturing and re-annealing VcA1 DNA likewise revealed "split ends" similar to those of phage Mu (Fig. 5), but the presence of a "G loop" characteristic of phage Mu DNA (3), has not yet been established. It thus appears that phage VcA1 is functionally and structurally similar to phage Mu. However, because sequence relatedness between them was not detected by colony hybridization, the two phages do not appear to be genetically related.

We have confirmed by colony hybridization that all classical strains contain the VcA1 prophage and that none of the El Tor strains are lysogenic for phage VcA1. The reasons for this extreme biotype specificity are not clear, since it seems likely that frequent encounters between susceptible El Tor strains and phage VcA1 should have occurred, especially in regions where these two biotypes have co-existed. That El Tor strains

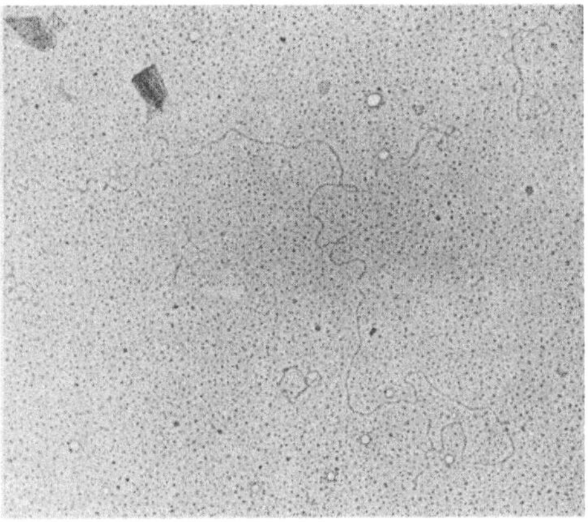

Fig. 5. Heteroduplex of phage VcA1 DNA. Molecule shows "split-ends" characteristic of phage Mu (3) arising from heterogeneous bacterial DNA. Marker plasmid is pAH113, 7000 bp, provided by Arnold Horwitz, UCLA.

have not become lysogenized may be because the VcA1 prophage is defective in most classical strains and consequently, few infectious phage are present in the environment. However, this explanation does not account for the observed presence of the dVcA1 prophage in all classical strains, unless it is assumed that the strains present today are the widely distributed descendents of a defectively lysogenic progenitor. Although this possibility seems unlikely, our preliminary evidence that the dVcA1 prophage occupies the same chromosomal site in all classical strains is consistent with this assumption, especially when it is recalled that phage VcA1 appears to integrate promiscuously into the chromosome of El Tor strains.

Our studies indicate that phage VcA1 can be used to generate a random array of auxotrophic mutations in *V. cholerae* strains that it lysogenizes. These mutations occur at high frequencies and appear to result from a single mutational event. The VcA1 insertion mutations are highly stable and are advantageous because, after acquiring plasmid pSJ15, mutants that contain them are converted into Hfr donors whose transfer origins lie within the mutated gene. Our results show that these kinds of Hfr strains are efficient donors, and indicate that similar kinds of donors could probably be constructed in other VcA1-susceptible strains of interest.

The fact that VcA1 and VcA2 prophages appear to be indefinitely stable in classical strain NIH 41 and El Tor strain RJ1 raises the question of why both prophages are generally defective in classical strains. Their defectiveness does not seem to result from a changed host range similar to that controlled by the G segment in phage Mu (20). Instead they appear to be defective because of a block in morphogenesis that leads to the production of incomplete phage structures (4,13). This block is probably not in a host function, since classical strains cured of defective prophage VcA2 support the replication of VcA2 or other kappa type phages (4). Without further experimentation, speculations on the possible role of these prophages and the reasons for their defectiveness are probably premature. However, regardless of the eventual explanation for the different activities of phages VcA1 in classical and El Tor biotypes, it is likely that continued characterization of these phages should lead to better insights into the biology of *V. cholerae*.

This investigation was supported by the United States–Japan Cooperative Medical Science Program administered by the National Institute of Allergy and Infectious Disease. We thank Larry and Agda Simpson, UCLA, for continued help and advice with the hybridization experiments.

REFERENCES

1. Bhaskaran, K. 1974. Vibrio genetics, pp. 41-59. *In* D. Barua and W. Burrows (ed.), Cholera, W. B. Saunders Co., Philadelphia.
2. Brenner, D. J., G. R. Fanning, K. E. Johnson, R. V. Citarella and S. Falkow. 1969. Polynucleotide relationships among members of *Enterobacteriaceae.* J. Bacteriol. **98**:637-650.
3. Bukhari, A. K. 1976. Bacteriophage Mu as a transposition element. Annu. Rev. Genet. **10**:389-412.
4. Gerdes, J. C., and W. R. Romig. 1975. Complete and defective bacteriophages of classical *V. cholerae*: Relationship to the Kappa type bacteriophage. J. Virol. **15**:1231-1238.
5. Gerdes, J. C., and W. R. Romig. 1975. Genetic basis of toxin production and pathogenesis in *Vibrio cholerae*: evidence against phage conversion. Inf. Immun. **11**:445-452.
6. Grunstein, M., and D. S. Hogness. 1975. Colony hybridization, a method for the isolation of cloned DNAs that contain a specific gene. Proc. Natl. Acad. Sci. U. S. A. **72**:3961-3965.
7. Johnson, S. R., and W. R. Romig. 1979. Transposon-facilitated recombination in *Vibrio cholerae* Mol. Gen. Genet. **170**:93-101.
8. Johnson, S. R., and W. R. Romig. 1979. *Vibrio cholerae* hybrid sex factor that contains ampicillin transposon Tn *1*. J. Bacteriol. **137**:531-536.
9. Johnson, S. R., B. C. S. Liu, and W. R. Romig. 1981. Auxotrophic mutations induced by *Vibrio cholerae* mutator phage VcAl. FEMS Microbiol. Letters **11**:13-16.
10. Johnson, S. R., and W. R. Romig. 1981. *Vibrio cholerae* conjugative plasmid pSJ15 contains transposable prophage dVcAl. J. Bacteriol. **146**:632-638.
11. Kleckner, N., J. Roth, and D. Botstein. 1977. Genetic engineering *in vivo* using translocatable drug-resistance elements: new methods in bacterial genetics. J. Mol. Biol. **116**:125-159.
12. Miller, J. H. 1972. Experiments in molecular genetics. Cold Spring Harbor Laboratory, Cold Spring Harbor, NY.
13. Parker, C., S. H. Richardson and W. R. Romig. 1970. Production of bacteriophage-associated materials by *V. cholerae*: possible correlation with pathogenicity. Infect. Immun. **1**:417-420.
14. Parker, C., and W. R. Romig. 1972. Self-transfer and genetic recombination mediated by P, the sex factor of *Vibrio cholerae.* J. Bacteriol. **112**:707-714.
15. Parker, C., D. Gauthier, A. Tate, K. Richardson and W. R. Romig. 1979. Expanded linkage map of *Vibrio cholerae.* Genetics. **91**:191-214.
16. Rigby, P. W. J., M. Dieckmann, C. Rodes, and P. Berg. 1977. Labelling deoxyribonucleic acid to high specific activity *in vitro* by nick-translation with DNA polymerase I. J. Mol. Biol. **113**:237-251.
17. Southern, E. M. 1975. Detection of specific sequences among DNA fragments separated by gel electrophoresis. J. Mol. Biol. **98**:503-517.
18. Takeya, K. 1967. El Tor cholera, with special reference to kappa-type choleraphage. Jpn. J. Trop. Med. **8**:5-9.
19. Taylor, A. L. 1963. Bacteriophage-induced mutation in *Escherichia coli.* Proc. Natl. Acad. Sci. U. S. A. **50**:1043-1051.
20. van de Putte, P., S. Cramer, and M. Giphart-Gassler. 1980. Invertible DNA determines host specificity of bacteriophage Mu. Nature. **286**:218-222.
21. Weston, L., Drexler, and S. H. Richardson. 1973. Characterization of vibriophage VA-1. J. Gen. Virol. **21**:155-158.

Advances in Research on Cholera and Related Diarrheas, eds., S. Kuwahara, N. F. Pierce, 183–191.

ISOLATION OF ENTEROTOXIN STRUCTURAL GENE DELETION MUTATIONS IN *VIBRIO CHOLERAE* INDUCED BY TWO MUTAGENIC VIBRIOPHAGES

John J. Mekalanos, Steve L. Moseley†, John R. Murphy and Stanley Falkow†

Department of Microbiology and Molecular Genetics, Harvard Medical School, Boston, Massachusetts 02115, U. S. A.
†Department of Microbiology and Immunology, University of Washington, Seattle, Washington 98195, U. S. A.

Introduction

Colonization of the upper bowel of man by toxinogenic *Vibrio cholerae*, the etiologic agent of Asiatic cholera, results in a diarrheal syndrome due primarily to the action of cholera toxin, which stimulates fluid secretion by activating adenylate cyclase in intestinal epithelial cells (1). The toxin is a multimeric protein (M_r 84,000) composed of one A Subunit (M_r 28,000) and five B Subunits (M_r 11,600) (2). The B subunits mediate binding to ganglioside cell surface receptors and perhaps also facilitate entry of the A subunit into the eukaryotic cell (2, 3). The A subunit promotes the activation of adenylate cyclase in target cells by catalyzing the transfer of the ADP-ribosyl moiety of NAD to a GTPase-regulatory component of the cyclase complex (4, 5).

Recently, the heat-labile enterotoxin (LT) of *E. coli* has been shown to be highly similar to cholera toxin in both structure and mode of action (6, 7). While the LT A and B subunit genes have been found to exist on a variety of plasmids, the gene(s) encoding cholera toxin has not been definitely located, although there are data to suggest that it resides on the *V. cholerae* chromosome (8, 9, 10). While several laboratories have reported isolation of toxin (Tox) mutations that affect the production of one or both of the toxin subunits, none of these mutants have been shown to produce structurally altered polypeptides (11-17).

The isolation of deletion mutations in the toxin structural gene(s) would facilitate its unambiguous genetic mapping. Furthermore, the high stability of deletion mutations would have practical value in the construction of stably attenuated strains of *V. cholerae* for use as live oral vaccines against cholera. In this communication, we report the isolation of deletion mutations in the cholera toxin structural gene. Furthermore, several mutants with complete deletions of the toxin gene(s) exhibit little impairment of growth in adult rabbit intestine. These strains may be useful as stable and safe prototypes for a live oral cholera vaccine.

Materials and Methods

1. *Bacterial strains and bacteriophage.* Phage VcA1 was grown and partially purified as described (18). Phage VcA2cts1 is a thermoinducible mutant of phage VcA2 (R.H. Hudson and W.R. Romig; unpublished results) which displayed better virion stability and plaque morphology than the parental phage (18).
2. *Mutant isolation and toxin assays.* Mutagenesis of strain RV79 with VcA1 and VcA2cts1 was performed by preparing a lysogen population from plate lysates (10^4 plaques per plate) grown at 30°C in Tryptone-yeast extract medium (18). Colonies from these lysogen populations were screened for loss of toxin production by the ganglioside filter assay (13), or for auxotrophic mutations on M63 minimal medium (19).

Toxin production in liquid culture was measured with the S49 mouse lymphosarcoma cell assay (15). Toxin antigen was measured with an enzyme linked immunosorbent assay performed essentially as described by Harris *et al.* (20). Purified cholera toxin (21) served as the standard in the above assays. Toxin production and growth *in vivo* was performed using the ligated intestinal loop model in rabbits as described (13). For each strain, approximately 10^7 cells were injected in a 5 cm intestinal loop, and 18 h later the loops were scored for fluid accumulation and for viable counts after homogenization of the tissue. Serial passage of bacteria was performed as above without intermediate culturing of the test strains (e.g., intestine to intestine transfer).
3. *DNA preparation and analysis.* DNA was prepared from bacterial cells by the method of Brenner *et al.* (22). DNA was prepared from partially purified phage by extraction with phenol equilibrated with 50mM Tris, 50mM EDTA, pH 8.0 followed by ethanol precipitation of the aqueous phase. Digestion of bacterial and phage DNA with restriction endonucleases was performed under the conditions suggested by the manufacturer.

Preparation of LT sequence probes from plasmid EWD299 (23) was performed by the methods of Moseley and Falkow (9). A 1,275 base pair Hinc II fragment and 590 base pair Eco RI-Hind III fragment were used as the LT-A and LT-B subunit sequence probes, respectively. Labelling of these LT fragments and purified VcA1 DNA with ^{32}P-dCTP (New England Nuclear, Boston, MA) to a specific activity of about 10^7 cpm/ug was performed by nick translation (24). Electrophoresis in 0.7% agarose gels and Southern blot hybridization was performed as described (9, 25).

Results

I. Mutagenic Properties of Bacteriophage VcA1 and VcA2cts1.

Early work focusing on the isolation of toxin mutations in *V. cholerae* had largely utilized nitrosoguanidine as a mutagen (11–17), which usually induces point mutations of the transition variety. Since we were interested in isolating deletion mutations in the cholera toxin structural gene, we decided to investigate other means of mutagenesis. Ultraviolet light and nitrous acid which are deletionogenic in *E. coli* (19), were in effective mutagens in *V. cholerae* due primarily to a high level of cell killing by these agents.

Recent observations in another laboratory suggested that the *V. cholerae* bacteriophage VcA1 had properties consistent with it being capable of transposition and insertion into many different sites on the *V. cholerae* chromosome (26). These properties

Table 1. Frequency and type of auxotrophic mutants induced by VcA1 and VcA2cts1.

	Frequency	*Types*
VcA1	0.6%	*ilv*, *cys*, *his*, *arg* (2), asn (2), met (2), thr (2), aro (4), undetermined (6).
VcA2cts1	0.2%	*thr*, *arg*, *thy*, undetermined (3).
RV79	<0.05%	–

suggested that VcA1 might have biological properties similar to those of bacteriophage Mu in *E. coli* (27). Consistent with this prediction, Johnson *et al.* (29) have recently observed the induction of auxotrophic mutations by VcA1. Independently, we have also observed that both VcA1 and VcA2, a serologically related, heteroimmune kappa-type vibriophage (18), were capable of inducing auxotrophic mutations coincident with lysogenization in *V. cholerae* strain RV79.

As shown in Table 1, phage VcA1 and VcA2cts1 (a thermoinducible mutant of VcA2) induced auxotrophic mutations at frequencies of about 0.6% and 0.2% respectively, in lysogen populations of RV79. The frequency of spontaneous auxotrophy in untreated cultures was below detectable levels (less than 0.05%). Furthermore, the frequency of auxotrophy induced by both of the two phages increased to about 1–2% when colonies were picked from rich media to minimal plates, suggesting that cross-feeding on the replica plates resulted in failure to identify a large fraction of auxotrophic mutants. The frequency of auxotrophy induced by lysogeny with these vibriophages is therefore comparable to that seen with bacteriophage Mu in *E. coli* (27).

The variety and multiplicity of auxotrophies observed suggests that these phages are capable of random insertion in the cholera chromosome (26, 28). We have obtained physical evidence that at least one of the two phages (VcA1) is indeed integrated at different sites in different lysogens of *V. cholerae* strain RV79. P-VcA1 DNA prepared by nick translation was used as probe in the Southern blot analysis of chromosomal DNA derived from several independent VcA1 lysogens. This analysis (data not shown) demonstrated that in different lysogens, the VcA1 prophage was integrated at different positions relative to chromosomal restriction enzyme sites (J.J. Mekalanos, unpublished results). These results are consistant with recent independent genetic evidence which indicate that the VcA1 prophage is located vary close to phage induced mutations (29). Similar analysis of VcA2cts1 mutations has been precluded by our inability to obtain enough sufficiently pure VcA2cts1 DNA to do these experiments.

The high stability observed for both VcA1 and VcA2cts1 induced mutations is consistent with their being Mu-like in nature. No detectable reversion (less than 10^{-10}) of several tested VcA1 or VcA2cts1 induced auxotrophic mutations was observed, suggesting that these vibriophages might also resemble wild-type Mu in being essentially incapable of precise excision (27).

II. Isolation of phage induced nontoxinogenic mutants of *V. cholerae*.

The high stability of the phage-induced auxotrophic mutations suggested that mutagenesis of *V. cholerae* with VcA1 and VcA2cts1 might be an excellent means of

Table 2. Toxin production by wild-type and mutant strains of *V. cholerae.*[a]

	Toxin Equivalents (μg/ml)	
Strain	*Toxicity*[b]	*Toxin Antigen*[c]
569B	15	15
M13	0.016	0.05
RM3	0.008	0.02
RM6	0.005	0.02
RV79	0.1	0.1
M7922	<0.001	<0.01
M7923	<0.001	<0.01
M7928	<0.001	<0.01
M7929	<0.001	<0.01
M7930	<0.001	<0.01

[a] Wild-type and mutant strains were grown as described (17).

[b] Determined in the S49 lymphosarcoma cell culture assay (15).

[c] Determined by enzyme-lined immunosorbant assay as described by Harris *et al.* (20).

generating stable mutations in the toxin structural gene. VcA1 and VcA2cts1 lysogen populations of *V. cholerae* strain RV79 were therefore screened for nontoxinogenic mutants by the ganglioside filter assay (13). Phenotypically nontoxinogenic clones were present in VcA1 and VcA2cts1 lysogen pools at a frequency of about 0.05%.

Five nontoxinogenic mutants were analyzed for toxin production by the S49 lymphosarcoma cell assay (15) and for toxin antigen production by an enzyme-linked immunosorbent assay (20). Table 2 shows that no toxin (<1 ng/ml) or toxin antigen (<10 ng/ml) was detectable by either assay in culture supernatant fluids of any of these five mutants. In contrast, the toxin produced by three nitrosoguanidineinduced, hypotoxinogenic mutants (M13, RM3, and RM6) of strain 569B was detected by both assays. The phage-induced nontoxinogenic mutants described here are therefore highly defective in production of active or immunologically detectable toxin gene products.

III. Identification of deletion mutations in the cholera toxin structural gene.

Moseley and Falkow (9) recently reported that ^{32}P-labelled probes derived from the cloned genes for the A and B subunits of the heat-labile enterotoxin (LT) of *E. coli* would hybridize to chromosomal fragments of *V. cholerae* DNA under conditions of reduced stringency. The *V. cholerae* restriction enzyme fragments showing homology with these LT probes were predicted to be those containing part or all of the structural gene(s) for cholera toxin. We have used these LT A and B subunit gene probes to analyze the structure of the cholera toxin gene in RV79 and in the five nontoxinogenic, phage-induced mutants described above.

Southern blot analysis of Hind III digested DNA prepared from these strains is shown in Figure 1. Unexpectedly, VcA1-induced mutant M7922 and the two VcA2cts1-induced mutants, M7928 and M7930, had lost all detectable sequences hybridizing to the LT-A subunit gene probe. In contrast, VcA1-induced mutant M7923 like the parental strain RV79, displayed a single 20 kilobase fragment that hybridized to the LT-A subunit gene probe. VcA2cts1-induced mutant M7929 had also lost most of the hybridization signal orginally present in RV79 but displayed a weak signal of about 23 kilobases in size.

A similar analysis utilizing the LT-B subunit probe produced the same hybridization signals seen using the A-subunit probe for all strains, with the exception that M7929 was completely unreactive with the LT-B subunit probe (data not shown). This result indicates that, as in the case of other strains of *V. cholerae* (9, 10), the DNA sequences coding for cholera toxin's A and B subunits are located within 20 kilobases of each other in strain RV79.

The above data indicate that mutants M7922, M7928, and M7930 have deletion mutations that have removed the structural gene(s) coding for cholera toxin. Mutant M7923 may be an insertion or deletion mutant which has inactivated a toxin regulatory element required for expression of the toxin structural gene(s). These results also suggest that none of the toxin mutants appear to have sustained a simple point insertion of either the VcA1 or VcA2cts1 prophages into a toxin structural gene. Such an insertion should have manifested itself as a change in the number and/or molecular weight of the bands hybridizing to the LT probes. Indeed, mutant M7922 appears to have lost its VcA1 prophage (assuming it was orginally lysogenized), since this strain was found to be VcA1 sensitive and negative for the VcA1 sequence in Southern blots. Perhaps the toxin gene deletion event in M7922 was associated with loss of the VcA1 prophage from this strain. In contrast, M7928, M7929, and M7930 were all lysogenic for VcA2cts1. The absence of spontaneously occurring nontoxinogenic mutants of strain RV79 (frequency less than 0.02%) argues that the toxin gene deletion events we have observed are directly related to infection and lysogenization of this strain with VcA1 and VcA2cts1.

Since all the toxin gene deletion mutants were prototrophic and grew with normal division rates, the deletion events responsible for loss of the toxin gene have been confined to DNA sequences that are nonessential for growth of these strains *in vitro*. The mutants were also motile and sensitive to a variety of *V. cholerae* typing phages, showing

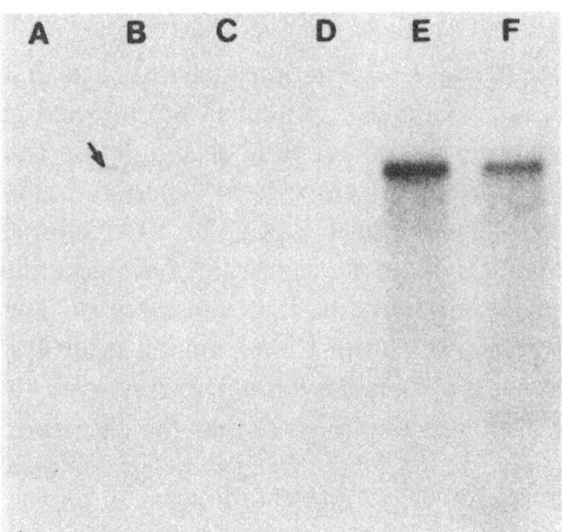

Figure 1: Autoradiograph of Southern blot analysis of *V. cholerae* DNA from wild-type and nontoxinogenic mutant strains analyzed with ^{32}P-labelled LT-A probe. (A) M7928; (B) M7929; (C) M7930; (D) M7922; (E) M7923; (F) RV79. Arrow indicates position of a weak band of 23 kilobases in size.

that no major alterations in the cell surface occurred concomitantly with the toxin gene(s) deletion mutations.

IV. Intestinal colonization by toxin gene deletion mutants.

The availability of isogenic wild-type and toxin gene deletion mutants has allowed us to begin evaluation of the role of the toxin in intestinal colonization of *V. cholerae.* The three strains known to have total toxin gene deletion mutations were selected for these studies (M7922, M7928, and M7930). With the latter two it was necessary to cure the VcA2cts1 prophage, to eliminate the temperature-sensitive phenotype from these strains. This was accomplished simply by isolating clones resistant to 42°C which had regained sensitivity to VcA2cts1 phage. Two cured derivatives were selected by this procedure (M7941 and M7942); these remained prototrophic.

Table 3. Growth of wild-type and mutant strains *in vivo.*[a]

Strain	*Cell density*[b]	*Fluid response*[c]
RV79	16	0.96
M7922	7.8	<0.05
M7941	3.6	<0.05
M7942	2.6	<0.05
569B	10	1.4

[a] Measured in the rabbit ileal loop assay as described (13).

[b] The average bacterial cell density attained in 16-18 hr expressed in colony forming units x 10^{-9} per cm intestine (three determinations). One cm of intestine was equivalent to approximately 0.4 g of tissue.

[c] The average fluid response in 16-18 hr expressed in ml per cm of intestine (three determinations).

Table 3 shows the result of serial intestinal passage of these mutant strains in rabbits. For each strain, approximately 10^7 cells were injected in a 5 cm intestinal loop, and 18 hr later the loops were scored for fluid accumulation and for viable counts after homogenization of the gut tissue. All three toxin deletion mutants multiplied 10^2-10^3 fold, attaining average cell densities *in vivo* of 2–8 x 10^9 colony forming units per cm of intestine. The three mutants induced no significant fluid accumulation, and as expected for total toxin gene(s) delection mutants, they generated no Tox+ revertants detectable by the ganglioside filter assay. In contrast, the parental strain RV79 attained only a 2 - 6 fold higher average cell density than the mutant strains, even though it induced a large secretory response. These experiments suggest that the cholera toxin gene does not play an essential role in the process of intestinal growth and survival of *V. cholerae* in this animal model.

Discussion

Mutations altering toxin production in *V. cholerae* have been previously described (11-17) but the molecular mature of these have not been determined. Analysis of VcA1 and VcA2cts1 induced nontoxinogenic mutants of *V. cholerae* strain RV79 has led us to conclude that several of these clones possess deletion mutations in the structural gene encoding cholera toxin. This represents the first definitive demonstration of a deletion mutation of the cholera toxin structural gene. As such, it will eventually allow us to map genetically the location of the toxin gene in *V. cholerae* strain RV79. The demonstration that the toxin deletion mutants show no major defect in their ability to grow in the laboratory, or in the gut of susceptible animals, argues strongly that the cholera toxin gene is nonessential in *V. cholerae*. Growth defects in other toxin mutant strains, which have been attributed to possible physiological roles for the toxin in *V. cholerae* (16), may more likely represent pleiotropic effects of repeated mutagenesis with nitrosoguanidine. Several of the mutations we characterized proved to be complete deletions of the toxin gene. However, we also found that one mutant (M7929) retained some DNA homologous to the LT-A subunit probe but had lost all sequences hybridizing to the LT-B subunit probe. Thus, the methods described here can also be used to construct partial deletions of the toxin gene. Whether these methods are generally applicable to other strains of *V. cholerae* would depend mainly on the sensitivity of these strains to VcA1 and VcA2cts1.

The induction of toxin deletion mutations by the two vibriophages used in this study is curious in light of the fact that at least one of them (VcA1) is likely to induce mutations via the insertion of its DNA into random sites on the *V. cholerae* chromosome (26, 29). The event responsible for deletion of the toxin gene(s) concomitant with VcA1 and VcA2cts1 lysogenization is at present unclear. Daniell *et al.* (30) have reported that a approximately 15% of *lacZ* mutants induced by phage Mu in *E. coli* repressed for *lac* expression were deletion mutations. In contrast, Mu lysogenization concomitant with active transcription of the *lac* operon, produced either by induction with IPTG or via the use of a *lacI* constitutive mutant, increased the frequency of deletions observed among *lac* Z mutations to 57% and 93%, respectively. These investigators concluded that active transcription of *lac* reduced the ability of Mu to insert its DNA into the *lacZ* gene but did not alter its ability to cause complete deletions of this gene. Since RV79 produces toxin in the phage growth medium used here, active transcription of the toxin gene(s) may have similarly interfered with the point insertion of the VcA1 and VcA2cts1 phages into this gene(s). As with Mu and *lac*, phage-induced deletion events would then become responsible for a large fraction of the mutations isolated. Experiments are in progress to examine the influence of transcription on the target specificity of VcA1 and VcA2cts1 in *V. cholerae*.

Finally, we have characterized several mutant strains of *V. cholerae* which might have practical value as prototype live oral cholera vaccines. Strains previously developed for this purpose have displayed instability *in vivo*, as evidenced by the appearance of toxinogenic revertant clones in the stools of animals (12, 13) and human volunteers (31). The toxin gene deletion mutants described here would be predicted to be stably attenuated since they have lost the genetic information encoding the toxin. In addition, these deletion mutants can colonize the mucosal surface and multiply within the gut in the rabbit ligated-loop model. It remains to be determined whether the mutants will colonize as well in other animal models in which the gut remains open (e.g., chinchillas [32]). Colonization of man by such mutants should induce protective, secretory IgA antibody that would inhibit bacterial attachment to the mucosa, motility, chemotaxis, protease and neuraminidase activity, and other undefined activities required by *V. cholerae* for virulence (33, 34, 35). Antitoxin, of course, would not be induced by these mutants. However, it role in immunity to cholera is currently in dispute and it may actually be of little protective value (36). Moreover, in the event that an antitoxin response is a significant component of immunity to cholera, the methods described her could be used to construct strains with deletion mutations in the A subunit gene, but which continue to produce the highly antigenic B subunit of the toxin (16). Alternatively, the deletion mutants we have characterized could also serve as hosts for the reintroduction of an altered *tox* gene (constructed by recombinant DNA methods) that codes for an immunologically crossreactive nontoxic analogue of the toxin.

We thank S.R. Johnson, B.C.S. Liu, and W.R. Romig for the communication of their unpublished results. We also thank J. Felton for the critical reading of the manuscript and J. Segal for its preparation. J.J.M. thanks J. Costa for his help in settingup the Southern blotting method.

This investigation was supported by U.S. Public Health Service Grants R22 AI-13938 to J.R.M. and AI-10885 to S.F. from the National Institute of Allergy and Infectious Disease. It was also supported by contract DADA 17-72-C2149 to S.F. from the U.S. Army Research and Development Command. J.R.M. is recipient of Public Health Service Career Development Award AI00146 from the National Institute of Allergy and Infectious Diseases. J.J.M. is recipient of Postdoctoral Fellowship 1F32 AI05816-01A1 from the National Institute of Allergy and Infectious Disease. S.L.M. is recipient of National Research Service Award AI-07149.

REFERENCES

1. Collier, R. J. and Mekalanos, J. J. (1980) *Multifunctional Proteins* eds. Bisswanger, H. and Schmincke-Ott E. (John Wiley and Sons, New York), pp. 261-291.
2. Gill, D. M. (1976) Biochemistry **15**, 1242-1248.
3. Cuatrecases, P. (1973) Biochemistry **12**, 3577-3581.
4. Cassel, D. and Pfeuffer, T. (1978) Proc. Natl. Acad. Sci. U. S. A. **75**, 2669-2673.
5. Gill, D. M. and Meren, R. (1978) Proc. Natl. Acad. Sci. U. S. A. **75**, 3050-3054.
6. Clements, J. D., Yancey, R. J. and Finkelstein, R. A. (1980) Infect. Immun. **29**, 91-97.
7. Gill, D. M., Evans, D. J. and Evans, D. G. (1976) J. Infect. Dis. **133**, S103-S107.
8. Vasil, M. I., Holmes, R. K. and Finkelstein, R. A. (1975) Science **187**, 849-850.
9. Moseley, S. L. and Falkow, S. (1980) J. Bact. **144**, 444-446.
10. Kaper, J. B., Moseley, S. L. and Falkow, S. (1981) Infect. Immun. **32**, 661-667.
11. Howard, B. D. (1971) Nature **230**, 97-99.
12. Finkelstein, R. a., Vasil, M. L., Holmes, R. K. (1974) J. Infect. Dis. **129**, 117-123.
13. Mekalanos, J. J., Romig, W. R. and Collier, R. J. (1978) Proc. Natl. Acad. Sci. U. S. A. **75**, 941-945.
14. Mekalanos, J. J., Sublett, R. and Romig, W. R. (1979) J. Bact. **139**, 859-865.
15. Ruch, F. E., Murphy, J. R., Graf, L. H. and Field, M. (1978) J. Infect. Dis. **137**, 747-755.
16. Honda, T. and Finkelstein, R. A. (1979) Proc. Natl. Acad. Sci. U. S. A. **76**, 2052-2056.
17. Mekalanos, J. J. and Murphy, J. R. (1980) J. Bact. **141**, 570-576.
18. Gerdes, J. C. and Romig, W. R. (1975) J. Virol. **15**, 1231-1238.
19. Miller, J. H. (1972) Experiments in molecular genetics. Cold Spring Harbor Laboratory, Cold Spring Harbor, New York.
20. Harris C. C., Yolken, R. H., Krokan, H. and Hsu, I. C. (1979) Proc. Natl. Acad. Sci. U. S. A. **76**, 5336-5339.

21. Mekalanos, J. J., Collier, R. J. and Romig, W. R. (1978) Infect. Immun. **20**, 552-558.
22. Brenner, D. J., Fanning, G. R., Johnson, K. E., Citarella, R. V. and Falkow, S. (1969) J. Bact. **98**, 637-650.
23. Dallas, W. S., Gill, D. M. and Falkow, S. (1979) J. Bact. **139**, 850-858.
24. Maniatis, T., Jeffry, A. and Kleid, A. G. (1975) Proc. Natl. Acad. Sci. U. S. A. **72**, 1184-1188.
25. Southern, E. M. (1975) J. Mol. Biol. **98**, 503-517.
26. Johnson, S. R. and Romig, W. R. (1981) J. Bact. **146**, 632-638.
27. Bukhari, A. I. (1976) Ann. Rev. Genet. **10**, 389-412.
28. Parker, C. D., Gauthier, D., Tate, A., Richardson, K. and Romig, W. R. (1979) Genetics **91**, 191-214.
29. Johnson, S. R., Liu, B. C. S. and Romig, W. R. (1981) *in press.* FEMS Letters **11**, 13-16.
30. Daniell, E., Roberts, R. and Abelson, J. (1972) J. Mol. Biol. **69**, 1-8.
31. Woodward, W. E., Gilman, R., Hornick, R., Libonati, J. and Cash, R. (1975) Proc. 11th Joint Conference on Cholera. N. I. H., p. 330.
32. Blackman, U., Graboff, S. R., Haag, G. E., Gottfeld, E., and Pickett, M. J. (1974) Infect. Immun. **10**, 1098-1104.
33. Freter, R. (1972) Infect Immun. **6**, 134-141.
34. Guentzel, M. N., and Berry, L. J. (1975) Infect Immun. **11**, 890-897.
35. Baselski, V. S., Upchurch, S., and Parker, C. D. (1978) Infect. Immun. **22**, 181-188.
36. Cash, R. A., Music, S. I., Libonati, J. P., Craig, J. P., Pierce, N. F. and Hornick, R. B. (1974) J. Infect. Dis. **130**, 325-333.

Advances in Research on Cholera and Related Diarrheas, eds., S. Kuwahara, N. F. Pierce, 193–199.

PLASMIDS AND THE HEAT-LABILE ENTEROTOXIN OPERON ORIGINATING IN A CLINICALLY ISOLATED STRAIN SEROTYPE 078:H11 OF ENTEROTOXIGENIC *ESCHERICHIA COLI*

Tatsuo Yamamoto[1], Takeshi Yokota[1], and Shogo Kuwahara[2]

Department of Bacteriology, School of Medicine, Juntendo University 2-1-1, Hongo, Bunkyo-ku, Tokyo, Japan[1], and Department of Microbiology, School of Medicine, Toho University, Tokyo[2]

Enterotoxigenic *Escherichia coli* is one of the important agents of diarrheal illness, whose pathogenic mechanism is well understood; it adheres to the epithelial cells of the small intestine and produces enterotoxins such as heat-labile toxin (LT) and heat-stable toxin (ST). Evans *et al.* (3) showed that a clinically isolated enterotoxigenic *E. coli* H10407 (serotype 078:H11) specifies both colonization factor antigen I (CFA/I) and enterotoxin (LT and ST) production. These genetic traits of the pathogenicity are plasmid-born (2-4, 6, 7, 9). A 56-60 million molecular weight plasmid specifying CFA/I and ST production, a 42 million molecular weight plasmid specifying "LT production" and a cryptic plasmid with 3.7-3.8 million molecular weight have been identified in *E. coli* H10407. In this communication, we show that *E. coli* H10407 carries at least four distinct species of plasmid: a CFA/I-and ST-coding plasmid, an LT- and ST-coding plasmid, a self-transmissible plasmid and a cryptic plasmid(s). Thus, *E. coli* H10407 carries two ST genes. We also analyzed the LT region, and succeeded in construction of recombinant plasmids which produced toxoids of LT.

Plasmids of E. coli H10407.

(i) Isolation of plasmids. In a previous experiment (11), we isolated an LT- and ST-coding plasmid (pJY11) from *E. coli* H10407, which was kindly provided by M. Ohashi and originated from the laboratory of D. G. Evans. In such experiments, we also obtained an ampicillin (Ap) resistant, self-transmissible plasmid (designated pJY12), which carried an Ap transposon Tn*1*, from the above *E. coli* H10407 carrying RP4.

In this experiment, pJY12 was introduced into another *E. coli* H10407 which was kindly provided by Y. Takeda and originated from the laboratory of S. Donta. The Ap resistant *E. coli* H10407 strain (designated *E. coli* TY201) was mated with *E. coli* 20S0, and the LT- or CFA/I-coding plasmid of *E. coli* TY201 was transferred into *E. coli* 20S0 by mobilization with pJY12. As expected, the LT- and CFA/I-coding plasmids (designated pJY11b and pCS1, respectively) tested all specified ST production as well. Next, pJY12 was eliminated from the clones, and *E. coli* 20S0 carrying pJY11b or pCS1 was obtained.

Table 1. Plasmids of *E. coli* H10407 (serotype 078:H11).

Plasmid designation	Relevant phenotype	Molecular weight X 10^6 (size in kb)
pCS1	CFA/I, ST	62 (94)
pJY11	LT, ST	42 (64)
pTRA1	Tra	42 (64)
a cryptic plasmid (s)	–	3-4

In a separate experiment, pMK1 (ColE1 carrying a kanamycin, Km, transposon Tn*5*, 10) was introduced into *E. coli* H10407, which was the same strain as that used for the isolation of pJY11b or pCS1, by genetic transformation. The resultant Km resistant *E. coli* H10407 strain (designated *E. coli* TY202) was mated with *E. coli* 20S0. Many of the Km resistant transconjugants carried a self-transmissible plasmid (designated pTRA1) in addition to pMK1. The pMK1 plasmid was eliminated from the clones, and *E. coli* 20S0 carrying pTRA1 was obtained. This method is based on the fact that pJY12 can mobilize the ColEl plasmid as well. pJY12 was shown to be pTRAl::Tn*1*.

(ii) Characterization of plasmids. Molecular weight and restriction endonuclease digestion pattern of the plasmids were analyzed (Table 1 and 2). pJY11 and pJY11b were identical in molecular weight as well as in *Eco*RI or *Pst*I digestion patterns, indicating that *E. coli* H10407 does actually carry the LT- and ST-coding plasmid (pJY11). As reported with the "LT-coding plasmid" of *E. coli* H10407 by McConnell *et al.* (6) and Willshaw *et al.* (9), pJY11 (and pJY11b) manifested T5 (and T6) phage restriction as well. Although pJY11 and pTRA1 were not distinguishable from each other in molecular weight, the *Eco*RI and *Pst*I digestion patterns were quite different.

Table 2. Restriction endonuclease-generated fragments and the toxin genes.

Restriction endonuclease	Plasmid	Fragment*[1]
*Eco*RI	pCS1	25.5, 19, 16, 12, 9.4, 8.3 (ST), 2.1, 1.4, 0.74
	pJY11	26, 25 (LT-B), 13 (LT-A, ST), 0.67
	pTRA1	23.5, 16, 10.5, 8.5, 3.0, 2.8, 0.64, 0.58, 0.46
*Pst*I*[2]	pCS1	1.7 (ST)
	pJY11	5.3 (LT), 1.5 (ST)

*1 Numbers represent fragment size in kb. ST, LT, LT-A and LT-B indicate fragments carrying the ST gene, the LT genes (*toxA, B*), the LT subunit A gene (*toxA*) and the LT subunit B gene (*toxB*), respectively. Detailed location of the *toxA* and *toxB* genes is described in Fig. 1.

*2 Only fragments carrying the toxin genes are indicated.

Toxin gene-containing fragments were identified by cloning techniques; the LT and ST genes of pJY11 were described previously (11, 12, 14). It can be noted that the ST^+ *Eco*RI and *Pst*I fragments of pJY11 differ from those of pCS1. In addition, a heterogeneity of ST levels of the two ST genes was confirmed (Table 3). The ST gene of pCS1 produced approximately 16-32 times as much ST as did that of pJY11. Preliminary experiments showed that although both STs were completely neutralized by excess amounts of antiserum to STa (kindly provided by Y. Takeda), the pJY11-ST was more resistant to the serum treatment than the pCS1-ST. These results clearly indicate that the two ST genes (and probably the two ST peptides) are different.

(iii) Conjugal transfer among E. coli K12 strains. Although pJY12 (pTRA1::Tn*1*) was transferred at a frequency of 10^{-1} to 10^{-2} (transconjugants per donor) among *E. coli* K12 strains, no conjugal transfer was observed with pJY11 or pCS1 or even with the derivative plasmids carrying drug resistance markers. When pJY12 was present in pCS1 or pJY11 containing *E. coli* cells, transfer of pCS1 and pJY11 was observed at a frequency of 65% and 3% of the pJY12 transfer, respectively. Simultaneous transfer of the three plasmids from *E. coli* cells carrying pCS1, pJY11 and pJY12 was demonstrated at a frequency of 1.5% of the pJY12 transfer. Similar results were obtained even when pTRA1 was employed instead of pJY12.

The LT operon (toxA, B). pJY11 has four *Eco*RI sites. The LT operon (11, 14) straddles the two *Eco*RI fragments, E1 and E2 (Fig. 1). The entire LT region was cloned as a 5.3 kb *Pst*I fragment (Pa-Pb) or as a 2.4 kb *Hind*III fragment (Ha-Hc). The *Xba*I site was located within LT subunit A gene (*toxA*) (12, 14). When the Pa-Ea region or the E2 fragment was cloned into a cloning vehicle, the recombinant plasmids (e. g., pJY23) produced a smaller LT-A derivative (designated LT-A′) with 24,500 molecular weight (12, 14). This unambiguously indicates that the C terminus of *toxA* is located downstream (right side in Fig.1) of the *Eco*RI site. A lack of a promoter for LT subunit B gene (*toxB*) is evident from the experiments (14) in which the *toxB* fragment (Hb-Hc in Fig. 1) is cloned, in both orientations, into a downstream region within an operon on a vector, as shown in Fig. 2.

Products of cloned LT regions synthesized in *E. coli* minicells were analyzed on

Table 3. Comparison of ST levels as detected in suckling mice of *E. coli* 20S0 carrying pJY11, pCS1 and their cloned ST genes.

Plasmid	Relative ST activity (fold) in the culture supernatant.
pJY11	1
pCS1	16
pJYS101	8
pJYS201	256

pJYS101 is a pBR322 recombinant plasmid carrying the 1.5 kb ST^+ *Pst*I fragment of pJY11(11), and pJYS201 is a pBR322 recombinant plasmid carrying the 1.7 kb ST^+ *Pst*I fragment of pCS1.

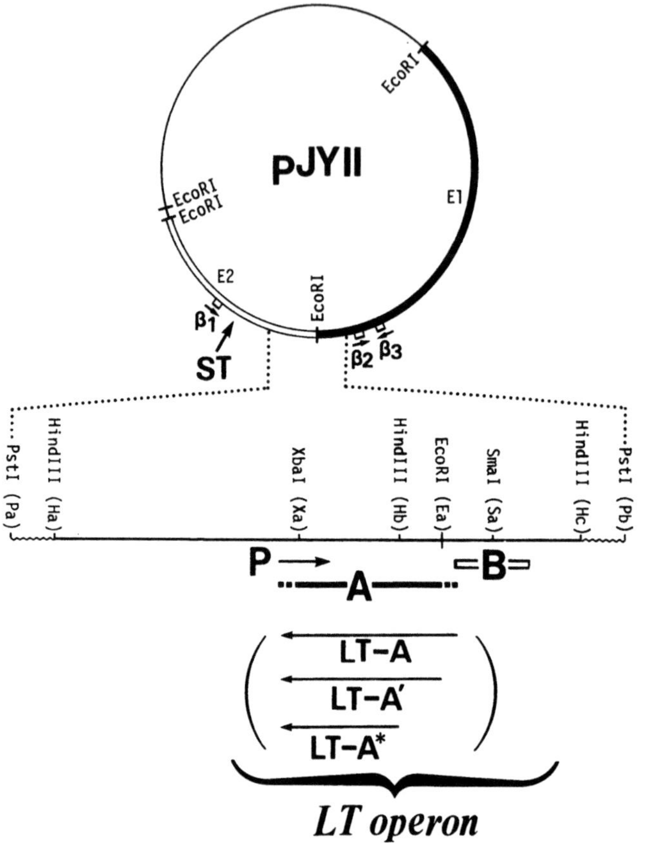

Fig. 1. Location of the LT operon (*toxA, B*) on pJY11. P, A and B represent the LT promoter, the LT subunit A gene (*toxA*) and the LT subunit B gene (*toxB*), respectively. The arrow adjacent to P indicates the direction of transcription. LT-A′ and LT-A* are peptides produced from deleted *toxA* lacking carboxy terminal regions. E1 and E2 represent *Eco*RI fragments of 25 kb and 13 kb, in size, respectively. β represents repeating sequences.

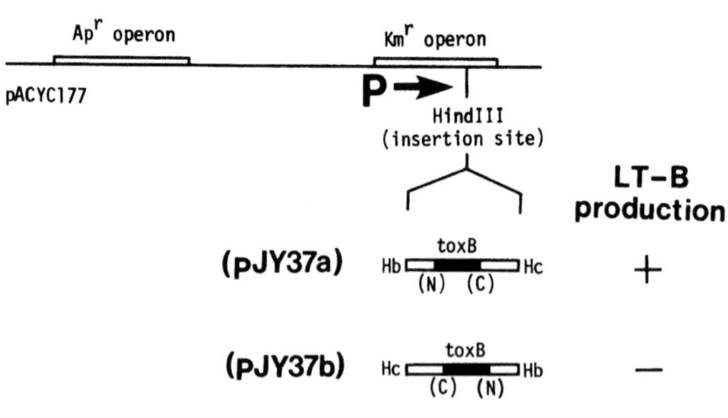

Fig. 2. Evidence for a lack of a promoter for *toxB.* N and C represent the amino and carboxy termini of *toxB*, respectively. Restriction endonuclease cleavage sites Hb and Hc are shown in Fig. 1.

SDS-polyacrylamide gels, by using antisera to cholera toxin subunit A or B (12). As shown in Fig. 3, only three peptides were confirmed as major products from the LT operon: LT-A with 26,800-27,000 molecular weight, LT-Al (?) with 22,000 molecular weight and LT-B with 11,800-12,000 molecular weight. LT-B was apparently larger than cholera toxin subunit B (11,590 molecular weight, 5).

The LT region of a porcine *E. coli* has also been shown to be a polycistronic operon (1).

Recombinant plasmids which produce toxoids of LT. LT-B and LT-A derivatives, lacking the ability to form LT activity but retaining immunological properties, are toxoids of LT which we hope may be useful as vaccines to protect against diarrheal diseases caused by enterotoxigenic (LT^+) *E. coli* or possibly even by *V. cholerae*. We succeeded in the construction of recombinant plasmids which produce the intact LT-B as well as LT-A* (12, 14), as summarized in Table 4. Although LT-A′ (Fig. 1) formed LT activity in the presence of LT-B, LT-A* (Fig. 1 and Table 4) did not form LT activity even in the presence of LT-B. Recently, Spicer *et al.* (8) reported the location of the LT-Al and LT-A2 loci of the LT operon originating in a porcine *E. coli*. If our LT-A1 and LT-A2 loci (originating in a human *E. coli*) are similar to those of porcine *E. coli* origin, LT-A* may lack the LT-A2 portion. LT-A* is coded for by the LT promoter. In contrast, LT-B is coded for by a promoter on a vector such as that of the Km resistance operon or the chloramphenicol (Cm) resistance operon.

Trans-complementation of the LT genes. Two separate LT genes (*toxA* and *toxB*), which were placed on two compatible plasmids, did produce LT (12), as shown in Fig. 4 (2). This suggests that clustering of the two genes is not essential for the synthesis of LT.

Release of LT subunits by E. coli. In *E. coli*, a majority of LT synthesized is cell-associated. However, a small portion (approximately 10%) is released into the culture

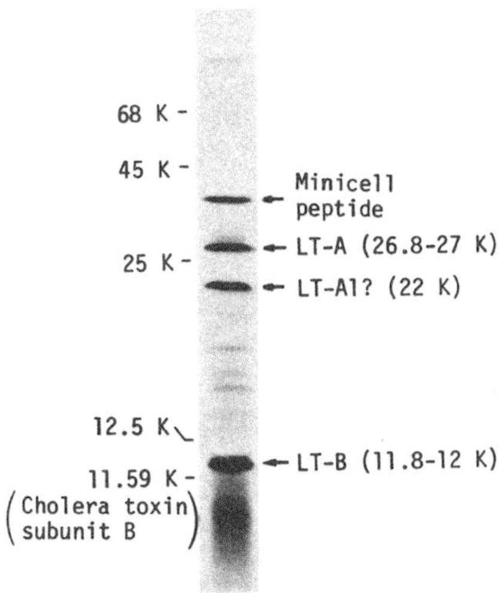

Fig. 3. Products of the LT operon in *E. coli* minicells. ^{14}C-labeled products of pJYL2299 (a pBR322 recombinant plasmid carrying the 5.3 kb LT^+ *Pst*I fragment, Pa-Pb in Fig. 1), synthesized in *E. coli* minicells, were analyzed on SDS-polyacrylamide (15%) gels.

Table 4. Toxoid-producing recombinant plasmids.

Toxoid production	Plasmid	Cloned region	Cloning vector	The cloned LT region is transcribed by using a promoter of:
LT-B	pJY24	Ea-Pb	pBR322	(pBR322)
	pJY26	E1	pGA24	(pGA24)
	pJY35	Ea-Hc	pGA24	the Cm resistance operon of pGA24
	pJY37a	Hb-Hc	pACYC177	the Km resistance operon of pACYC177
LT-A*	pJY34b	Ha-Hb	pACYC177	the LT operon

Abbreviations for restriction endonuclease cleavage sites are described in Fig. 1. LT-B production from pJY37a is also shown in Fig. 2.

supernatant. By using cloned LT genes as shown in Table 4 and reference (14), we showed that (i) LT-B is released into the culture supernatant; (ii) LT-A or its derivatives (LT-A′ and LT-A*) can not be released into the culture supernatant; (iii) introduction of LT-B into the LT-A (or LT-A′) producing *E. coli* cells results in release of LT-A (or LT-A′); however, (iv) LT-A* can not be released into the culture supernatant even in the presence of LT-B (13). Based upon these observations, we speculate a release-mechanism of LT subunits (and LT) as summarized in Fig. 4. Thus, LT-A (and LT-A′) requires LT-B to be released into the culture supernatant. With LT-A*, we speculate that the peptide can not

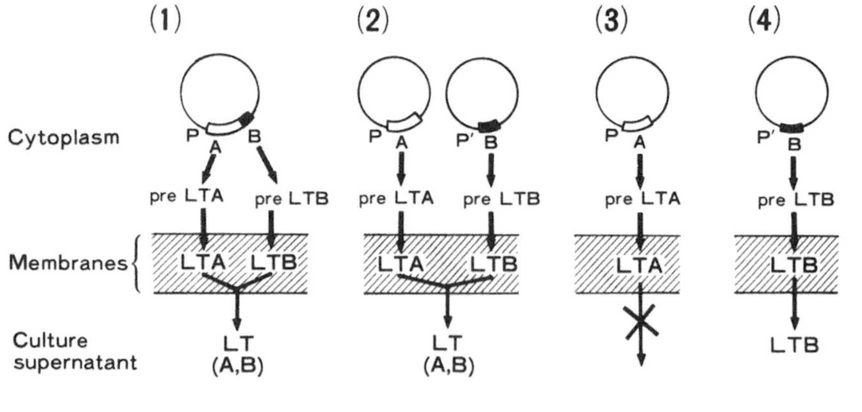

Fig. 4. A possible model for the release of LT subunits and LT by *E. coli*. A, B, P and P′ represent the LT subunit A gene (*toxA*), the LT subunit B gene (*toxB*), the LT promoter and a promoter on a vector, respectively. preLT-A and preLT-B are precursors (signal peptide + mature LT-A or mature LT-B) to LT-A and LT-B, respectively. (1) *E. coli* cell with a plasmid carrying the entire LT operon; (2) *E. coli* cell with two compatible plasmids carrying the two LT genes on each plasmid; (3) *E. coli* cell with a plasmid carrying a cloned *toxA*; and (4) *E. coli* cell with a plasmid carrying a cloned *toxB*.

interact with LT-B (presumably because it lacks the LT-A2 portion) and therefore remains inside the cells. Recently, we analyzed the signal sequence of *toxB*. This sequence is considered to be necessary for secretion of LT-B through the bacterial inner membrane.

REFERENCES

1. Dallas, W. S., D. M. Gill, and S. Falkow. 1979. Cistrons encoding *Escherichia coli* heat-labile toxin. J. Bacteriol. **139**:850-858.
2. Evans, D. G., and D. J. Evans, Jr. 1978. New surface-associated heat-labile colonization factor antigen (CFA/II) produced by enterotoxigenic *Escherichia coli* of serotype 06 and 08. Infect. Immun. **21**:638-647.
3. Evans, D. G., R. P. Silver, D. J. Evans, Jr., D. G. Chase, and S. L. Gorbach. 1975. Plasmid-controlled colonization factor associated with virulence in *Escherichia coli* enterotoxigenic for humans. Infect. Immun. **12**:656-667.
4. Glyes, C., M. So, and S. Falkow. 1974. The enterotoxin plasmids of *Escherichia coli*. J. Infect. Dis. **130**:40-49.
5. Kurosky, A., D. E. Markel., J. W. Peterson, and W. M. Fitch. 1977. Primary structure of cholera toxin β-chain: a glycoprotein hormone analog? Science **195**:299-301.
6. McConnell, M. M., H. R. Smith, G. A. Willshaw, S. M. Scotland, and B. Rowe. 1980. Plasmids coding for heat-labile enterotoxin production isolated from *Escherichia coli* 078: a comparison of their properties. J. Bacteriol. **143**:158-167.
7. Smith, H. R., A. Cravioto, G. A. Willshaw, M. M. McConnell, S. M. Scotland, R. J. Gross, and B. Rowe. 1979. A plasmid coding for the production of colonization factor antigen I and heat-stable enterotoxin in strains of *Escherichia coli* of serogroup 078. FEMS Microbiol. Letts. **6**: 255-260.
8. Spicer, E. K., W. M. Kavanaugh, W. S. Dallas, S. Falkow, W. H. Konigsberg, and D. E. Schafer. 1981. Sequence homologies between A subunits of *Escherichia coli* and *Vibrio cholerae* enterotoxins. Proc. Natl. Acad. Sci. U. S. A. **78**:50-54.
9. Willshaw, G. A., E. A. Barclay, H. R. Smith, M. M. McConnel, and B. Rowe. 1980. Molecular comparison of plasmids encoding heat-labile enterotoxin isolated from *Escherichia coli* strains of human origin. J. Bacteriol. **143**:168-175.
10. Yamamoto, T, and T. Yokota. 1980. Construction of a physical map of a kanamycin (Km) transposon, Tn*5*, and a comparison to another Km transposon, Tn*903*. Mol. Gen. Genet. **178**: 77-83.
11. Yamamoto, T., and T. Yokota. 1980. Cloning of deoxyribonucleic acid regions encoding a heat-labile and heat-stable enterotoxin originating from an enterotoxigenic *Escherichia coli* strain of human origin. J. Bacteriol. **143**:652-660.
12. Yamamoto, T., and T. Yokota. 1981. *Escherichia coli* heat-labile enterotoxin genes are flanked by repeated deoxyribonucleic acid sequences. J. Bacteriol. **145**:850-860.
13. Yamamoto, T., and T. Yokota. 1982. Release of heat-labile enterotoxin subunits by *Escherichia coli*. J. Bacteriol. **150**:1482-1484.
14. Yamamoto, T., T. Yokota, and A. Kaji. 1981. Molecular organization of heat-labile enterotoxin genes originating in *Escherichia coli* of human origin and construction of heat-labile toxoid-producing strains. J. Bacteriol. **148**:983-987.

Advances in Research on Cholera and Related Diarrheas, eds., S. Kuwahara, N. F. Pierce, 201–206.

EXPRESSION OF PLASMID GENES ENCODING *ESCHERICHIA COLI* HEAT-LABILE ENTEROTOXIN IN BACTERIAL STRAINS WITH DIFFERENT GENETIC BACKGROUNDS

Roger J. Neill and Randall K. Holmes

Department of Microbiology, Uniformed Services University of the Health Sciences, Bethesda, Maryland

Although rapid progress has been made in understanding the ecology and molecular biology of Ent plasmids and in defining the structure, mode of action, and immunochemistry of *E. coli* heat-labile enterotoxin (LT), little is known concerning the factors that control the synthesis of this plasmid-coded toxin. In an initial effort to identify genetic factors that might control production of LT, we have compared the expression of plasmid-coded LT structural genes in bacterial with known regulatory mutations and in strains representing a variety of bacterial genera found among the aerobic gram negative flora of the intestinal tract. The role of each of the following genetic variables has been evaluated: defects in cyclic-3′, 5′-adenosine monophosphate (cAMP) metabolism in *E. coli,* a chromosomal hypertoxinogenic (*htx*) mutation in *E. coli,* and genera other than *Escherichia* as hosts for Ent plasmids.

Cyclic AMP was reported to stimulate the *in vitro* synthesis of LT coded by the porcine *E. coli* plasmid P307 (3). Moreover, cAMP metabolism has been implicated in the *in vivo* control of heat-stable toxin (ST) (6), and structural genes for ST and LT are often found on the same plasmids. To test the possibility that cAMP was required for the synthesis of LT *in vivo,* the porcine *E. coli* plasmid pCG86 was transferred by conjugation into isogenic *E. coli* strains containing wild type or deletion mutant alleles of adenylate cyclase (Δ *cya*) or cAMP receptor protein (Δ *crp*) genes. These strains were grown at 37°C with or without 1 mM cAMP. Samples were taken during exponential growth, and cell-associated LT was measured by a solid-phase radioimmunoassay (1).

The results presented in Table 1 show that neither the Δ *cya* nor Δ *crp* mutations prevented synthesis of LT. The addition of cAMP had no effect on the yields of toxin in the wild type and Δ *crp* strains, although the 1 mM cAMP supplement was sufficient to affect other cAMP dependent functions. The reduced growth rate characteristic of *cya* strains was reversed by the cAMP supplement. In addition, the rate of induction of β-galactosidase in the wild type strain was stimulated two-fold in comparison with unsupplemented conditions (data not shown). The reason for the high specific activity of LT in the Δ *cya* strain without added cAMP is unknown.

Table 1. Production of the heat-labile enterotoxin coded by plasmid pCG86 in *E. coli* strains with mutations affecting cyclic AMP metabolism.

Bacterial strain	Genotype	Generation time (minutes)		Cell-associated LT[a)] (μg/mg protein)	
		–cAMP	+cAMP[b)]	-cAMP	+cAMP[b)]
CA8000(pCG86)	wild type	50	46	1.37	1.41
CA8306(pCG86)	Δ*cya*	80	55	4.53	1.28
CA8445.1(pCG86)	Δ*crp*	90	90	1.20	1.49

a) In bacteria harvested from log phase cultures (A_{590} ≅1.0–1.7). LT antigen in sonic extracts was measured by a solid phase radioimmunoassay (1). Concentrations of LT were calculated by using a standard curve determined with purified LT.

b) 1 mM cAMP added to culture at time of inoculation in glucose-Syncase medium containing thiamine (10 μg/ml) and tetracycline (25 μg/ml).

In conclusion, neither cAMP nor the cAMP binding protein is essential for synthesis of LT in *E. coli* strains harboring pCG86.

Previous work in our laboratory (5) has described hypertoxinogenic (*htx*) mutants of *E. coli* KL320 (pCG86). The *htx* mutations in these strains were chromosomal. One of the *htx* mutants (HE12) was charcterized by a 3-6 fold increase in the amount of cell--associated LT and a slight increase in the amount of extracellular LT. We wished to determine if the hypertoxinogenic phenotype reflects a specific interaction of *htx* with plasmid pCG86 or if it is also expressed with other Ent plasmids.

For this purpose Ent plasmids labeled with antibiotic resistance markers were transferred by conjugation into strain HE22, a derivative of HE12 cured of pCG86. As controls, the same plasmids were introduced into the parent strain KL320. Ent plasmids were derived from *E. coli* strains collected from patients from widely separated geographic locations. In addition, the LT structural gene from the porcine *E. coli* plasmid P307 cloned into a multicopy plasmid (EWD299) was transformed into HE22 and into KL320. Cells were grown in glucose-Syncase medium containing additional necessary nutrients and appropriate selective antibiotics. A solid phase radioimmunoassay was used to measure extracellular LT in samples of the culture fluid and cell-associated LT in sonic lysates of bacterial cells.

The results of these studies are summarized in Table 2. The yields of cell-associated LT were approximately 2-3 times greater in HE22 strains than in KL320 control strains harboring each of the plasmids tested. Extracellular LT represented 1% or less of total LT for all strains tested except those containing the multicopy plasmid EWD299. In strains with EWD299 extracellular LT represented 5-10% of the total toxin produced.

These results indicate that the effect of this *htx* mutation is not specific for pCG86. Therefore, the *htx* mutation may affect a common regulatory mechanism involved in the expression of LT genes coded by many different LT plasmids.

Antigenically related heat-labile enterotoxins have been detected in a variety of gram-negative enteric bacteria. In *E. coli* the structural genes for LT are often located on

Table 2. Effect of an *E. coli htx* mutation on production of LTs coded by Ent plasmids from several different sources.

Plasmid[a)]	Characteristics	Yield of LT (μg/ml culture)			
		E. coli KL320 (wild type)		*E. coli* HE22 (*htx*)	
		Cell-associated	Extra-cellular	Cell-associated	Extra-cellular
pCG86	LT, ST; Porcine	1.8	<0.03	4.3	0.06
EWD299	Cloned LT; Porcine	11.6	1.2	23.3	1.2
pTD2Tc	LT; Human	1.3	<0.03	3.6	<0.03
TP213Tc	LT, ST; Human	0.58	<0.03	0.97	<0.03
TP235Km	LT; Human	3.3	<0.03	9.0	0.07
TP236Tc	LT; Human	4.2	0.04	7.1	0.04
TP237Tc	LT; Human	1.5	<0.03	4.0	<0.03
TP252Km	LT; Human	2.2	<0.03	4.2	<0.03

a) These plasmids are described in the following references: pCG86 (7); EWD299 (2); and TP213Tc, TP235Km, TP236Tc, TP237Tc, and TP252Km (8). pTD2 is a plasmid from *E. coli* Throop D (4) that was identified in our laboratory. pTD2Tc is pTD2 with transposon Tn10 and was constructed for this study.

conjugative or nonconjugative plasmids. We wished to determine if conjugative LT plasmids from *E. coli* can be transferred into a variety of other enteric bacteria and if their LT genes can be expressed in the new bacterial hosts.

We selected the porcine *E. coli* plasmid pCG86 and the human *E. coli* plasmid TP237Tc for these studies. Each plasmid was transferred from an *E. coli* K12 donor into appropriate recipient strains by conjugation on a gar plates. The recipients, none of which produced heat-labile enterotoxin before plasmid transfer, included a prototrophic strain of *S. typhimurium* (LT2) and a purine and thiamine auxotroph derived from it (*purF*-145), avirulent derivatives of *S. sonnei* and *S. flexneri*, and clinical isolates of *E. cloacae*, *K. pneumoniae*, and *C. freundii*. Concentrations of LT in sonic lysates of transconjugant bacterial cells and culture fluids were measured by solid phase radioimmunoassays.

Each plasmid was successfully transferred by conjugation into all of the recipient strains. Each plasmid directed synthesis of LT in all of the recipient strains (Table 3). Using the Y-1 adrenal cell assay, enterotoxin activity was also detected in culture supernatants and in sonic lysates of bacterial strains harboring either LT plasmid. Thus, LT was produced in biologically active form in each of the transconjugant strains.

The amounts of LT produced by these transconjugant bacterial strains varied over a range of approximately 100 fold. Only *S. typhimurium* produced more LT than *E. coli*. The amounts of toxin produced by specific bacteria harboring plasmid pCG86 or TP237Tc were usually similar except for *S. flexneri* and the *purF*145 derivative of *S. typhimurium*. *S. flexneri* with plasmid pCG86 produced much more LT than *S. flexneri* with TP237Tc, whereas the reverse was observed in *purF*145. These results suggest

Table 3. Production of plasmid-coded LT by several different enteric bacteria after introduction of plasmid pCG86 or TP237Tc.

Bacterial species[a)]	Yield of LT (μg/ml culture)[b)]			
	pCG86		TP237Tc	
	Cell–associated	Extra–cellular	Cell–associated	Extra–cellular
Escherichia coli	2.0	0.03	1.8	<0.03
Enterobacter cloacae	0.63	0.07	0.54	<0.03
Shigella sonnei	0.13	<0.03	0.15	<0.03
Shigella flexneri	1.1	0.25	0.10	0.05
Citrobacter freundii	0.07	<0.03	0.14	<0.03
Klebsiella pneumoniae	0.04	<0.03	0.04	<0.03
Salmonella typhimurium LT2	4.3	0.06	11.6	0.30
*Salmonella typhimurium pur*F145	0.10	<0.03	4.4	0.14

a) Control experiments demonstrated that these strains did not produce LT or cross-reacting antigens that were detectable in our solid phase radioimmunoassay for LT.

b) In stationary phase, overnight cultures grown in supplemented glucose-Syncase medium containing tetracycline HCl at 5 μg/ml. Bacterial growth was similar for all strains tested (final $A_{590} \cong 5$-8).

functional differences in control of LT production by these plasmids, although the mechanisms for the observed differences are not known.

Because LT and cholera enterotoxin (CT) are closely related with respect to structure and mode of action, we wished to investigate the possibility that their biosynthesis might be subject to control by the same regulatory functions if both toxins were produced by a single bacterial host. As an approach for studying this question, plasmid pCG86 was transferred by conjugation from *E. coli* into the classical *V. cholerae* strain 569B Inaba and two of its hypotoxinogenic mutant derivatives M13 and M14. Although transfer of pCG86 from *E. coli* into *V. cholerae* by conjugation occurred at very low frequencies, the plasmid was stably maintained in *V. cholerae* 569B for at least 30 generations of growth in liquid culture in the absence of antibiotics.

CT and LT were measured with two different competitive binding radioimmunoassays that permitted independent quantitation of the two toxins in each cell extract or culture fluid (5). Cultures were grown in glucose-Syncase medium at 37°C. Media for strains containing pCG86 were supplemented with 5 μg/ml tetracycline-HCL. The results of these experiments are summarized in Table 4. No LT antigen was produced by the parent strain 569B, but LT was synthesized in the derivative strain 569B(pCG86). Approximately 99% of LT produced in *E. coli* remains cell-associated. In contrast, more than 95% of the CT produced by *V. cholerae* 569B is extracellular. In cultures of *V. cholerae* 569B(pCG86), more than 95% of the LT was found to be extracellular, similar to the distribution of CT. The presence of pCG86 had no significant effect on the total amount of CT produced by 569B(pCG86), however, it did alter the distribution of CT, causing a larger proportion to remain cell-associated. The mechanism by which pCG86 affects the distribution of CT in 569B(pCG86) has not been determined.

V. cholerae M13 is a severely hypotoxinogenic mutant of 569B. The *tox*-1 allele in M13 determines the hypotoxinogenic phenotype and is linked to the *his*-1 locus. The *tox*-1 mutation had no effect on production or localization of LT. Therefore, the regulatory function altered in M13 does not control the synthesis of pCG86-coded LT. In contrast, the presence of pCG86 in M13 was associated with a slight increase in CT production, suggesting that the plasmid may provide a function which partially suppresses *tox*-1.

Compared to the parent 569B, the mutant M14 produces less CT, most of which remains cell-associated. The amount of LT produced by M14(pCG86) was similar to 569B(pCG86), but the mutation in M14 caused approximately half of the LT to remain cell-associated. Thus, the genetic defect in strain M14 has similar effects on release of CT and LT, suggesting that these two enterotoxins may be secreted by a common pathway in *V. cholerae.*

In summary we have assessed the role of a variety of genetic variables on the expression of the plasmid-coded structural genes for LT:

1) Neither cAMP nor cAMP binding protein is essential for synthesis *in vivo* of LT coded by plasmid pCG86.

2) A chromosomal mutation (*htx*) increases yields of LT coded by a variety of Ent plasmids from *E. coli* strains of human and porcine origin, suggesting a common regulatory feature controlled by the *htx* locus.

3) The porcine plasmid pCG86 and the human plasmid TP237Tc were transferred into a number of gram-negative enteric bacteria in which the LT genes were expressed. This wide host range of Ent plasmids from *E. coli* may have significant ecologic implica-

Table 4. Genetic control of CT and LT production in *V. cholerae* strains harboring plasmid pCG86.

Bacterial strain	Yield of CT[a] (μg/ml culture)		Yield of LT[a] (μg/ml culture)	
	Cell–associated	Extra–cellular	Cell–associated	Extra–cellular
569B	0.01	7.5	<0.004	<0.04
569B(pCG86)	0.28	9.9	0.08	1.6
M13	<0.004	<0.004	<0.004	<0.004
M13(pCG86)	<0.004	0.02	0.07	1.4
M14	1.0	0.24	<0.004	<0.04
M14(pCG86)	2.2	0.52	0.6	0.5

a) Specific assays for CT and for LT were performed with competitive-binding radioimmunoassay methods described previously (5). Under the conditions used there were no detectable cross-reactions between CT and LT. Limits of sensitivity (<0.04 or <0.004 μg/ml) were determined by the use of either unconcentrated or concentrated samples of culture supernatant or sonic extracts of bacteria in individual experiments.

tions. Enterotoxigenic bacteria of many genera have been associated with diarrheal diseases both in humans and in animals, but the role of plasmids in controlling production of heat-labile enterotoxins and the functions that determine dissemination of specific plasmids in these bacteria require further study.

4) Finally, *V. cholerae* strains harboring the Ent plasmid pCG86 were able to synthesize both CT and LT. Most of the LT synthesized by 569B(pCG86) was extracellular, in contrast to the cell-associated localization of LT in most other bacteria included in our study. Secretion of LT was affected in a *V. cholerae* mutant that was altered in the ability to secrete CT, but the *tox*-1 mutation that controls CT synthesis had no effect on LT production. These results suggest that LT and CT may share a common pathway of secretion in *V. cholerae* but their biosynthesis is not controlled by identical regulatory elements.

We are indebted to M. McConnell, W.K. Maas, D. Kopecko, R.A. Finkelstein, B. Ames, and J. Beckwith for many of the bacterial strains used in this study.

This study was supported in part by Public Health Service research grant 5 R22 AI14107 from the National Institute of Allergy and Infectious Diseases and in part by the Uniformed Services University of the Health Sciences. The opinions expressed are the private views of the authors and should not be construed as official or as necessarily reflecting the views of the Department of Defense.

REFERENCES

1. Bramucci, M. G., E. M. Twiddy, W. B. Baine, and R. K. Holmes. 1981. Isolation and characterization of hypertoxinogenic (*htx*) mutants of *Escherichia coli* KL320(pCG86). *Infect. Immun.* **32**: 1034-1044.
2. Dallas, W. S., D. M. Gill, and S. Falkow. 1979. Cistrons encoding *Escherichia coli* heat-labile toxin. *J. Bacteriol.* **139**:850-858.
3. Dorner, F., C. Hughes, G. Nahler, and G. Hogenauer. 1979. *Escherichia coli* heat-labile Enterotoxin: DNA directed *in vitro* synthesis and structure. *Proc. Nat. Acad. Sci. USA.* **76**:4832-4836.
4. Finkelstein, R. A., M. J. Vasil, J. R. Jones, R. A. Anderson, and T. Barnard. 1976. Clinical cholera caused by enterotoxigenic *Escherichia coli. J. Clin. Microbiol.* **3**:382-384.
5. Holmes, R. K., M. G. Bramucci, and E. M. Twiddy. 1980. Genetic and biochemical studies of heat-labile enterotoxin of *Escherichia coli*, p. 189-201. *In* Proceedings of the 15th Joint Conference on Cholera. NIH Publication 80-2003. National Institutes of Health, Bethesda, MD.
6. Martinez-Cadena, M. G., L. M. Guzman-Verduzco, H. Stieglitz, and Y. M. Kupersztoch-Portnoy. 1981. Catabolite repression of *Escherichia coli* heat-stable enterotoxin activity. *J. Bacteriol.* **145**:722-728.
7. Mazaitis, A. J., R. Maas, and W. K. Maas. 1981. Structure of a naturally occurring plasmid with genes for enterotoxin production and drug resistance. *J. Bacteriol.* **145**:97-105.
8. McConnell, M. M., H. R. Smith, G. A. Willshaw, S. M. Scotland, and B. Rowe. 1980. Plasmids coding for heat-labile enterotoxin production isolated from *Escherichia coli* 078: Comparison of properties. *J. Bacteriol.* **143**:158-167.

Advances in Research on Cholera and Related Diarrheas, eds., S. Kuwahara, N. F. Pierce, 207–216.

DETECTION OF ENTEROTOXIGENIC *ESCHERICHIA COLI* BY COLONY DNA HYBRIDIZATION: USE OF A SECOND HEAT STABLE ENTEROTOXIN GENE PROBE

Steve L. Moseley, Peter Echeverria, and Stanley Falkow

Department of Medical Microbiology, Stanford University, School of Medicine, Stanford, California, and Armed Forces Research Institute of Medical Sciences, Bangkok, Thailand

Introduction

Enterotoxigenic *Escherichia coli* (ETEC) pathogenic for humans and animals produce two classes of enterotoxins. The heat labile toxin (LT) is of high molecular weight, consists of two subunits, is functionally, structurally and genetically related to the enterotoxin of *Vibrio cholerae*, and is homologous among different strains of LT producing *E. coli* (5, 14). Its mechanism of action involves the activation adenylate cyclase (8). The heat stable toxin (ST) is of low molecular weight and acts by stimulating guanylate cyclase (9).

Biological, biochemical and genetic evidence suggests that STs from different strains of *E. coli* represent a heterologous group of toxins. There are at least two distinct types of ST (3, 10). STa is methanol soluble and is active in the infant mouse model. STb is methanol insoluble, and is not active in the infant mouse model, but can be detected in ligated pig ileal loops. A gene encoding STa from an *E. coli* strain of bovine origin has been shown to reside on a bacterial transposon, and its nucleotide sequence has been determined (23, 24). An isolated fragment of DNA from a homologous porcine *E. coli* gene encoding ST was utilized as a genetic probe in a study attempting to identify ETEC from patients with diarrhea by colony DNA hybridization (16). While all LT producing strains were identified by an LT gene probe, many STa producing strains (as determined by the infant mouse assay) did not possess DNA homologous to the ST gene probe, suggesting the existence of heterologous genes encoding STa. Similar results were subsequently reported by So *et al.* (21).

This study describes the isolation of a gene encoding STa from a human isolate of *E. coli*, and preliminary use of this gene as a probe for the detection of ETEC in patients with diarrhea in Thailand.

MATERIALS AND METHODS

Bacterial strains and plasmids. E. coli 153837-2 is a strain of *E. coli* which produces ST and was isolated from the diarrheal stool of a human in Bangladesh. *E. coli* strain HB101 and plasmid pBR322 have been described previously (2). EWD299 is a recombinant plasmid encoding LT production, and has been described previously (5). pRIT10036 is a recombinant plasmid encoding ST production, and has been described previously under the designation CLS-2 (16). This plasmid consists of a *Pst* I insert of approximately 1.1 megadaltons from a porcine strain of *E. coli* into pBR322 (11). pSLM004 is described in the present study.

ETEC were isolated from children and adults with diarrhea at Children's Hospital, and Bamrasnaradura Infectious Disease Hospital, Bangkok, Soongnern Hospital, Soongnern, and Peace Corps volunteers at four different locations in rural Thailand. Strains from animals were isolated in a rural village in Soongnern district. Ten lactose positive colonies, selected from a MacConkey agar culture of stool, had been stored on nutrient agar slants and tested for LT and ST in the Y-1 adrenal cell (19), and suckling mouse assays (6).

Plasmid DNA isolation. Plasmid DNA was isolated as described by So *et al.* (22).

Restriction of DNA. Restriction endonucleases were obtained from New England Biolabs, Inc., Boston, MA. Digestion of DNA was carried out under conditions specified by the supplier.

Ligation and transformation of DNA. Bacteriophage T4 DNA ligase was a gift from Walter Dallas, Cetus Corporation, Berkeley, Ca. Ligation reaction conditions were 20mM Tris, pH 7.5, 10mM $MgCl_2$, 5mM NaCl, 10 mM dithiothreitol, and 40 mM adenosine triphoshate. pBR322 DNA (approximately 0.01 ug) was cleaved with the appropriate restriction endonucleases and mixed with the DNA fragments to be ligated at an approximate ratio of one pBR322 molecule to 100 insertion fragments. The ligation was carried out in a reaction volume of 10 ul at 0 C for two hours. The entire ligation mixture was used to transform *E. coli* K12 HB101. Two ml of an overnight stationary culture of HB101 in L broth were diluted into fresh L broth and incubated for 100 min at 37 C with agitation. The cells were washed once in 20 ml 10mM $CaCl_2$, 10mM MOPS (Sigma), pH 6.5. The cells were resuspended in 2 ml 75mM $CaCl_2$, 10mM MOPS pH 6.5, 0.5% glucose. The entire ligation mixture was then added to 0.2 ml of the cell suspension, and the cells kept on ice for 45 min. The transformation mixture was then incubated at 42 C for 10 min. A volume of 0.5 ml fresh L broth was added and the mixture was incubated for 2 hours at 37 C. The mixture was then plated on media containing the appropriate antibiotic.

Southern blot hybridization analysis of restricted DNA. The procedure of Southern (25) was used with modifcation (15). Plasmid DNA (0.1 ug) was digested with the appropriate restriction endonuclease, and the resulting fragments separated by electrophoresis in 2% agarose. The DNA was transferred to nitrocellulose and hybridized to radiolabeled probe DNA under conditions of low stringency as described previously (15). The formamide concentration in the hybridization solution was 25%.

Nucleotide sequence analysis. The method of Maxam and Gilbert (13) was used. pSLM004 DNA was cleaved with *Eco* RI+*Hind* III and the resulting fragments separated by electrophoresis in a 10% polyacrylamide gel. The fragment containing the ST gene was isolated by electroelution from the acrylamide followed by DEAE-cellulose chromatography (DE-52, Whatman). This fragment and smaller fragments obtained by restriction of this fragment were analyzed as shown in Fig. 1. The 5 'termini were labeled with gamma-^{32}P-ATP (New England Nuclear) by a T4 polynucleotide kinase reaction (Behtesda

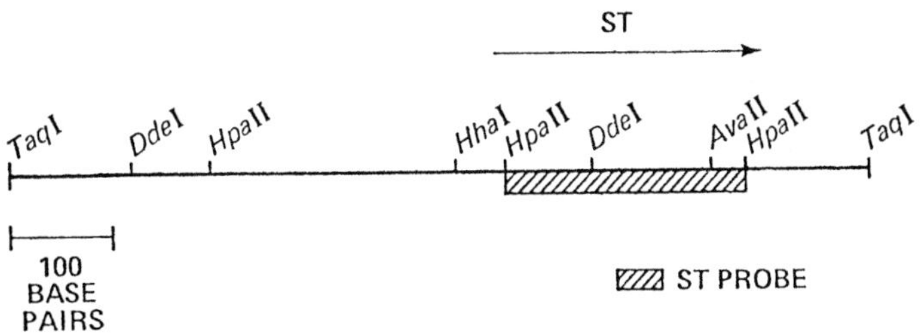

Figure 1. Restriction map of the *Taq* I insert of pSLM004. The *Hpa*II fragment used as a hybridization probe was also subjected to sequence analysis, with portions of the adjacent fragments. Polarity of the ST gene was determined by sequence analysis.

Research Laboratories) (13). The 3 'termini were labeled with alpha-^{32}P deoxynucleotide triphosphates (New England Nuclear) by *an E. coli* DNA polymerase I-Klenow fragment reaction (Bethesda Research Laboratories).

Colony DNA hybridization. Preparation of probe DNA for LT and ST genes has been described previously (16). The gene encoding ST from a porcine isolate is referred to as ST-P. A probe for a heterologous ST gene of human origin, ST-H, consisted of a 215 base pair *Hpa* II fragment of pSLM004 (Fig. 1). This fragment was obtained by cleavage of pSLM004 DNA with *Eco* RI+*Hind* III, isolation of the ST gene-containing fragment as described above, cleavage with *Hpa* II, and subsequent isolation of the appropriate fragment. The probe DNA was labeled with alpha-^{32}P deoxynucleotides (New England Nuclear) by nick translation (12).

Colony hybridization with growth from spotted stools was performed as described previously (16), with the exception that the nitrocellulose filters were neutralized with 1M ammonium acetate, 0.02 M NaOH, rather than with Tris-NaCl.

Comparison of standard assays with spotted stool colony DNA hybridization for the detection of ETEC. Stools or rectal swabs were collected from children less than two years of age with watery diarrhea of less than 72 hours duration at Children's Hospital, Bangkok during one week in April 1981. Specimens were cultured simultaneously on MacConkey agar and spotted in triplicate on nitrocellulose filters. After overnight incubation at 37 C, ten lactose-positive colonies were selected from the MacConkey plate and tested within two weeks of isolation for LT with the Y-1 adrenal cell and ST with the suckling mouse assays. The nitrocellulose filters were hybridized with the LT, ST-P and ST-H probes.

RESULTS

Construction of a recombinant plasmid expressing ST encoded by a gene from a human isolate of ETEC (ST-H). Purified plasmid DNA from *E. coli* strain 153837-2 was cleaved with the restriction endonuclease *Bam* HI, and the resulting fragments ligated to *Bam* HI-cleaved pBR322 plasmid DNA. The ligation mixture was used to transform *E. coli* strain HB101. Ampicillin-resistant transformants were screened for sensitivity to tetracycline, and ampicillinresistant, tetracycline-sensitive colonies were screened for the production of ST by the infant mouse assay. One transformant was found to produce ST. Restriction analysis of plasmid DNA from this strain revealed that a *Bam* HI Fragment of aproximately 1.9 kilobase pairs had been inserted into pBR322. This recombinant plasmid was designated pSLM003.

Demonstration of partial homology between the ST-H gene and a gene encoding ST isolated from a porcine ETEC (ST-P). The existence of heterologous ST genes was demonstrated by the failure of an ST-P gene probe to detect homologous DNA squences in some ST producing strains of *E. coli* (16). These hybridization studies were carried out under conditions of high stringency, so that only highly homologous DNA was detected. pSLM003 was examined for partial homology to a gene encoding ST-P by hybridization under conditions of reduced stringency, allowing detection of sequences of incomplete homology. The ST-P probe consisted of a 157 base pair *Hinf* I-generated DNA fragment isolated from plasmid pRIT10036 as described previously (16). The ST-P probe was radiolabelled with ^{32}P and hybridized under conditions of low stringency to *Taq* I-restricted pSLM003 DNA which had been separated by electrophoresis in a 2% agarose slab gel and transferred to nitrocellulose. The results are shown in Fig. 2. Among the inserted sequences from strain 153837-2, partial homology was detected between the ST-P probe and a *Taq* I fragment of pSLM003 of approximately 840 base pairs (size data not shown).

Nucleotide sequence of the gene encoding ST-H. The 840 base pair *Taq* I fragment containing partial homology with the ST-P probe was recloned into the *Cla* I site of pBR322. This plasmid was designated pLSM004. *E. coli* strain HB101 (pSLM004) was found to produce ST as detected in the infant mouse assay. The ST-encoding *Taq* I fragment of pSLM004 was mapped with regard to several restriction endonucleases by analysis of partial and double digests (Fig. 1). The four *Hpa* II fragments were isolated, spotted on nitrocellulose, and hybridized to the ST-P probe at low stringency. A *Hpa* II

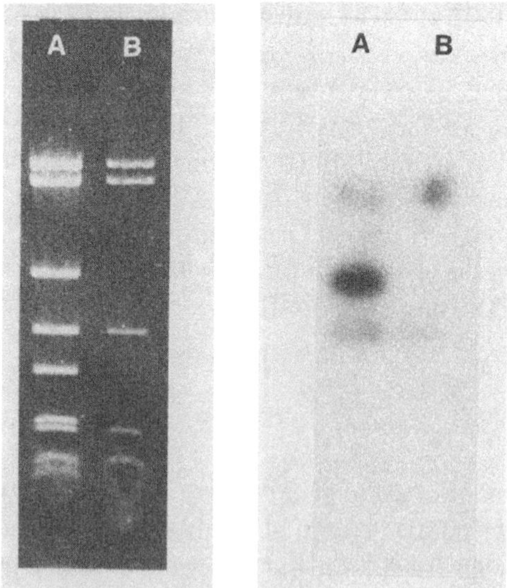

Figure 2. Partial homology between ST-P and ST-H genes. Plasmid DNA was digested with *Taq*I, transferred to nitrocellulose and hybridized to the ST-P probe under conditions of reduced stringency. Left: Agarose gel electrophoresis of *Taq*I digested plasmid DNA. Right: Autoradiograh of blot after hybridization to ST-P probe. (A) pSLM003, (B) pBR322.

fragment of approximately 215 base pairs displayed partial homology to the ST-P probe. This fragment and portions of the adjacent fragments were subjected to nucleotide sequence analysis. Analysis of the nucleotide sequence (to be published elsewhere) revealed a gene encoding 72 amino acids. The gene is preceded by a 5 base pair sequence encoding a ribosome binding site (20) and ends with a translational stop codon (TAA). The stop codon is followed by a 15 base pair region of dyad symmetry encoding a transcript with a predicted secondary structure characteristic of a transcriptional terminator (1).

Homology of Thai ETEC with DNA probes. Twenty-four LT+ST+, 17 LT+ST− and 22 LT−ST+ *E. coli* were examined for homology with the LT, ST−P and ST−H DNA probes. The sources of these isolates are given in Table 1. All 41 LT+ST+ and LT+ST− *E. coli* were homologous with the LT probe. Five *E. coli*, not included in the analysis, were initially considered to be positive in the Y-1 adrenal cell assay, but were not identified with the LT probe. Sterile culture filtrates of the *E. coli* isolates caused rounding of Y-1 adrenal tissue cultures which was not inhibitd by *V. cholera* human convalescent serum (NIH Research Reagent Cat. No. G005-501-572). These isolates presumably produced a cytotoxin rather than LT.

All of the LT+ST+ and LT−ST+ *E. coli* were detected with either the ST-P and/or the ST-H probes. Among LT+ST+ isolates, eleven were homologous with ST-P, eleven with ST-H and two with both. Of 22 LT−ST+ *E. coli* examined, 13 were detected with the ST−H, six with the ST−P and three with both probes.

Table 1. Source of Enterotoxigenic *Escherichia coli* isolated from individuals with diarrhea.

No. of ETEC	Source	
24 LT+ST+	10+	Children, Children's Hospital, Bangkok
	6	Children, Soongnern Hospital, Soongnern
	4	Adults, Bamrasnaradura Hospital, Nonthaburi
	3	Peace Corps volunteers, rural Thailand
	1	Adult, Soongnern Hospital, Soongnern
17 LT+ST−	7	Children, Children's Hospital, Bangkok
	3	Children, Soongnern Hospital, Soongnern
	3	Adults, Soongnern Hospital, Soongnern
	2	Peace Corps volunteers, rural Thailand
	1	Buffalo, Soongnern
	1	Pig, Soongnern
2 LT−ST+	10	Adults, Bamrasnaradura Hospital, Nonthaburi
	5	Children, Soongnern Hospital, Soongnern
	3	Adults, Soongnern Hospital, Soongnern
	2	Children, Children's Hospital, Bangkok
	1	Peace Corps volunteers, rural Thailand
	1	Pig, Soongnern

\+ Number of individuals from whom ETEC were isolated (one ETEC/individual)

Genes homologous with either the ST–P or ST–H probes were distributed among isolates of LT+ST+ *E. coli* from patients from differnt sources. LT–ST+ *E. coli*, homologous with ST–H but not ST–P, were only found in individuals with diarrhea in rural Thailand. The difference between the proportion of LT–ST+ *E. coli* homologous with the ST–P probe from rural vs urban Thiland (9/9 vs 4/12) was significant (p=0.03 [Fisher's exact test]), Table 2. All seven of the LT–ST+ strains isolated from children with diarrhea in urban or rural Thailand were homologous with only the ST-H probe.

Detection of ETEC infections in patients with diarrhea. One hundred and ten stools were examined simultaneously with the DNA hybridization assay and by testing ten lactose-positive colonies for LT and ST. The same eight children were found to be infected with ETEC by both methods. Two children were infected with LT+ST+, five with LT+ST–, and one with LT–ST+ *E. coli.* The number of ETEC detected by the Y-1 adrenal and suckling mouse assays varied from one to ten. In three stools the LT probe detected DNA coding for LT when only one of ten isolates tested from the stool culture was positive in the Y-1 adrenal cell assay. The ST–H probe which detected all of the stools containing ST producing colonies was also able to detect a stool in which only one of ten colonies tested produced ST. None of the stools were positive with the ST–P probe. An example of these results is shown in Fig. 3.

DISCUSSION

The present study has confirmed the existence of heterologous genes encoding STa and reports the isolation and characterization of one of these genes from a strain of *E. coli* of human origin. So and McCarthy (24) have reported the isolation and sequence

Table 2. Homology of ST–P and ST–H with LT+ST+ and LT–ST+ *E. coli* isolated from patients with diarrhea in urban and rural Thailand.

Source	No. of ETEC isolated	No. of colonies homologous with ST–P	ST–H	ST–P + ST–H
Urban †	14 LT+ST+	5	8	1
	12 LT–ST+	5	4	3
Rural △	10 LT+ST+	6	3	1
	9 LT–ST+	0	9	0
Total	24 LT+ST+	11	11	2
	21 LT–ST+	5	13	3

LT+ = produce heat-labile toxin
ST+ = produce heat-stable toxin
† Urban refers to metropolitan Bangkok
△ Rural refers to specimens collected from Thais in Soongnern and American Peace Corps volunteers at U'thong, Pranburi, Inburi, and Sri Prachan

One LT–ST+ *E. coli* isolated from a pig in rural Thailand was only homologous with ST–P.

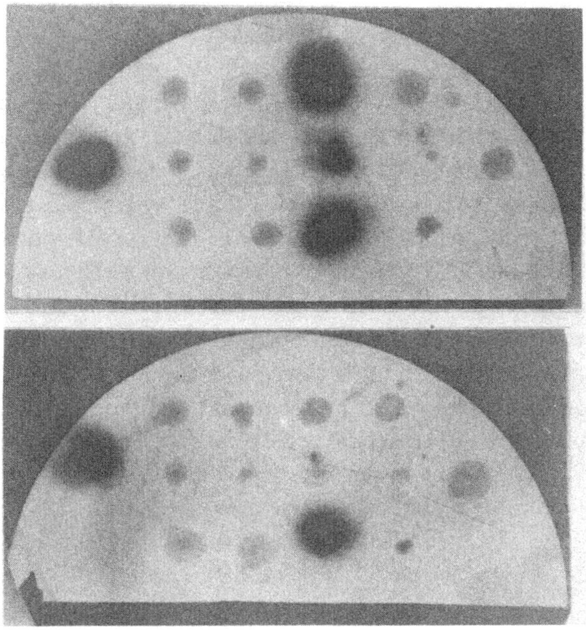

Figure 3. Colony hybridization with bacterial growth from directly spotted diarrheal stools. The nitrocellulose filters have been overlayed with the resulting autoradiographs. Top: four of 14 stools were detected with the LT probe. Bottom: a duplicate filter of the same fouteen stools after hybridization with the ST-H probe. Two were detected.

determination of a gene encoding STa from a strain of bovine origin. An apparently homologous STa gene from an *E. coli* strain of porcine origin has also been isolated, and the product of that gene was characterized using an *in vitro* transcription-translation system (11). The nucleotide sequence and gene product analyses suggest that the ST molecule is initially synthesized as a 72 amino acid precursor of a molecular weight of 8,000, and is subsequently processed to a protein of a molecular weight of 5,000 (11, 24). However, biochemical studies on ST preparations have resulted in reports of an ST from a porcine strain consisting of 33 amino acids with a molecular weight of 3,580 (18) and an ST from a human strain consisting of 18 amino acids of a molecular weight of 1,972 (4). Recent studies utilizing isolated fragments of DNA encoding ST as genetic hybridization probes have demonstrated that STa and STb are genetically distinct, and furthermore that there appear to be at least two geneticaly distinct forms of STa (16, 21).

Hybridization studies with a porcine ST gene probe (ST–P) homologous to the bovine gene sequenced by So and McCarthy (24) reveals that the ST–H gene isolated in the present study shares partial homology with the bovine-porcine ST gene (Fig. 2). Nucleotide sequence analysis of the ST–H gene (sequence to be published elsewhere) confirms the evolutionary relatedness of the two genes. All changes that occur between the two genes are nucleotide substitutions, there are no deletions or insertions. There are a total of 67 nucleotide changes out of a total of 216 nucleotides in each gene, resulting in an overall sequence divergence of 31%. These changes result in 29 amino acid changes out of 72 amino acids encoded by each gene, with most changes (18/29) being non-conservative.

The divergence observed between the bovine ST and ST–H genes is in marked contrast to the observed evolutionary divergence of other genes, such as the genes of the *trp* operon of *E. coli* and *Salmonella typhimurium* (17). Among these genes, the majority of nucleotide differences are synonymous with regard to amino acid sequence, and the majority of amino acid changes that do occur are conservative. It would therefore appear that the constraints demanded by the biological function of ST on the structure of the molecule are not as severe as with other proteins, such as the products of the *trp* operon. The result is a greater degree of divergence within a smaller gene among members of a single species than is observed within a larger gene among different species. The high degree of divergence is also evidenced by the amino acid sequence of an 18 amino acid peptide which displays the full biological activity of STa (4). While this sequence is very similar to that predicted by the bovine ST gene nucleotide sequence, it does differ in two amino acids. Furthermore, preliminary nucleotide sequence data of yet another gene encoding ST from a human *E. coli* isolate suggests the existence of an ST very similar, but not identical to that encoded by the ST–H gene described here (7).

Despite the divergence observed between the genes encoding ST–P and ST–H, a great deal of structural similarity between their products remains. Analysis of the ST–P gene products suggests that the initial protein is processed for trans-membrane transport (11). The nucleotide sequence of the homologous bovine ST gene supports this interpretation, predicting that 13 of the first 18 amino acids are hydrophobic, and that this portion of the molecule is related to other signal peptides involved in transmembrane transport of a protein (24). A similar structure is predicted for the ST–H product, with 13 of the first 19 amino acids hydrophobic. Another similarity is the number and position of cysteines. The identical position of seven cysteins in the two gene products suggests that similar intramolecular associations may take place in the two molecules resulting in similar secondary structures. The greatest degree of homology among the two genes occurs between codons 53 and 68, suggesting that this region may play an essential role in the function of the molecule. This interpretation is supported by the existence of the 18 amino acid peptide with ST activity corresponding to codon positions 55-72 (4).

The preliminary data reported here regarding use of the ST–H gene as a probe for the detection of ETEC suggests that most ST producing *E. coli* which are not detected by the ST–P gene probe are in fact detected by the ST–H gene probe. All LT+ST+, ST+ST–, and LT–ST+ *E. coli* isolated in Thailand were detected with either the LT, ST–P, or ST–H probes. As in a previous study (16) the LT probe was homologous with all LT producing *E. coli* suggesting that the structural genes coding for LT are homologous in strains from a variety of sources. So *et al.* (21) employing a probe from an ST gene homologous to the ST–P used in this study, identified 27% (3/11) of LT+ST+ and 72% (21/29) of LT–ST+ *E. coli*. Moseley *et al.* (16), using a similar probe for ST, detected 11% (3/26) of LT+ST+ and 71% (12/17) of LT–ST+ *E. coli*. These results indicated that at least two genes code for ST synthesis as detected in the suckling mouse assay. By using both ST–P and ST–H probes, all strains which were positive in the suckling mouse assay were identified. Among 24 LT+ST+ *E. coli* examined in this study, 50% were homologous with ST–P, while the rest were detected with the ST–H probe.

Two were homologous with both. 27% of 22 LT–ST+ *E. coli* were detected with the ST–P probe, 59% with the ST–H probe, and 14% with both. Although only 63 ETEC isolated from five populations were examined, these results indicate that the three probes employed could identify all ETEC which were positive in the Y-1 adrenal and suckling mouse assays in Thailand.

The observation that some strains of ETEC were detected with both the ST–P and ST–H probes indicate that these strains possess two genes encoding ST production. Preliminary data (S. Moseley, unpublished observations) suggest that in some of these strains, the two genes reside on different plasmids. The use of the ST gene probes should therefore be of value in the study of the molecular epidemiology and disemination of plasmids encoding enterotoxins.

By examining ETEC from different sources in Thailand with the ST–P and ST–H probes, it was recognized that this technique would be useful in defining the epidemiology of ETEC. LT–ST+ strains in rural Thailand were homologous with only the ST–H and not the ST–P probe while strains in Bangkok were homologous with either one or the other, or both. Furthermore, all LT–ST+ *E.coli* isolated from children were homologous with ST–H. In Bangladesh, (16) 70% of LT–ST+ *E. coli* compared with 27% of strains from Thailand were homologous with the ST–P probe ($p<.001$) (chi-square). Although the number of strains examined were not sufficient to draw firm conclusions, examining more strains in different populations and environments should help clarify the epidemiology of this enteric pathogen.

The DNA hybridization assay should serve as a useful tool in defining the epidemiology of ETEC infections. A major advantage of this assay is that it differentiates between the two heterologous genes encoding ST which, in addition to serotyping of the *E. coli*, offers another epidemiological marker.

In the future, we plan to use the DNA hybridization assay to characterize the genomes coding for enterotoxin, and to identify environmental sources of ETEC in an attempt to define the epidemiology of ETEC infections in Thailand.

REFERENCES

1. Adhya, S. and M. Gottesman. (1978). Control of transcription termination. Ann. Rev. Biochem. **47**:967-996.
2. Bolivar, F. and K. Backman. (1979). Plasmids of *Escherichia coli* as cloning vectors. In R. Wu (Ed.), *Methods in enzymology,* Vol. 68, p. 245-267. Academic Press, New York.
3. Burgess, M. N., R. J. Bywater, C. M. Cowley, N. A. Mullan, and P. M. Newsome. (1978). Biological evaluation of a methanol-soluble, heat-stable *Escherichia coli* enterotoxin in infant mice, pigs, rabbits, and calves. Infect. Immun. **21**:526-531.
4. Chan, S. -K., and R. A. Gianella. (1981). Amino acid sequence of heat stable enterotoxin produced by *Escherichia coli* pathogenic for man. J. Biol. Chem. **256**:7744-7746.
5. Dallas, W. S., D. M. Gill, and S. Falkow. (1979). Cistrons encoding *Escherichia coli* heat-labile toxin. J. Bacteriol. **139**:850-858.
6. Dean, A. G., Y. C. Ching, R. G. Williams, and L. B. Harden. (1972). Test for *Escherichia coli* enterotoxin using infant mice: application in a study of diarrhea in children in Honolulu. J. Infect. Dis. **125**:407-411.
7. DeWilde, M., M. Ysebaert, and N. Harford. (1981). DNA sequence at the ST_{A2} enterotoxin gene from an *E. coli* strain of human origin. In S. B. Levy, R. C. Clowes, and E. L. Koenig (Eds.), *Molecular Biology, Pathogenicity, and Ecology of Bacterial Plasmids,* p. 596. Plenum Press, New York.

8. Evans, D. J., L. C. Chen, G. T. Curlin, and D. G. Evans. (1972). Stimulation of adenyl cyclase by *Escherichia coli* enterotoxin. Nature N. Biol. **236**:137-138.
9. Field, M., L. Graf, W. Laird, and P. Smith. (1978). Heat stable enterotoxin of *Escherichia coli* : *in vitro* effects on guanylate cyclase activity, cyclic GMP concentration, and ion transport in small intestins. Proc. Natl. Acad. Sci. USA **75**:2800-2804.
10. Gyles, C. L. (1979). Limitations of the infant mouse test for *Escherichia coli* heat-stable enterotoxin. Can. J. Comp. Med. **43**:371-379.
11. Lathe, R., P. Hirth, M. DeWilde, N. Harford, and J. P. Lecoq. (1980). Cell free synthesis of enterotoxin of *Escherichia coli* from a cloned gene. Nature **284**:473-474.
12. Maniatis, T., A. Jeffrey, and A. G. Kleid. (1975). Nucleotide sequence of the rightward operator of phage lambda. Proc. Natl. Acad. Sci. USA **72**:1184-1188.
13. Maxam, A. M., and W. Gilbert. (1980). Sequencing end-labeled DNA with base-specific chemical cleavages. In L. Grossman, and K. Moldave (Eds.), *Methods in Enzymology,* Vol. 65. Academic Press, New York.
14. Moseley, S. L., W. S. Dallas, and S. Falkow. (1979). Molecular homology among heat labile enterotoxin genes of *Escherichia coli* and the enterotoxin gene of *Vibrio cholerae.* In The US-Japan Cooperative Medical Science Program. Proceedings of the fifteenth joint conference on cholera, p. 266-278. NIH publication No. 80-2003. Bethesda, MD.
15. Moseley, S. L., and S. Falkow. (1980). Nucleotide sequence homology between the heat labile enterotoxin gene of *Escherichia coli* and *Vibrio cholerae* deoxyribonucleic acid. J. Bacteriol. **144**:444-446.
16. Moseley, S. L., I. Huq, A. R. M. A. Alim, M. So, M. Samadpour-Motalebi, and S. Falkow. (1980). Detection of enterotoxigenic *Escherichia coli* by DNA colony hybridization. J. Infect. Dis. **142**: 892-898.
17. Nichols, B. P., and C. Yanofsky. (1979). Nucleotide sequences of *trpA* of *Salmonella typhimurium* and *Escherichia coli*: an evolutionary comparison. Proc. Natl. Acad. Sci. USA **76**:5244-5248.
18. Rao, M. C., S. A. Orellana, M. Field, D. C. Robertson, and R. A. Giannella. (1981). Comparison of the biological actions of three purified heat stable enterotoxins: effects on ion transport and guanylate cyclase activity in rabbit ileum in vitro. Infect. Immun. **33**:165-170.
19. Sack, D. A., and R. B. Sack. (1975). Test for enterotoxigenic *Escherichia coli* using Y-1 adrenal cels in miniculture. Infect. Immun. **11**:334-336.
20. Shine, J., and L. Dalgarno. (1974). The 3′-terminal sequence of *Escherichia coli* 16S ribosomal RNA: Complementarity to nonsense triplets and ribosome binding sites. Proc. Natl. Aad. Sci. USA **71**:1342-1346.
21. So, M., R. Atchison, S. Falkow, S. Moseley, and B. J. McCarthy. (1981). A study of the dissemination of Tn1681: a bacterial transposon encoding a heat-stable toxin among enterotoxigenic *Escherichia coli* isolates. In Cold Spring Harbor Symposia on Quantitative Biology, Vol. XLV, p. 53-58. Cold Spring Harbor Laboratory.
22. So, M., W. S. Dalls, and S. Falkow. (1978). Characterization of an *Escherichia coli* plasmid encoding for synthesis of heat-labile toxin; molecular cloning of the toxin determinant. Infect. Immun. **21**:405-411.
23. So, M., F. Heffron, and B. J. McCarthy. (1979). The *Escherichia coli* gene encoding heat stable toxin is a bacterial transposon flanked by inverted repeats of Isl. Nature **277**:453-456.
24. So, M., and B. J. McCarthy. (1980). Nucleotide sequence of bacterial transposon Tn1681 encoding a heat stable toxin (ST) and its identification in enterotoxigenic *Escherichia coli* strains. Proc. Natl. Acad. Sci. USA **77**:4011-4015.
25. Soutern, E. M. (1975). Detection of specific sequences among DNA fragments separated by gel electrophoresis. J. Molec. Biol. **98**:503-517.

ENTEROTOXINS

Advances in Research on Cholera and Related Diarrheas, eds., S. Kuwahara, N. F. Pierce, 219–225.

A NEW IMMUNO ASSAY OF CHOLERA TOXIN WITH STABLE POLYSTYRENE LATEX PARTICLES

Takeshi Yokota, Teruyo Ito, and Shogo Kuwahara*

*Department of Bacteriology, School of Medicine Juntendo University, Tokyo 113 and * Department of Microbiology, School of Medicine, Toho University, Tokyo 143, Japan.*

Abstract:

Automatic and manual latex agglutination tests were employed to measure cholera toxin (CT), and their subunits A and B. Dow polystyrene latex particles with an average diameter of 0.22 μm and stable polystyrene- chlorostyrene latex particles with a diameter of about 1 μm, both of which were sensitized by purified rabbit specific immunogloblin corresponding to each antigen, were employed for the former and latter methods, respectively. Automatic agglutination was carried out by a nephelometric assay system, in which portions of the suspension of sensitized latex particles and samples were mechanically mixed and the time-dependent differences of light scattering due to agglutination were recorded. Manual latex agglutination was performed in microtiter plates.

As low as 1,000 and 31 pg/ml of purified CT were estimated by the automatic and manual latex agglutination tests, respectively. Using the latex agglutination method, we measured the amounts of CT produced by clinical isolates of *Vibrio cholerae.* Furthermore, fine estimation of CT in numbers of cyclic AMP- deficient mutants of *V. cholerae* revealed that cyclic AMP is not essential for the production of the toxin.

Introduction

Accurate measurement of amounts of enterotoxins produced by *Vibrio cholerae* or enterotoxigenic *Escherichia coli* is frequently required. This is essential for the identification of nontoxigenic strains of *V. cholerae*, for the comparison of toxigenicities of the clinical isolates obtained in different decades, and for confirmation of transformants of *E. coli* by cloned LT genes (13).

Conventional assay methods for enterotoxins, however, are complex and time-consuming. It is almost impossible to estimate accurately CT or LT in one hundred strains by the tissue culture method with the CHO-Kl cells even though this method is sensitive enough. Conversely, the reverse passive hemagglutination test is insensitive and may be interfered with by non-specific reactions (7).

After the latex agglutination test was first introduced by Singer and Plotz (12) for measurement of rheumatoid factors, it quickly became popular for measurement of various antigens and antibodies (10, 11). To ensure accurate and rapid determination of the end point of agglutination reaction, instrumental reading methods such as scattering spectroscopy were also devised (1).

This paper deals with automatic and manual latex agglutination tests for cholera toxin.

Materials and Methods

Bacteria. Three nontoxigenic and four toxigenic clinical isolates and four cyclic AMP-deficient mutants of *V. cholerae* were used.

Chemicals. Purified cholera toxin (Choletox), Freund's complete adjuvant, Freund's incomplete adjuvant, and bovine albumin fraction V were purchased from The Chemo-Sero-Therapeutic Institute, Kumamoto, Iatron Co. Ltd., Tokyo, Difco laboratories, Detroit, Mich., and Armour pharmaceutical Co., Chicago.I11., respectively. Sephadex G-75, cyanbromide-activated Sepharose 4B were purchased from Pharmacia Fine Chem Inc., Uppsala, Sweden. Polystyrene-chlorostyrene stable latex particles (1 μm of diameter) were manufactured by Takeda Chemical Industry, Osaka and a gift from S. matsuzawa, Department of Forensic Medicine, Juntendo University, Tokyo. Dow polystyrene latex particles (0.22 μm of diameter) were obtained from the Dow Chemical Co., Indianapolis, Ind.

Separation of CT to subunits A and B. The purified CT was split into subunits A and B according to the method of Ohtomo (9). The subunits were separated by gel-filtration with Sephadex G-75 after treatment of the CT with 6 M urea in propionic acid buffer (pH 4.0) at 37°C for 60 min.

Preparation of antisera. Rabbit antisera to CT, subunits A and B were prepared by the method of Heiningen (6). Twenty-five micrograms of purified CT or each subunit, dissolved in 0.5 ml phosphate buffered saline (pH 7.2), was injected subcutaneously twice with an equal volume of complete adjuvant, and additionally 2 times with incomplete adjuvant at one week intervals. The aminal were sacrificed one week after the final injection and the sera collected. The specific IgG to CT or each of its subunits was purified according the method of Kudoh *et al.* (7).

Sensitization of latex particles. A one percent suspension of the stable poly-styrene-chlorostyrene particles or 0.1% Dow latex suspension in 0.05 M glycine-NaOH buffer (pH 8.2) containing 0.05 M sodium chloride was mixed with 10 μg or 40 μg of specific IgG per mg latex particles at room temperature for 60 min with gentle shaking, followed by the addition of one drop per ml of 30 % bovine serum albumin solution for stabilization and thorough washing with glycine buffer containing 0.05 M sodium chloride and 0.1 % bovine serum albumin. The sensitized latex particles were resuspended in the same buffer to make a final concentration of 0.5 %.

Automatic agglutination test. A latex agglutination nephelometric system (LANAS) automatic immuno-chemistry analyzer (Eiken Chemical Co., Ltd., Tokyo) was employed for this purpose. Four-hundred μl of a 0.1 % suspension of the sensitized latex particles and 80 μl of samples were mechanically mixed in the analyzer, and scatterd light caused by the agglutinated reaction mixture was recorded from 35 sec. after the mixing at 100 sec intervals. The amounts of CT were estimated from the standard curve of purified CT.

Manual agglutination test. Microtiter plates with U-type bottoms were used. Twenty-five microliters of a 0.05% suspension of the sensitized latex particles was poured into each well, followed by the addition of the same volume of samples which were serially diluted with glycine-NaOH buffer (pH 8.2). The plates were sealed with plastic tape and kept at room temperature overnight. The amounts of CT were estimated from the end point of agglutinated latex particles.

Preparation of culture filtrates of V. cholerae. Purified test strains of *V. cholerae* were inoculated into 10 ml of liquid medium consisting of 30 g Bacto-peptone, 5 g Bacto-yeast extract, 5 g sodium chloride, and 1,000 ml distilled water adjusted to pH 7.2. The microbes were cultured at 37°C overnight with a Monod-type shaker (Taiyo Bussan Co., Tokyo). For cyclic AMP-deficient mutants of *V. cholerae*, the medium was supplemented with or without 0.5 mM cyclic AMP. The culture filtrates were obtained by refrigerated centrifugation at 10,000 X G for 30 min. followed by passing through a Millipore filter (0.3 μm) (Millipore Corporation, Bedford, Mass.).

Preparation of sonicated cell-free extracts. Cell-free extracts were prepared as the supernatant of the cell suspension sonicated at 10 kc for 4 x 15 sec at 0°C.

Bioassay of CT with the CHO-Kl cells. Activities of the enterotoxins in the culture fluids or cell-free extracts were assayed by the tissue culture method with chinese hamster ovary cells, CHO-Kl (6).

Results

Optimum conditions for the manual latex agglutination test.

Purified CT (Choletox) was used as the standard. The lyophilized toxin was dissolved in the original volume of distilled water and kept at 4°C. Before use, the toxin was diluted with the medium employed for the cultivation of test microbes adjusted pH to 6.0 to make a final concentration of 1 μg/ml. The use of a weakly acidic medium was critical to get a stable working reference. If an alkaline medium was employed, the end point of the reference test was unsatisfactory as shown in Table 2.

The optimum amount of specific IgG and pH for the sensitization of latex particles were determined to be 10 to 40 micrograms per mg of latex and pH 8.2, respectively. Poor sensitization was observed when the IgG was added to latex at a pH lower than 6.2. For stabilization, the source of bovine serum albumin was important. As indicated on Table 3, The product of Armour Pharmaceutical Co., Chicago gave the best result.

When the density of the sensitized latex particles was decreased, the sensitivity increased conversely. However, since it was difficult to read the end point at low densities, a 0.05 % suspension was selected for routine work. Stable results were obtained when the reaction was carried out at room temperature rather than at 37°C.

Table 1. Influence of pH of medium* used for preparation of standard working toxin solution.

pH	Amount of CT detectable by the manual latex agglutination test
6.0	31 pg/ml
7.0	31-63 "
8.0	250 "

* Peptone-yeast extract-NaCl medium.

Table 2. Influence of source of bovine serum albumin on the sensitivity of the manual latex agglutination.

Source	Minimum amount of CT determined
Armour Co.	31 pg/ml
X Co.	4,000. 〃
Y Co.	8,000. 〃

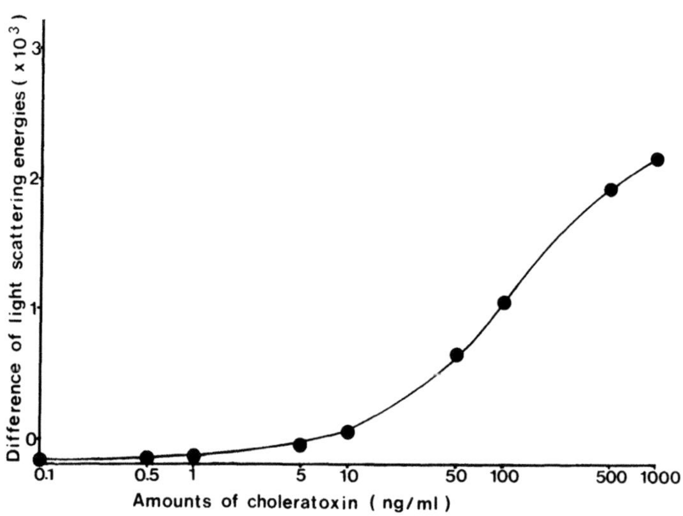

Fig. 1. Standard curve for CT quantitation by automatic latex agglutination. The intensity of agglutination was expressed as △ LSE (difference of light scattering energy), which was automatically calculated from the difference of the scattering light from 35 sec. to 135 sec. after mixing with latex particles.

Table 3. Amounts of CT in culture fluids of *V. cholerae* measured by the automatic and manual latex agglutination tests and by the tissue culture method using CHO-K1 cells.

			Amount of CT measured by		
Biotype	strain	source	Automatic method	Manual method	CHO-Kl method
	BR1074	river	<1 ng/ml	<0.01 ng/ml	<0.01*ng/ml
eltor	BR2633	〃	<1	<0.01	<0.01
	JR290	〃	<1	<0.01	<0.01
	S249	patient	38	128	10
	K20	〃	1.8	2	1
cholerae	CC4560	〃	70	64	10
	569B	〃	1700	2048	1,000.

*Approximate toxin concentration.

In contrast to the acidic medium used for the preparation of the standard working solution of the toxin, the optimum pH for further dilution of the standard toxin and for reaction mixtures was found to be 8.2 (0.05 M glycine-NaOH buffer).

Based upon the result obtained, the latex agglutination test for CT was routinely carried out as follows: Two-fold serial dilutions of the working standard toxin solution prepared with medium at pH 6.0 were placed in wells of microtiter plates with glycine-NaOH buffer (pH 8.2) (25 μl each). The same volume of the sensitized latex particles suspended in the same buffer was added to each well followed by thorough mixing, and the end point of the reaction was read macroscopically after 18 hrs at room temperature. Concentrations as low as 31 pg/ml of CT could be estimated by this method.

Automatic latex agglutination test.

A rapid measurement of CT was possible using the automatic latex agglutination test with a nephelometric assay system. Since an autosampler and autochanger were connected to the system, accurate time difference of light scattering energies in each tube was determined as shown in Fig. 1. The method, however, was rather insensitive when compared to the manual method. The lowest toxin concentration which could be measured by the automatic method was found to be about 1ng/ml.

Measurement of amounts of CT in culture filtrates of V. cholerae.

Amounts of CT in culture filtrates of 7 strains of *V. cholerae* isolated in different years and places were measured by the manual and automatic latex agglutination tests and by the tissue culture method using CHO-Kl cells as indicated in Table 3. All three strains of *V. cholerae* isolated from rivers were confirmed to be nontoxigenic by the three different methods, whereas four clinical isolates of the same microbe were recognized as toxin-producers though the amounts varied from one strain to another.

While some discrepancies were found among the amounts of CT measured by the three methods, all the methods were in agreement regarding the toxigenicity of each strain.

Amounts of CT produced by cyclic AMP-deficient mutants of V. cholerae.

Amounts of CT, and subunits A and B produced by 4 cyclic AMP deficient mutants of *V. cholerae* were estimated by latex agglutination tests. Amounts of CT in the culture supernatant are presented in Table 4. Although excretion of CT, especially that of subunits B seemed to be stimulated in the presence of exogenous cyclic AMP in some mutants, it seemed to be difficult to conclude that cAMP is essential for the toxin production. The amounts of intracellular toxin were estimated using supernatant of sonic disrupted cells. No marked differences in the toxin production were observed in the presence or absence of cAMP (Data was not shown). From these results, it has been concluded that cyclic AMP is not an essential factor for the production of choleratoxin.

Discussion

Although the ligated intestinal test (3), skin permeability test (2), and tissue sulture methods with tumor-type cells (4,6) have been widely used for the measurement of cholera toxin (CT) and heat-labile enterotoxin (LT) of *E. coli*, the necessity of more convenient methods is obvious, since conventional methods are complex and time-consuming. For this purpose, automatic and manual latex agglutination tests were devised.

The automatic latex agglutination test is capable of estimating concentrations of CT

Table 4. Amounts of CT measured by the manual latex agglutination test in culture fluids of *V. cholerae* grown in the presence or absence of cyclic AMP.

strain	Presence of 0.5 mM cyclic AMP	Amount of Holotoxin	Subunit A	Subunit B
IK, cya^+	–	<0.1	<0.1	<0.1
IK12, *cya*[a)]	–	<0.1	<0.1	<0.1
	+	0.13	<0.1	0.13
IK23, *cya* [a)]	–	2.0	0.5	4.0
	+	1.0	1.0	8.0
E2, cya^+	–	4.0	4.0	32.0
E2511, *cya* [b)]	–	1.0	4.0	2.0
	+	2.0	8.0	8.0
569B cya^+	–	100.	100.	100.
B42, *cya* [c)]	–	200.	100.	100.
	+	400.	100.	200.

a). *cya* mutant of Ikenohata strain (14).
b). *cya* mutant of E2 strain (15).
c). *cya* mutant of 569B (14).

as low as 1 ng/ml. Although the method is rather insensitive as compared with the tissue culture method which can measure 10 pg/ml of CT, it is more accurate and more rapid than the latter and routinely sensitive enough to estimate CT in culture fluids of toxigenic strains of *V. cholerae.* Concentration of CT can be determined in 100 sample, within 1 hour by the automatic method, so that the method may be a useful tool for a large scale epidemiological survey.

The manual latex agglutination test is less expensive and more sensitive than the automatic method, although over-night reaction was required. Since the reagents for the latex agglutination tests are stable for at least 6 months, it is more convenient than the reverse passive hemagglutination test for measurement of the enterotoxins.

It was surprising to have found that cyclic AMP is not an essential factor for the production of cholera toxin. We had previously reported that cyclic AMP deficient mutants of *V. cholerae* E2 required cyclic AMP for the production of toxin as measured by the skin permeability test (8). This conclusion might have resulted from the absence of an accurate immunochemical method for measuring small amounts of CT.

The automatic and manual latex agglutination test, for measurement of CT may find various uses in the study of *V. cholerae.* The latex agglutination test for measurement of LT is now under investigation, and will be published later.

REFERENCES

1). Blume, P. and L. J. Greenberg. 1975. Application of different light scattering to the latex agglutination assay for rheumatoid factor. Clin. Chem. **2**: 1234-1237.
2). Craig, J. P. 1965. A permeability factor (toxin) found in cholera stool and culture filtrates and its neutralization by convalescent cholera sera. Nature (London) **20**: 614-616.

3). De, S. N. and D. N. Chatterjee. 1953. An experimental study of the mechanism of action of *Vibrio cholerae* on the intestinal mucous membrane. J. Pathol. Bacteriol. **66**: 153-159.

4). Donta, S. T., H. W. Moon, and S. C. Whipp. 1974. Detection of heat-labile *Escherichia coli* enterotoxin with the use of adrenal cells in tissue culture. Science **183**: 334-336.

5). Guerrant, R. L., L. L. Brunton, E. C. Schneitman, L. I. Rebhun, and A. G. Gilman. 1974. Cyclic adenosine monophosphate and alteration of chinese hamster ovary cell morphology: a repid, sensitive *in vitro* assay for the enterotoxins of *V. cholerae* and *Escherichia coli.* Infect. Immun. **10**: 320-327.

6). Heyningen, S. Van. 1976. The subunits of cholera toxin : structure, stoichiometory, and function. J. Infect. Dis. **133** (Suppl.):S5-13.

7). Kudoh, Y., S. Yamada, S. Matsushita, K. Ohta, M. Tsuno, T. Muraoka, N. Ohtomo, and M. Ohashi. 1978. Detection of heat-labile enterotoxin of *Escherichia coli* by reversed passive hemagglutination test with specific immuno-globulin against cholera toxin. Fourteenth Joint Conference on Cholera, The U. S. Japan Cooperative Medical Science Program: 266-273.

8). Ohashi, M., T. Shimada, H. Fukumi, and T. Yokota. 1973. Enterotoxin production by an adenosine 3', 5'-cyclic monophosphate-deficient mutant of *Vibrio cholerae.* Nineth Joint Conference on Cholerae, The U. S. Japan Cooperative Medical Science Program : 25-32.

9). Ohtomo, N., T. Muraoka, A Tashiro, Y. Zinnaka and K. Amako. 1976. Size and structure of the cholera toxin molecule and its subunits. J. Infect. Dis. 133(Suppl.) S31-40.

10). Quash, G., A. M. Rosh, A Niveleau, J. Grange, T. Keolouangkhot and J. Huppert. 1978. The preparation of latex particles with covalently bound polyamines, IgG and measles agglutinins and their use in visual agglutination tests. J. Immunol. Methods. **22**: 165-174.

11). Robbins, J. L., G. A. Hill, B. N. Carle, J. H. Carlquist and S. Marcus. 1962. Latex agglutination between human chorionic gonadotropin and rabbit antibody. Proc. Soc. Exp. Biol. Med. **109**: 321-325.

12). Singer, J. M. and C. M. Plotz. 1956. The latex fixation test. 1. application to the serologic diagnosis of Rheumatoid Arthritis. Am. J. Med. **21**: 888-892.

13). Yamamoto, T., T. Yokota and S. Kuwahara. 1981. The heat-labile enterotoxin genes originating in a clinically isolated *E. coli* strain. Seventeenth Joint Conference on Cholerae, The U. S. Japan cooperative Medical Science Program.

14). Yokota, T., T. Ito, R. Sekiguchi and S. Kuwahara. 1980. Role of cyclic AMP in the evolution of *Vibrio cholerae.* The sixteenth Joint Conference on Cholera, The U. S. Japan Cooperative Medical Science Program.

15). Yokota, T. and S. Kuwahara. 1974. Adenosine 3′, 5′-cyclic monophosphatedeficient mutants of *Vibrio cholerae.* J. Bacteriol. **120**: 106-113.

Advances in Research on Cholera and Related Diarrheas, eds., S. Kuwahara, N. F. Pierce, 227–231.

FURTHER EVIDENCE SHOWING THAT SUBUNIT B OF CHOLERA TOXIN ENTERS THE CELL

Yutaka Zinnaka, Sumiaki Tsuru, Nobuya Ohtomo*, Toyoharu Muraoka* and Kenji Takeya**

*Department of Bacteriology, National Defense Medical College, Tokorozawa, Saitama 359, *the Chemo-Sero-Therapeutic Research Institute, Kumamoto 860 and **Department of Microbiology, Kyushu University School of Medicine, Fukuoka 812, Japan*

Lymphocyte has been known to bind cholera toxin (CT) on its surface (7, 13, 16). Since the subsequent accumulation of intracellular cyclic AMP is observed (9, 19), it is believed that the A subunit (SA) of CT penetrates the cell membrane after binding of CT to the receptor ganglioside with the B subunit (SB) to stimulate intracellular adenylate cyclase as suggested in other CT-cell system [reviews see 3, 6, 11, 18]. There has been a speculative model for the internalization of CT into cell (2), in which SA penetrates the cell membrane through the channel constructed by SB's extending themselves into the bilayer of the membrane. In such a model, it is expected that SA disappears from the surface after absorption, although SB remains on the surface. We have started the present study with an intention to give a substantial basis for CT-cell interaction. Mouse thymus cells have been chosen for this study because these cells are easily obtainable in large numbers with minor contamination of other type of cells and suitable for the analysis with a fluorescence-activated cell sorter, which facilitates to determine the relative amount of specific antigen on the cell surface.

In the previous report (20, 21), it was demonstrated that both SA and SB were detected on the surface of these cells immediately after adsorption, and the surface-bound SA decreased with time, as expected, but SB also disappeared from the surface in the same manner when the cells were incubated at 37 C. These subunits were then detected within the cell by fluorescent antibody staining after permeabilization of the cytoplasmic membrane with a critical concentration of saponin. Such findings suggest that not only SA but also SB is internalized within the cell. Three alternative explanations are possible, [1] endocytosis, [2] simple penetration of both subunits through the cell membrane and [3] incorporation of SB within the cell membrane itself. In the last case, the positive antibody-binding after saponin treatment is explained to be the uncovering of the corresponding subunit by the solubilization of some constituent of the membrane. The following experiment has been arranged to provide further approach to these questions (17).

The rate of binding of CT and its subunits on the cell surface was determined by a fluorescence-activated cell sorter (FACS-II, Becton Dickinson Electronics Laboratory, Mountain View, Calif., U.S.A.) (1). Thymus cells were harvested from 5-week-old mice (strain ddN) and pelleted cells (1×10^7) were treated with 0.1 ml of purified CT (1 μg/ml) for 10 min at 4 C. After removing unbound CT by a brief centrifugation at 4 C, the cells were incubated at 4 C and at appropriate intervals, 0.1 ml of either fluorescein isothiocyanate(FITC)-conjugated rabbit anti-SA or anti-SB immunoglobulin (0.5 mg/ml) was added and incubation was continued for 10 min at 4 C. The cells were then washed and analyzed with FACS.

When the FITC-conjugated anti-SB was added to the toxin-treated cells after 10 min of incubation, most cells (95% as calculated from the differential count with light scattering) were positively stained, but both the number of fluorescent cells and relative intensity of fluorescence decreased with time and the former reached the control level (20%) after 4 h of incubation. The experiment with anti-SA gave a similar result. The rate of fluorescent cells decreased from 90% to 18% during incubation at 4 C for 4 h.

To detect the possible existence of the subunits in the cytosol, these cells were treated with saponin (0.1 mg/ml) for 15 min in an ice bath to allow the fluorescent antibody to enter the cell immediately after interrupting incubation. Fluorescence was found to associate with cells which had been treated with CT followed by saponin but not with cells which had not been treated with CT before saponin. Ninety percent of the total cells treated with saponin immediately after CT treatment were labeled positively with FITC-conjugated anti-SB. Undoubtedly this fluorescence is due to surface labeling. After 4 h of incubation, when the surface fluorescence already disappeared in the cells which had not been treated with saponin, saponin-treated cells were still positively labeled, although the value decreased to about 50%. Control cells showed no such fluorescence. Another series of experiments with FITC-conjugated anti-SA resulted in a similar finding. These results are not distinguishable from those obtained with the cells incubated at 37 C in the previous experiment (20, 21).

To examine whether the subunits were incorporated in the bilayer of cell membrane itself, the membrane fraction was prepared (10) from the saponin-treated cells which had been treated with CT and incubated at 4 C for an appropriate time. These fractions were analyzed with FACS in the same manner as in the intact cell with anti-SB (17). The rate of fluorescence was about 90% after 10 min of incubation, but decreased with time, reaching about 5% in 4 h. It is suggested that SB was not associated with the membrane fraction at that time when the surface fluorescence had already disappeared. The above results are summarized in Table 1.

Table 1. Detection of CT subunits in mouse thymus cells treated with CT and incubated either at 4 C or 37 C. Result of FACS analysis (17, 21).

Time after CT	Detection of subunits				
	No saponin		Saponin-treated		
	Whole cell		Whole cell		Membrane
	SA	SB	SA	SB	SB
10 min	+++	+++	+++	+++	+++
1 h	++	++	NT	NT	NT
2 h	+	+	++	++	+
4 h	±	±	+++	+++	–

NT: not examined.

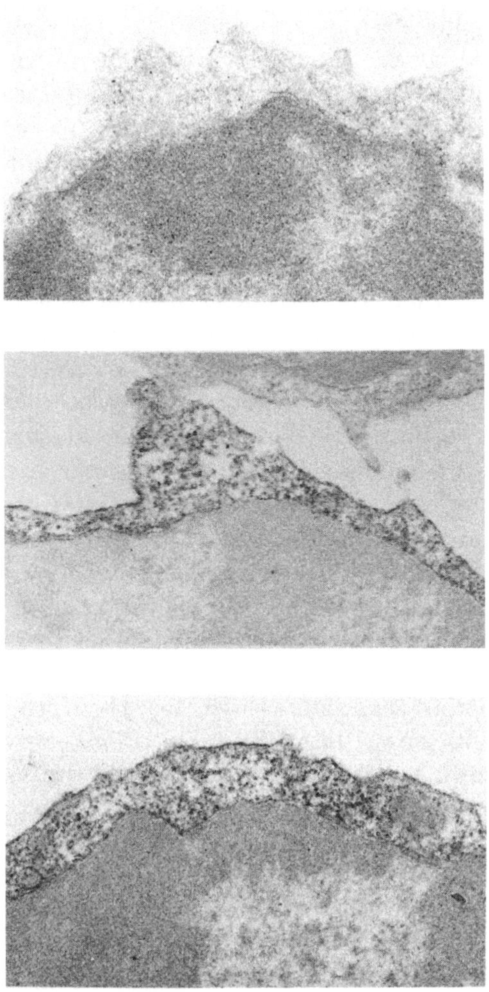

A

B

C

Figure 1. Electron micrographs of CT-treated mouse-thymus cell labeled with HRP-conjugated antibody. The cells were incubated with CT (1 μg/ml) at 4 C for 30 min. After removing unbound CT, incubation at 4 C was continued for 2 h. Then the cells were treated with saponin (0.1 mg/ml) together with 0.05 % glutaraldehyde in cacodylate buffer at 4 C for 15 min. After washing, the cells were labeled with anti-SA or -SB rabbit immunoglobulin (0.1 mg/ml) and HRP-conjugated antirabbit IgG goat serum successively (each for 45 min). The cells were then washed and processed for detection of HRP with diaminobenzidine (30 mg%) and hydrogen peroxide (0.01%) for 10 min at room temperature. The cells were pelleted and embedded in a droplet of 1.5% agar before fixation with osmium tetroxide. Other procedures were the same as in the standard technique. No contrast staining of sections with lead or uranyl salt was performed. [A] Control cell (no CT treatment) processed with anti-SB. Discontinuation of the cell membrane and leakage of cytosol constituent with only very weak reaction of HRP (probably non-specific) are observed (33,000x). [B] CT-treated cell labeled with anti-SA (26,400x). [C] CT-treated cell labeled with anti-SB (26,400x). Most HRP granules are in the cytoplasm although some HRP deposit is seen on the cell surface.

To demonstrate more directly the cytological localization of CT subunits, the cells were examined by immune electron microscopy with horseradish peroxidase(HRP)-conjugated antibody as a marker. In ordinary tissues, the frozen section technique is utilized to detect the antigen inside the cell, but for free cells such as thymus cells this technique is not feasible. Therefore, the cells treated with CT and incubated at 4 C were permeabilized with saponin to allow the marker antibody to enter the cell (12), and then processed for detection of HRP activity. The details will be published elsewhere (manuscript in preparation).

As shown in Fig. 1, the both subunits were found in the cytoplasm after 2 h of incubation. There was still some positive association of HRP with the surface membrane, but no positive association of HRP granule with Golgi region (not shown in the figure) was found. The presence of intracytoplasmic vesicles associated with such deposit was also exceptional. Since endocytosis is a temperature-dependent process, and may not occur or at least must be retarded at 4 C (14), we can conclude from all the above results that SB of CT is internalized into the cell by a mechanism other than endocytosis together with SA. This does not mean to exclude the presence of an endocytotic process at higher temperature, for instance, at 37 C.

Hansson *et al.* (5) examined structural localization of CT in the mouse thymus cell, and observed cap formation and presence of pinocytosed toxin after incubation for 30 min at 37 C, but the toxin remained on the cell surface below 18 C. Their result does not seem to be inconsistent with our observation, because they did not give the result of prolonged incubation at a low temperature nor did they try to detect the subunits within the cell. Joseph *et al.* (8) showed that HRP-linked CT and SB were endocytosed by murine neuroblastoma cells, and the endocytosed complex remained in the region near the Golgi apparatus. Their results are also not inconsistent with ours, since HRP itself is used as a marker for fluid-phase pinocytosis (4, 15), and the HRP-CT complex might not present the behavior of the native toxin or its subunits.

It is still unclear at present which physico-chemical mechanism is involved in these processes. Further study along such a line may be necessary to understand the phase of penetration in the cell-toxin interaction.

This study was supported by a grant from the U.S.-Japan Cooperative Medical Science Program, Cholera Panel.

REFERENCES

1. Bonner, W. A., H. R. Hulett, R. G. Sweet & L. A. Herzenberg (1972) Fluorescence-activated cell sorting. *Rev. Scient. Instrum.* **43**: 404-409.
2. Gill, D. M. (1976) The arrangement of subunits in cholera toxin. *Biochemistry* **15**: 1242-1248.
3. Gill, D. M. (1978) Seven toxic peptides that cross cell membranes. p. 291-332. *In* Jeljaszewicz, J. & T. Wadström (eds) *Bacterial toxins and cell membrane.* Academic Press, London, New York and San Francisco.
4. Goud, G., J.-C. Antoine, N. K. Gonatas, A. Stieber & S. Avrameas (1981) A comparative study of fluid-phase and adsorptive endocytosis of horseradish peroxidase in lymphoid cells. *Exp. Cell. Res.* **132**: 375-386.
5. Hansson, H. A., J. Holmgren & L. Svennerholm (1977) Ultrastructural localization of cell

membrane ganglioside by cholera toxin. *Proc. Natl Acad. Sci. USA.* **74**: 3782-3786.
6. Holmgren, J. (1978) Cholera toxin and the cell membrane. p. 333-366. *In* Jeljaszewicz, J. & Wadström (eds) *Bacterial toxins and cell membrane.* Academic Press, London, New York and San Francisco.
7. Holmgren, J., L. Lindholm & I. Lönnroth (1974) Interaction of cholera toxin derivatives with lymphocytes. I. Binding proporties and interference with lectin-induced cellular stimulation. *J. Exp. Med.* **139**: 801-819.
8. Joseph, K. C., S. U. Kim, A. Stieber & N. K. Gonatas (1978) Endocytosis of cholera toxin into neuronal GERL. *Proc. Natl Acad. Sci. USA.* **75**: 2815-2819.
9. Lönnroth, I. & C. Lönnroth (1977) Interaction of cholera toxin and its subunits with lymphocytes, the effects on intracellular cAMP. *Exp. Cell Res.* **104**: 15-24.
10. Misra, D. N., C. T. Ladoulis, L. W. Estes & T. J. Gill, III (1975) Biochemical and enzymatic characterization of thymic and splenic lymphocyte plasma membranes from inbred rats. *Biochemistry* **14**: 3014-3024.
11. Moss, J. & M. Vaughan (1979) Activation of adenylate cyclase by choleragen. *Ann. Rev. Biochem.* **48**: 581-600.
12. Ohtsuki, I., R. M. Manzi, G. E. Palade & J. D. Jamieson (1978) Entry of macromolecular tracers into cells fixed with low concentrations of aldehydes. *Biol. Cellul.* **31**: 119-126.
13. Révész, T. & M. Greaves (1975) Ligand-induced redistribution of lymphocyte membrane ganglioside GM1. *Nature* **257**: 103-106.
14. Silverstein, S. C., R. M. Steinman & Z. A. Cohn (1977) Endocytosis. *Ann. Rev. Biochem.* **46**: 669-722.
15. Steinman, R. M., S. E. Brodie & Z. A. Cohn (1976) Membrane flow during pinocytosis, a stereologic analysis. *J. Cell Biol.* **68**: 665-687.
16. Tsuru, S., Y. Zinnaka & K. Nomoto (1981) Decrease in cholera toxin-binding T cells in aged mice and human volunteers. *Int. Archs Allergy appl. Immun.* **64**: 217-221.
17. Tsuru, S., M. Matsuguchi, N. Ohtomo, Y. Zinnaka & K. Takeya (1982) Entrance of cholera enterotoxin subunits into cells. *J. Gen. Microbiol.* **128**: 497-502.
18. Vaughan, M. & J. Moss (1978) Mechanism of action of choleragen. *J. Supramol. Struct.* **8**: 473-488.
19. Zensser, T. V. & J. F. Metzger (1974) Comparison of the action of *Escherichia coli* enterotoxin on the thymocyte adenylate cyclase-cyclic adenosine monophosphate system to that of cholera toxin and prostaglandin E_1. *Infect. Immun.* **10**: 503-509.
20. Zinnaka, Y. & N. Ohtomo (1981) Entrance of cholera toxin subunits into cells (abstract). *Jpn. J. Med. Sci. Biol.* **34**: 56-57.
21. Zinnaka, Y., S. Tsuru, N. Ohtomo & K. Takeya (1981) Entrance of cholera toxin subunits into cells. p. 85-93. *In* Kuwahara, S. & Y. Zinnaka (eds) *Symposium on Cholera: Proceedings of the 16th Joint Conference, U.S.-Japan Cooperative Medical Science Program.* Japanese Cholera Panel, U.S.-Japan Cooperative Medical Science Program, Toho Univ., Tokyo.

Advances in Research on Cholera and Related Diarrheas, eds., S. Kuwahara, N. F. Pierce, 233–246.

PURIFICATION AND SOME PROPERTIES OF AN ENTEROTOXIN FROM *VIBRIO CHOLERAE* NON-O1 THAT IS IDENTICAL TO CHOLERA ENTEROTOXIN

Koichiro Yamamoto[1], Yoshifumi Takeda[1], Toshio Miwatani[1] and John P. Craig[2]

Department of Bacteriology and Serology, Research Institute for Microbial Diseases, Osaka University, Yamada-oka, Suita, Osaka 565, Japan[1] *and Department of Microbiology and Immunology, State University of New York, Downstate Medical Center, Brooklyn, New York 11203, USA*[2].

Vibrio cholerae non-O1 strains have been repeatedly isolated from a number of cholera-like cases and are now recognized as causative agents of diarrheal disease. Some cases of diarrhea due to non-O1 vibrios were very similar to cholera and production of cholera-like enterotoxin by some strains of non-O1 vibrios has been suggested.

Zinnaka and Carpenter (27) and Ohashi and his coworkers (19) independently reported that some strains of non-O1 vibrios produce an active substance which was biologically similar to cholera toxin. Last year at Gifu (7) we reported that a strain of *V. cholerae* non-O1, serovar O344, isolated from fresh water in Louisiana, produces an enterotoxin which is biologically similar to cholera toxin. We also demonstrated that this toxin was immunologically identical to cholera toxin in the Ouchterlony immunodiffusion test.

In this paper, we report the purification of enterotoxin from this non-O1 vibrio and conclude that the purified toxin cannot be distinguished from cholera toxin, not only in biological and immunological properties but also in molecular structure.

Materials and methods

Bacterial strains. Vibrio cholerae E8498 O344, Smith serovar (21)), isolated from surface water in the Dewitt canal in Louisiana, USA, was kindly supplied by Dr. P. Blake, Centers for Disease Control, Atlanta, Ga. (1). *V. cholerae* S7, isolated from a diarrhea patient in Sudan was supplied by Dr. Y. Zinnaka, Defense Medical College, Tokorozawa, Saitama, Japan. *V. Cholerae* 62058 was obtained from Dr. I. Huq, International Centre for Diarrhoeal Disease Research, Dacca, Bangladesh. *V. cholerae* WBDV-101E_1 was supplied by Dr. P. Echeverria, Armed Forces Research Institute of Medical Sciences, Bangkok, Thailand. As we reported previously (25) production of cholera-like enterotoxin by non-O1 vibrios was stimulated by lincomycin in culture medium. In order to obtain optimal growth in the presence of high levels of lincomycin we selected a lincomycin-resistant spontaneous mutant which was isolated from agar plates containing 300 μg/ml lincomycin (Lincocin®, Japan Upjohn, Tokyo) (25). This strain is designated E8498-Lin^r.

Cultivation. Organisms were cultivated for toxin production by the method previously described (7). A loopful of E8498-Lin^r organisms was inoculated into 5 ml of broth composed of 1% Trypticase peptone and 1% NaCl (T_1N_1). A 1.5-ml portion of a 6 h culture at 37° C was transferred to a 2-l Erlenmeyer flask containing 150 ml of medium containing casamino acid, 3%, yeast extract, 0.3%, K_2HPO_4, 0.05%, (pH 7.0) (CAYE) and incubated without shaking for 18 h at 37°C. One and a half ml of this culture was inoculated into 1-l Roux flasks each containing 150 ml of CAYE medium supplemented with 0.2% glucose and 300 μg/ml lincomycin, yielding a surface/volume ratio of 2 cm^2/ml. The Roux flasks were incubated without agitation, and the contents were pooled and centrifuged at 25,000 x g for 30 min at 4°C. The supernatant fluid was treated with 0.02% sodium azide and 0.05% disodium ethylenediaminetetraacetic acid (EDTA).

Reference cholera enterotoxin (CT). Purified CT prepared from *V. cholerae* strain 569B, serovar O1, prepared by the method of Ohtomo *et al.* (18) was obtained from Sanko junyaku Co. (Tokyo, Japan).

Vascular permeability factor (PF) assay. PF tests were carried out as previously reported (4,5,7). PF content was expressed as the number of 4 mm blueing doses (BD_4). One BD_4 was defined as the amount of PF producing a blue lesion 4 mm in diameter. Limit of blueing dose (Lb) of toxin was determined as previously described using U.S. Standard Cholera Antitoxin, NIH Lot 001, prepared against purified 569B enterotoxin (6).

Passive immune hemolysis (PIH). Passive immune hemolysis was carried out according to the method previously described (24) using rabbit anti-CT antibody purified by immunoaffinity chromatography and guinea pig complement. Hemolysis was measured by absorbance of the supernatant at 420 nm.

Chinese hamster ovary (CHO) cell assay. Ability to alter morphology of CHO cells was determined as previously described (13) using Lab-Tek® Tissue Culture Chamber (Miles Laboratories, Inc., Naperville, IL). Activity was expressed as the percentage elongated cells.

Mouse intestinal loop test. The intestinal loop test in mice was carried out as described previously (23). Fluid accumulation was measured by calculating the ratio of the weight of fluid, in mg, to the length of the loop, in cm (W/L ratio).

Polyacrylamide gel electrophoresis (PAGE). Conventional PAGE was carried out by the method of Davis (9) and SDS-PAGE by the method of Fairbanks (11) using 7% gel with 0.1% sodium dodecylsulfate (SDS) as detergent.

Agar gel immunodiffusion test. The method used was essentially that of Ouchterlony (20) using 1% noble agar in phosphate buffered saline containing 0.01% NaN_3.

Protein determination. Protein was determined by the method of Lowry *et al.* (17) using crystalline bovine serum albumin as standard.

Chromatography. Gel filtrations were carried out at 4°C using columns of Sephadex G-100, Bio-Gel A-5m, and Sephadex G-75 superfine. The columns were equilibrated with 50mM Tris-HCl buffer containing 3mM NaN_3, 1mM EDTA and 0.2M NaCl

(TEAN buffer) pH 7.8. The fractions were monitored for CT antigen by PIH.

Chemicals. Sephadex G-100 and G-75 gels were obtained from Pharmacia Fine Chemicals (Upsala, Sweden). Bio-Gel A-5m gel was obtained from Bio-Rad Laboratories (Richmond, Ca). Evans Blud, Coomasie Brilliant Blue, Dithiothreotol and crystalline bovine serum albumin were supplied by Sigma Chemical Co. (St. Louis, Mo). Casamino acids, yeast extract and Noble agar were obtained from Difco Laboratories (Detroit, Michigan). Trypticase was obtained form Baltimore Biological laboratories (Cockeysville, Maryland).

Results

Partial purificaton. Table 1 summarized the procedure for the purification of the toxin from E8498-Lin^r. The pH of the culture supernatant was adjusted to 5.0 with hydrochloric acid. Aluminum hydroxide powder was added at 0.1% and the mixture was stirred for 6 hours and allowed to stand for 18 hours at 4°C. After centrifugation, the precipitate was washed several times with 0.01M sodium formate pH 5.5, and then eluted with TEAN buffer, pH 8.5. The adsorption-elution procedure was repeated six times and the supernatants were pooled. The pooled eluates were concentrated by 50% saturation with solid ammonium and was designated as partially purified enterotoxin.

Gel filtration on Sephadex G-100 column. Partially purified toxin was applied to a column of Sephadex G-100 equilibrated with TEAN buffer, pH 7.8. As shown in Fig. 1,

Table 1

PURIFICATION PROCEDURE

V. cholerae E8498Lin^r, non-O1 48-hr stationary culture with 300 μg/ml lincomycin

↓

Culture supernatant

↓

$Al(OH)_3$ absorption at pH 5.0

↓

Washing

↓

Elution with TEAN buffer, pH 8.5

↓

50% Sat. $AmSO_4$ precipitation

↓

Column chromatography

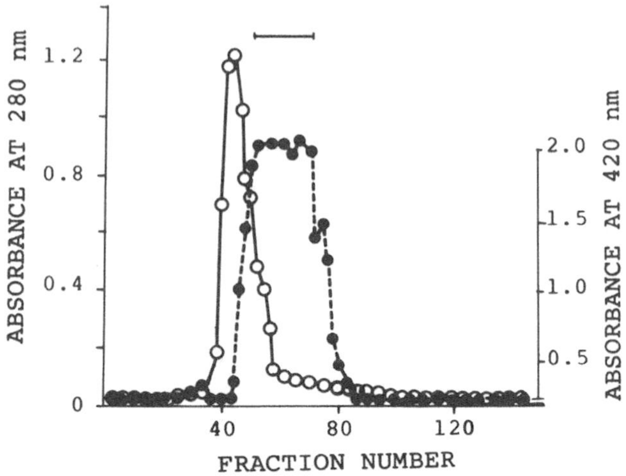

Fig. 1. Sephadex G-100 column chromatogram of non-O1 enterotoxin. Toxin partially purified by $Al(OH)_3$ was applied to the column. ○, A_{280}; ●, hemolysis by PIH(A420); ⊢—⊣, pooled active fractions.

the toxin, as monitored by PIH activity, was eluted after the single major protein peak. Tch active fractions were pooled and concentrated.

Gel filtration on Bio-Gel A-5m. The active fraction pool of the Sephadex G-100 eluates was applied to a Bio-Gel A-5m column and three protein peaks were obtained as shown in Fig. 2. CT-antigen was found in the third peak. The active fractions were concentrated and applied to a Sephadex G-75 column.

Gel filtration on Sephadex G-75. Two peaks of CT antigen were obtained by gel filtration of Sephadex G-75 (Fig. 3). The first peak was eluted simultaneously with the major absorbance peak at 280 nm. Since PF was found only in the first peak it was

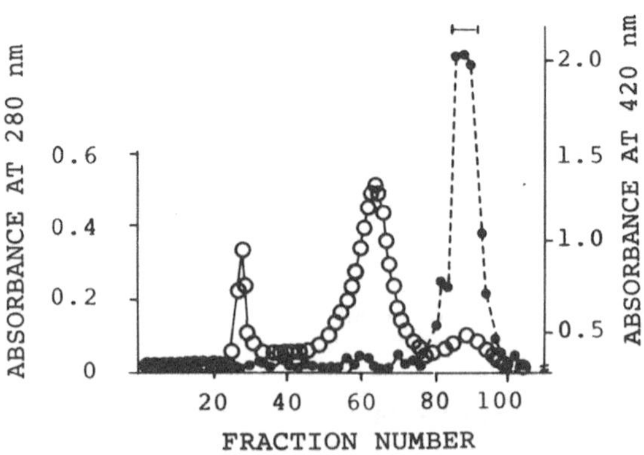

Fig. 2. Bio-Gel A-5m column chromatogram of non-O1 enterotoxin. Sample prepared by Sephadex G-100 (Fig. 1) was applied to the column, ○, A_{280}; ●, hemolysis by PIH(A_{420}); ⊢—⊣, pooled active fractions.

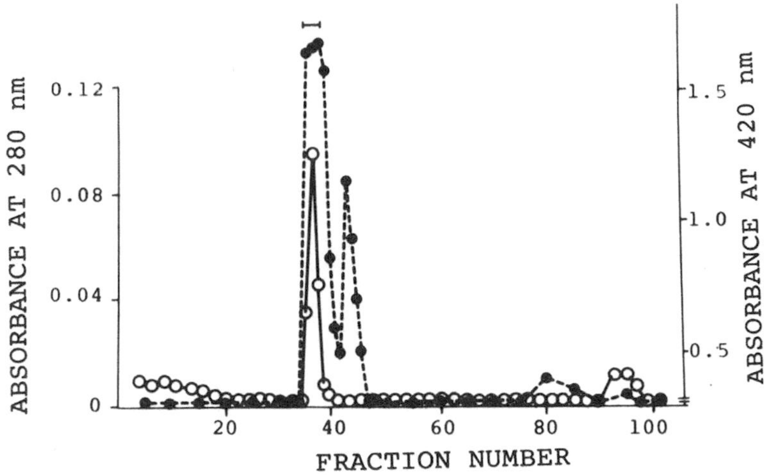

Fig. 3. Sephadex G-75 column chromatogram of non-O1 enterotoxin. Sample prepared by Bio-Gel A-5m (Fig. 2) was applied. ○, A_{280}; ●, hemolysis by PIH (A_{420}); ⊢—⊣, pooled active fractions.

considered likely that the second antigen peak might be a choleragenoid-like substance. The first peak was concentrated and rechromatographed on the same column (Fig. 4). The protein peak corresponded well with the peak of CT antigen. The antigen-containing fractions were concentrated and used as purified non-O1 toxin in further studies.

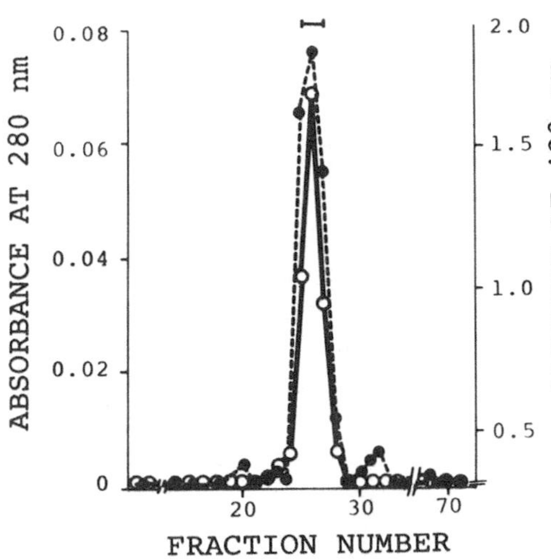

Fig. 4. Sephadex G-75 column chromatogram of non-O1 enterotoxin. Sample prepared by Sephadex G-75 was rechromatographed. ○; A_{280}; ●, hemolysis by PIH (A_{420}); ⊢—⊣, pooled active fractions.

Table 2. Purification of enterotoxin from *V. cholerae* E8498, O344.

Fraction	Total volume (ml)	Total protein (mg)	Total PF activity (BD_4)	Specific activity (BD_4/mg)	Relative activity	Yield of PF activity (%)
Partially purified enterotoxin	26	385	5.6×10^8	1.5×10^6	1	100
Sephadex G-100 column eluate	9.3	47	1.2×10^8	2.6×10^6	1.7	21
Bio-Gel A-5m column eluate	2.0	4.0	1.0×10^8	2.5×10^7	17	18
1st Sephadex G-75 column eluate	1.0	2.8	9.9×10^7	3.5×10^7	23	18
2nd Sephadex G-75 column eluate	1.2	0.68	6.4×10^7	9.4×10^7	63	11

The results of a typical purification procedure are summarized in Table 2. Biologic activity of each fraction was determined by vascular permeability in rabbit skin and expressed in BD_4. The toxin was purified about 65-fold from partially purified enterotoxin, with recovery of about 11%.

Disc electrophoresis The homogeneity of the purified toxin was examined on conventional PAGE (Fig. 5). The purified E8498 toxin gave a single disc and mobility indentical to that of purified CT from 569B.

Biological immunological activities of non-01 toxin We then carried out studies to determine whether or not E8498 toxin had biological and immunological properties similar to those of the reference CT.

Ability to cause elongation in Chinese hamster ovary cells was examined, and the dose-response curves are shown in Fig. 6. 50% of the CHO cells became elongated when about 1.3 ng/ml of E8498 toxin was added to the medium whereas about 4.2 ng/ml of CT was needed to give an equal activity.

E8498 toxin caused marked accumulation of clear fluid in mouse ligated intestinal loops. Fig. 7 shows that the W/L ratio of 140 mg/cm, which is about half of the mean maximal intensity, were essentially the same (70-80 ng) for both toxins.

Specific PF activity in rabbit skin was essentially identical for both purified toxins. Dose-response curves, with and without standard cholera antitoxin, are shown in Fig. 8. E8498 toxin contained 94 million BD_4/mg and cholera toxin, 98 million. Thus one BD_4 of cholera toxin was 10.2 pg and one BD_4 of non-1 toxin was 10.6 pg. Limit of blueing (Lb) titrations are shown on the right in Fig. 8. Graded doses of toxin were mixed with equal volumes of standard antitoxin at a concentration of 1 antitoxin unit per ml. One Lb of 569B toxin as 56.8 ng and one Lb of E8498 toxin was 57.8 ng. These results show that not only specific PF activity was the same for the two toxins but also the amount of antitoxin needed for neutralization was identical.

In PIH both toxins showed very similar dose-response curves (Fig. 9); 6.6 ng of

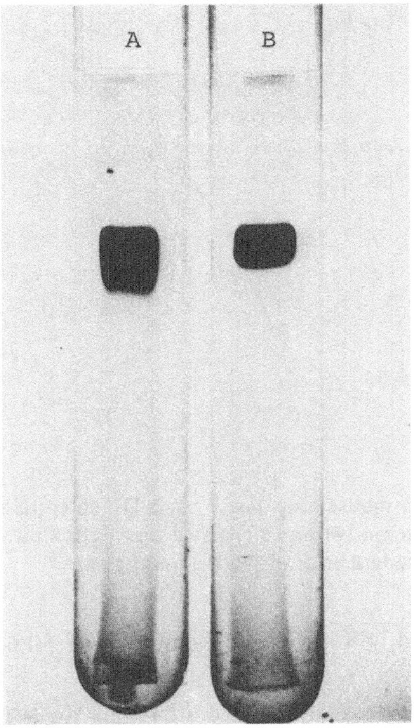

Fig. 5. Polyacrylamide gel disc electrophoresis of CT and E8498 enterotoxins. A, cholera toxin; B, purified E8498 enterotoxin; 100 μg of each toxin was applied.

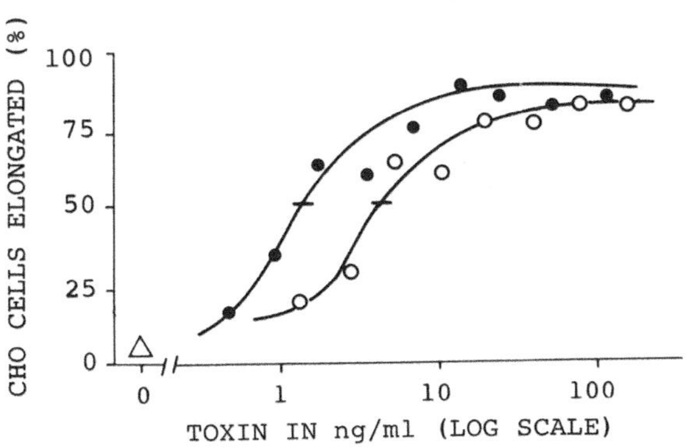

Fig. 6. Dose-response curve of morphological change in Chinese hamster ovary (CHO) cells by purified non-O1 enterotoxin and cholera toxin. ○, cholera toxin; ●, purified non-O1 enterotoxin. Each toxin was added to the culture medium of CHO cells at the final concentration indicated and percentages of elongated cells were enumerated after 18 h incubation. Each point indicates a mean of 8 determinations.

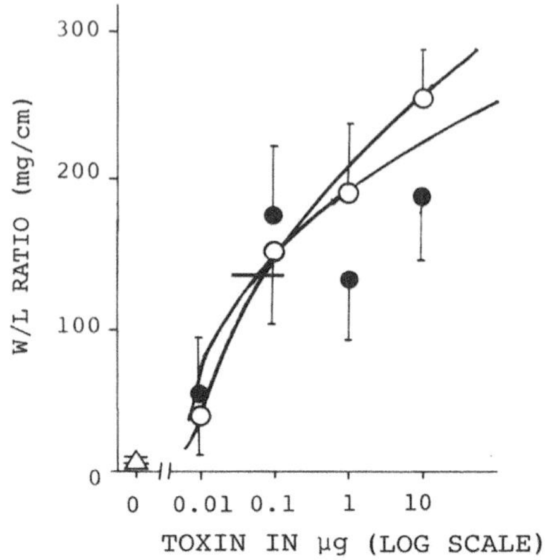

Fig. 7. Fluid accumulation in mouse loop test by non-O1 enterotoxin and cholera toxin. Cholera toxin (○) or non-O1 toxin (●) was inoculated into ligated intestine of mice. Each value represents mean ± one standerd error of five determinations.

E8498 toxin, and 9.5 ng of CT produced hemolysis of 50% of red blood cells in the system.

These findings all show that purified E8498 toxin is indistinguishable from CT prepared from 569B not only in biological activities but also in antigenic content, considering the experimental errors inherent in these systems.

Immunodiffusion test More evidence that both toxins were immunologically identical was obtained by Ouchterlony immunodiffuison tests using anti-569B toxin and anti-E8498 toxin as shown in Fig. 10. Each serum well (A and B) gave an identical single precipitation line against all three antigens with no spur. Purified E8498 toxin appears to be immunologically identical to CT preduced by 569B.

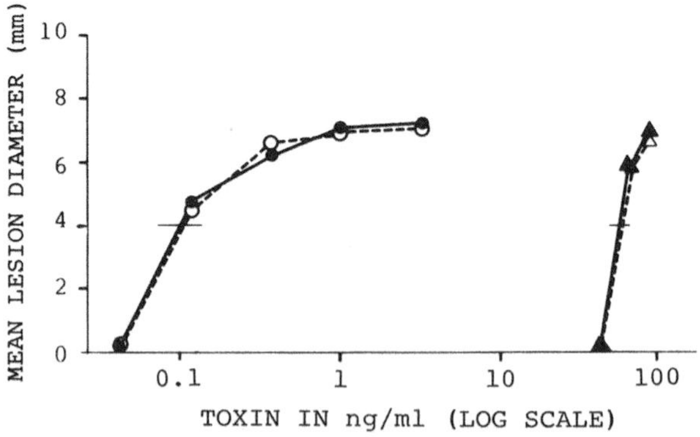

Fig. 8. Dose-response curve of PF activity of non-O1 enterotoxin and cholera toxin. BD_4 (●, ○) and Lb (▲, △) of cholera toxin (●, ▲) and non-O1 toxin (○, △) were determined for each curve. Each value represents the mean blueing lesion diameter (mm) observed 1 h after iv injection of blue dye given 24 h after intracutaneous injection of toxin.

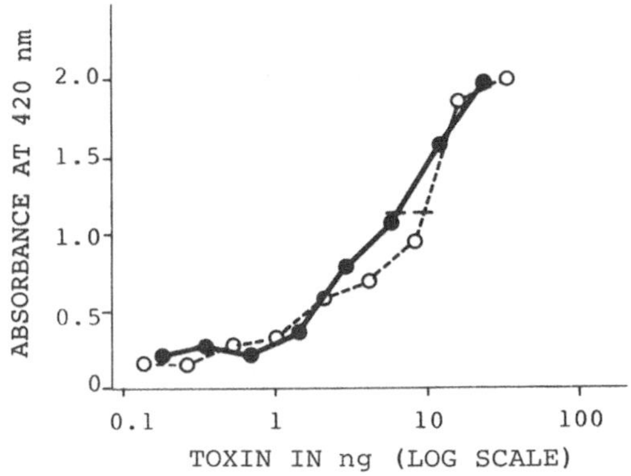

Fig. 9. Dose-response curves of non-O1 enterotoxin and cholera toxin by PIH. ○, cholera toxin; ●, non-O1 toxin.

SDS-PAGE In order to analyze the molecular structure of non-01 toxin SDS-PAGE was carried out. As shown in Fig. 11, in the second column purified E8498 toxin gave two bands with identical mobility to subunits A and B of cholera toxin. When the samples were reduced by DTT, the larger subunit of E8498 toxin which was coincident with subunit A of cholera toxin split into two band A_1 and A_2 as shown in column four. The four columns on the right (colums 5, 6, 7 and 8) serve as references. These patterns suggest that E8498 toxin is composed of the same subunits as cholera toxin, that is, A_1, A_2 and B.

Toxin from a non-O1 strain from a patient We also prepared purified enterotoxin from another strain of *V. cholerae*, non-01, S7, which was isolated from a diarrhea patient in Sudan. As shown in Fig. 12, S7 toxin yielded the same molecular weight components on SDS-PAGE as did cholera toxin.

Immunological properties of the toxin produced by several non-O1 strains were examined by Ouchterlony immunodiffusion tests. The strains used were all isolates from diarrhea patients. As shown in Fig. 13, the toxin preparations in the peripheral wells gave

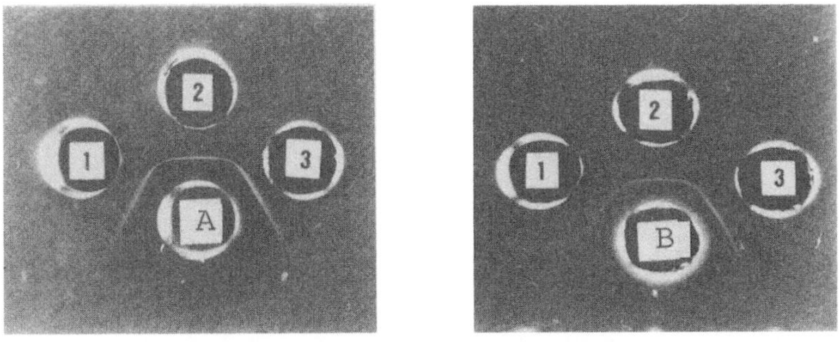

Fig. 10. Agar gel immunodiffusion test. Each well contains: (1) 5,000 x concentrated *V. cholerae* E8498 culture supernatant prepared by ultrafiltration and 50% saturation with ammonium sulfate. [7], (2) purified E8498 toxin, (3) cholera (569B) toxin, (A) anti-cholera toxin (569B), (B) anti-purified E8498 toxin.

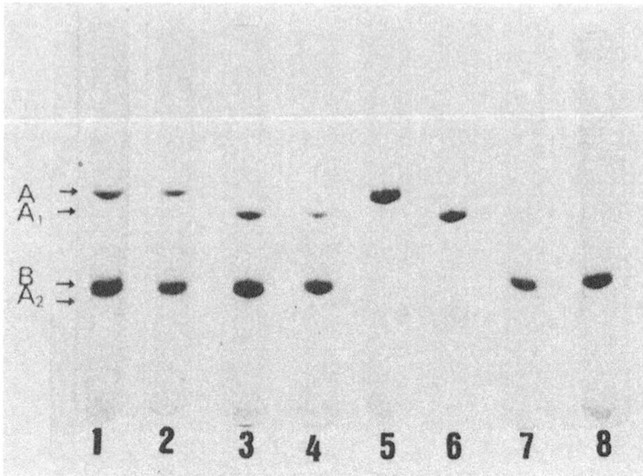

Fig. 11. SDS-PAGE of E8498 enterotoxin. Columns 1 and 3; cholera toxin; columns 2 and 4, purified E8498 toxin; columns 5 and 6, subunit A of cholera toxin; columns 7, 8, subunit B of cholera toxin; columns 2, 4, 6, 8, reduced with DTT.

single lines against both anti-cholera toxin (Fig. 12-A) and anti-E8498 toxin (Fig. 12-B). These findings indicate that toxins from two other non-O1 strains were immunologically identical to cholera toxin.

Discussion

We obtained highly purified cholera-like enterotoxin from a strain of *V. cholerae*,

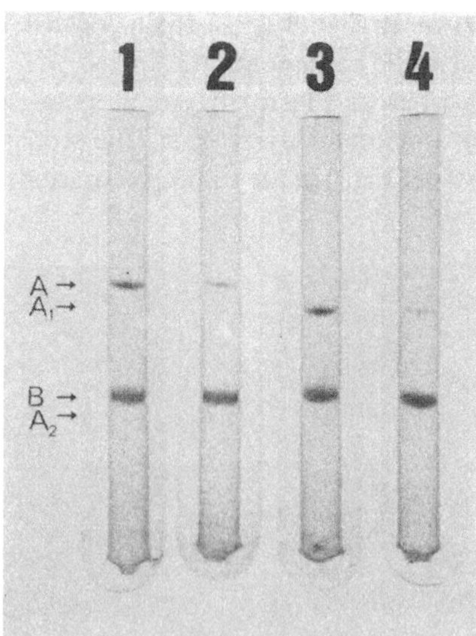

Fig. 12. SDS-PAGE of enterotoxin from a non-O1 strain from a human patient (*V. cholera*, non-O1 S7). Columns 1 and 3, cholera toxin; columns 2 and 4, purified S7 toxin; columns 3 and 4, reduced by DTT.

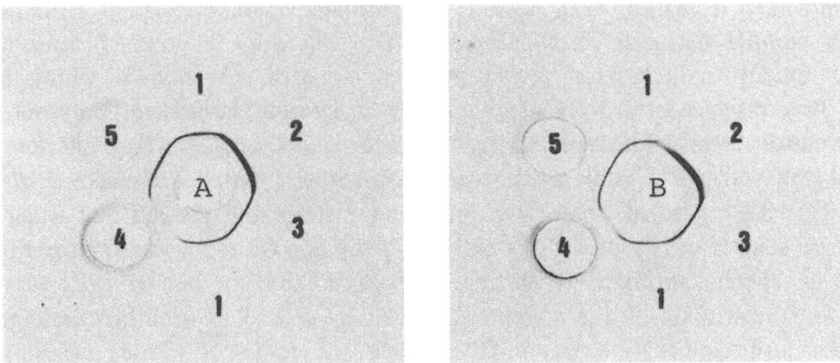

Fig. 13. Agar gel immunodiffusion test of enterotoxins for *V. cholerae* non-O1 strains from patients with diarrhea. Well 1, cholera toxin; well 2, purified E8498 toxin, well 3, partially purified S7 toxin; well 4, partially purified WBDV-101E_1 toxin; well 5, partially purified 62058 toxin; well A, anti-cholera toxin; well B, anti-purified E8498 toxin.

non-O1, E8498. This toxin exhibited specific activities almost identical to CT in several biologic and immunologic systems (Table 3). E8498 toxin was composed of the same A and B subunits as those found in cholera toxin (Fig. 11, 12). Ouchterlony agar immunodiffusion procedures also showed that E8498 toxin and cholera toxin had the same antigenic specificities. From these results we concluded that the cholera-like enterotoxin produced by this strain of *V. cholerae* non-O1 is indistinguishable from cholera toxin produced by the O1 strain 569B.

Table 3. Specific biological and immunological activities of enterotoxin produced by O1 and non-O1 strains of *V. cholerae*.

Assay	O1 Toxin (569B)		Non-O1 Toxin (E8498, 0344)	
CHO cell assay (Amount causing 50% elongation)	4.2		1.3	ng/ml
Mouse loop test (Amount producing W/L=140mg/cm)		70 - 80		ng
Rabbit skin test				
BD_4	10.2		10.6	pg
	(9.8 x 10^4		9.4 x 10^4	$BD_4/\mu g$)
Lb	56.8		57.8	ng
	(17.6		17.3	Lb/μg)
Passive immune hemolysis (Amount causing 50% hemolysis)	9.5		6.6	ng

Until now it has not been possible to determine whether cholera-like toxins produced by non-O1 strains are identical to the CT produced by O1 strains because highly purified non-O1 toxin has not previously been prepared. The non-O1 vibrios so far studied have produced relatively small amounts of enterotoxin in vitro. Moreover, they often produce several biologically active substances (7, 19, 26, 27) which interfere with or mask the activity of cholera-like enterotoxin in test systems. Zinnaka *et al.* (27) prepared partially purified toxin from one non-O1 strain and showed that when non-specific substances were removed the activity of the non-O1 toxin was completely neutralized by cholera antitoxin. Their report suggested that the non-01 toxin was very similar to cholera toxin. In the present work we were able to confirm their findings, and to further purify and analyze the non-O1 toxin directly, leading us to the conclusion that the toxins from E8498 and 569B are identical.

Enterotoxins composed of the same subunits as O1 cholera toxin were produced not only by the environmental non-O1 strain E8498, but also by a non-O1 strain isolated form a patient (S7). These findings suggest that perhaps all toxinogenic non-O1 and O1 strains produce toxic proteins of very similar or identical molecular structure. These data are consistent with the findings of Kaper *et al.* (15) that some strains of non-O1 vibrios possess genes which hybridize with DNA coding for the heat-labile enterotoxin (LT) from *Escherichia coli.* However, our findings with the non-O1 toxin from E8498 indicate that it is much more closely allied to CT from O1 strains than is *E. coli* LT. Although LT and CT share some common biological activities, molecular structure and enzymatic activities (2, 10, 12, 16), their antigenic (2) and amino acid composition (8, 22) are clearly distinguishable (3, 5, 6). Moreover, LT's of human and porcine origin are immunologically quite distinct (14, 16). Of course, since we have examined only a few non-O1 strains, and these toxins have been carefully compared with only one toxin from an O1 strain (569B), it is quite possible that differences in molecular structure will be found to exist among the enterotoxins produced by the species *Vibrio cholerae.*

Since the toxin produced by E8498, an environmental strain, has the same specific biologic activity as CT, it clearly provides this organism with the potential for being a causative agent of diarrhea. The amount of toxin produced in vitro by E8498 is relative small, but no less than that syntherized in vitro by many known virulent O1 strains of *V. cholerae* of the el tor biotype (unpublished observations). Since, however, other factors of virulence, in addition to the enterotoxin, are no doubt required to produce diarrhea in humans, the actual enteropathogenic potential of this non-O1 strain can be demonstrated only by oral challenge in volunteers.

REFERENCES

1. Blake, P. A., D. T. Allegra, J. D. Snyder, T. J. Barret, L. McFarland, C. T. Caraway, J. C. Feeley, J. P. Craig, J. V. Lee, N. D. Pur, and R. A. Feldman. 1980. Cholera -a possible endemic focus in the United States. New Engl. J. Med. **302**: 305-309.
2. Clements, J. D. and R. A. Finkelstein. 1978. Immunological cross-reactivity between a heat-labile enterotoxin(s) of *Escherichia coli* and subunits of *Vibrio cholerae* enterotoxin. Infect. Immun. **21**: 1036-1039.
3. Clements, J. D. and R. A. Finkelstein. 1979. Isolation and characterization of homogeneous heat-labile enterotoxin with highly specific activity from *Escherichia coli* culture. Infect. Immun. **24**: 760-769.

4. Craig, J. P. 1965. A permeability factor(toxin) found in cholera stool and culture filtrates and its neutralization by convalesent cholera sera. Nature (London) **207**: 614-616.
5. Craig, J. P. 1971. Cholera toxins. *In* Microbial toxins vol. IIA (Davis, S., Montie, T. and Ajl, S. J., eds), pp. 189-254, Academic Press, New York.
6. Craig, J. P., 1978. Toward the development of a standard reference cholera antitoxin. Report of Ad Hoc Commitee of the US cholera Panel. Develop. Biol. Standard, **41**: 415-422.
7. Craig, J. P., K. Yamamoto, Y. Takeda, and T. Miwatani. 1981. Production of cholera-like enterotoxin by a *Vibrio cholerae* non-O1 strain isolated from the environment. Infect. Immun. **34**: 90-97.
8. Dallas, W. S., and S. Falkow. 1980. Amino acid sequence homology between cholera toxin and *Escherichia coli* heat-labile toxin. Nature, **288**: 499-501.
9. Davis, B. J. 1964. Disc electrophoresis. II. Method and application to human serum proteins. Ann. N. Y. Acad. Sci. **212**: 404-427.
10. Evans, D. J., Chin, L. C., Curlin, G. T., and Evans, D. C. 1972. Stimulation of adenyl cyclase by *Escherichia coli* enterotoxin. Nature (London) New Biol. **236**, 137-138.
11. Fairbanks, G. 1971. Electrophoretic analysis of the major polypeptides of the human erythrocyte membrane. Biochemistry, **10**: 2606-2617.
12. Gyles, G. L. 1974. Immunological study of the heat-labile enterotoxins of *Escherichia coli* and *Vibrio cholerae.* Infect. Immun. **9**: 564-570.
13. Honda, T., M. Shimizu, Y. Takeda, and T. Miwatani. 1976. Isolation of a factor causing morphological changes of Chinese hamster ovary cells from the culture filtrate of *Vibrio parahaemolyticus.* Infect. Immun. **14**: 1028-1033.
14. Honda, T., T. Tsuji, Y. Takeda and T. Miwatani. 1981. Demonstration of immunological non-identity of heat-labile enterotoxins from human and porcine enterotoxigenic *Escherichia coli.* Infect. Immun. **34**: 337-340.
15. Kaper, J. B., S. L. Moseley, and S. Falkow. 1981. Molecular characterization of environmental and non-toxigenic strains of *Vibrio cholerae.* Infect. Immun. **32**: 661-667.
16. Kunkel, S. L. and D. C. Robertson. 1979. Purification and chemical characterization of the heat-labile enterotoxin produced by enterotoxigenic *Escherichia coli.* Infect. Immun. **25**: 586-596.
17. Lowry, O. H., N. J. Rosebrough, A. L. Farr, and R. F. Randall. 1951. Protein measurement with Folin phenol reagent. J. Biol. Chem. **193**: 265-275.
18. Ohtomo, N., T. Muraoka, H. Inoue, H. Sakaoka and H. Takahashi. 1974. Preparation of cholera toxin and immunization studies with cholera toxoid, p. 132-142. *In* Proceedings of the Ninth Joint Cholera Conference of the US-Japan Cooperative Medical Science Program, Grand Canyon, Arizona, Oct. 1-3, 1973. Department of State publication no. 8762, U.S. Department of State, Washington, D. C.
19. Ohashi, M., T. Shimada, and H. Fukumi. 1972. *In vitro* production of enterotoxin and hemorrhagic principle by *Vibrio cholerae*, NAG, Jpn. J. Med. Sci. Biol. **25**: 179-194.
20. Ouchterlony, O. 1969. Antigen-antibody reactions in gels. Acta Pathol. Microbiol. Scand. **26**: 507-515.
21. Smith, H. L., Jr. 1979. Serotyping of non-cholera vibrios. J. Clin. Microbiol. **10**: 85-90.
22. Spicer, E. K., W. M. Davanough, W. S. Dallas, S. Falkow, W. H. Donigsberg, and D. E. Schafer. 1981. Sequence homologies between A subunits of *Escherichia coli* and *Vibrio cholerae* enterotoxin. Proc. Natl. Acad. Sci. USA. **78**: 50-54.
23. Takeda, Y., T. Takeda, T. Yano, K. Yamamoto, and T. Miwatani. 1979. Purification and partial characterization of heat-stable enterotoxin of enterotoxigenic *Escherichia coli.* Infect. Immun. **25**: 978-985.
24. Tsukamoto, T., Y. Kinoshita, S. Taga, Y. Takeda, and T. Miwatani. 1980. Value of passive immune hemolysis for detection of heat-labile enterotoxin produced by enterotoxigenic *Escherichia coli.* J. Clin. Microbiol., **12**: 768-771.
25. Yamamoto, K., Y. Takeda, T. Miwatani, and J. P. Craig. 1981. Stimulation by lincomycin of production of cholera-like enterotoxin in *Vibrio cholerae*, non-O1 FEMS Microbiol. Letters, **12**:245-248.

26. Zinnaka, Y. and C. C. F. Carpenter. 1972. An enterotoxin produced by non-cholera vibrios. John Hopkins Med. J. **131**: 403-411.
27. Zinnaka, Y., S. Fukuyoshi, and Y. Okamura. 1973. Some observations on the NAG vibrio toxin, p. 116-123, *In* H. Fukumi and M. Ohashi (ed.), Proceedings of the Eighth Joint Conference on Cholera, US-Japan Cooperative Medical Science Program, Tokyo, Japan, August, 1972, The Japanese Cholera Panel, National Institute of Health, Tokyo.

Advances in Research on Cholera and Related Diarrheas, eds., S. Kuwahara, N. F. Pierce, 247–257.

HIGH AFFINITY RECEPTOR FOR HEAT-STABLE ENTEROTOXINS (ST_a) ON RAT INTESTINAL EPITHELIAL CELLS

Joseph C. Frantz and Donald C. Robertson

University of Kansas, Lawrence, KS 66045

Studies on the association of heat-stable enterotoxin (ST) produced by enterotoxigenic *E. coli* (ETEC) strain 431 with isolated rat intestinal epithelial cells and brush border membranes indicated that ST_as bind to a single class of specific high affinity receptor. Specific binding of radioiodinated ST (specific activity 600 to 900 Ci/mmole) was temperature dependent and reached a maximum between 5 and 10 minutes which correlated with increased activity of particulate guanylate cyclase. The rate of dissociation of 431 ST from either intestinal cells or brush border membranes was significantly less than the rate of association. The number of ST-specific receptors on rat intestinal cells determined by Scatchard analysis was 20,478± 6,185 per cell with an affinity constant (Ka) of 6.25 x 10^{11} L/M. The affinity constant determined for brush border membranes (Ka = 9.4 x 10^{11} L/M) agreed with the value obtained with whole cells. Binding experiments with ^{125}I-431 ST and brush border membranes showed that purified ST_as from ETEC strains 667 (class 1 porcine enteropathogen), B-41 (bovine enteropathogen), and human strains 213 C_2 (Mexico) and 153961-2 (Dacca, Bangladesh) exhibited similar patterns of competitive inhibition as homologous ST produced by strain 431 (class 2 enteropathogen). Further, purified LT (strain 286 C_2) did not inhibit binding of 431 ST. Digestion of brush border membranes showed the ST receptor to be resistant to lipases and glycosidases but somewhat sensitive to proteases. The putative ST binding protein radiolabeled with ^{125}I-431 ST was solubilized with sodium deoxycholate. One major radioactive band was detected by SDS-polyacrylamide gel electrophoresis followed by radioautography.

Introduction

Enterotoxigenic strains of *Escherichia coli* (ETEC) cause diarrhea in humans and other animals following colonization of the gut and production of 2 kinds of enterotoxins (20). The heat-labile (LT) toxin, has been shown to meditate secretion through stimulation of adenylate cyclase (6, 11, 12); whereas, the heat-stable low molecular weight toxin (ST), with biological activity in suckling mice and piglets (ST_a), provokes the loss of fluid and electrolytes through activation of quanylate cyclase (9, 10, 13, 19). Thus, both kinds of *E. coli* enterotoxins exert their action in the gut by modulating intracellular levels of cyclic nucleotides. It is not known if a second kind of ST with biological activity only in piglets (ST_b) acts through a mechanism involving either cAMP or cGMP (4).

The purpose of this investigation was to study the association of ST_as with rat intestinal cells and determine if a specific receptor is involved in the overall mechanism of action. Presumably, toxin binding is the first in a series of events leading to stimulation of guanylate cyclase and elevated levels of cGMP. In a previous study (9), we demonstrated an immunological similarity between ST_as of human, bovine and porcine origin; thus, it was of interest to determine if ST_as of different host origins bind to the same receptor which might suggest that all ST_as possess a common amino acid sequence involved in biological activity and immunological reactivity.

Materials and Methods

Cultures, Culture Conditions and Toxin Purification. Sources of human and porcine strains of enterotoxigenic *E. coli* (ETEC) and maintenance of stock cultures were as described previously (1). Preparation of media, growth conditions and purification of ST_as have been described elsewhere (1, 9). The heat-labile toxin (LT) produced by strain 286 C_2 was purified as described by Kunkle and Robertson (15).

Radioiodination of ST. Purified salt-free 431 ST was radiolabeled enzymatically using a reaction mixture which contained the following: ST, 1.0 ug; 0.2 M sodium phosphate, pH 7.2, 45 ul; Enzymobeads (Bio Rad Laboratories, Richmond, CA), 25 ul; $Na^{125}I$ (Amersham, Arlington Heights, IL), 1.0 mCi; and 1% D-glucose, 25 ul. Free ^{125}I was removed from ^{125}I-ST using XAD-2 adsorption chromatography (9). The labeled toxin preparation (specific activity of 600 to 900 Ci/mmol) retained biological activity in suckling mice for up to two weeks.

Intestinal Cells and Brush Border Membranes. Intestinal epithelial cells were isolated from female Sprague-Dawley rats (150 to 200 g) by the method of Weiser (22). Isolated cells were suspended in 24.5 mM HEPES, 2.5 mM NaH_2PO_4, 98 mM NaCl (pH 7.5) solution containing 1% bovine serum albumin (BSA). This solution hereafter is referred to as HPBS. The cell suspension was stored at 4°C until use with viability greater that 80% as judged by Trypan blue exclusion. Brush border membranes were prepared from isolated enterocytes as described by Hauser, *et al.* (14). Briefly, enterocytes were disrupted by ultrasonication followed by addition of solid $MgCl_2$ (20 mM). The preparation was subjected to differential centrifugation to separate brush border membranes from basal lateral membranes and other cell debris.

Binding Assay. Isolated rat epithelial cells (10^6) were incubated with a fixed amount of ^{125}I-431 ST (0.1 nM) in a final reaction volume of 200 ul for 10 min at the desired temperature. All experimental points were performed in triplicate. Following incubation, free ^{125}I-ST was separated from bound toxin by filtration using EAWP filters (Millipore Corp., Bedford, MA). Specific binding was calculated from the difference in total and nonspecific binding. Total binding was determined in those reaction mixtures which did not contain native toxin; whereas, nonspecific binding was estimated in reaction mixtures which contained a 100-fold excess of native toxin. Binding of ^{125}I-431 ST to rat brush border membranes was measured as described above except for the use of EGWP filters.

Enzymatic Digestion of Brush Border Membranes. Brush border membranes (100 ug) were incubated with various concentrations of lipases, proteases or glycosidases at 37°C for 20 minutes. The binding capacity of digested membranes was measured as described above.

Polyacrylamide Gel Electrophoresis of Brush Border Membranes. Reaction mixtures containing brush border membranes (400 ug) and ^{125}I-ST (1.0 nM) in the presence and absence of cold ST (1.0 uM) were incubated at 37°C for 10 minutes. Unbound ^{125}I-ST was removed by centrifugation. The pellet was resuspended in 100 ul TRIS-buffered saline-0.15% sodium deoxycholate and incubated for 18 h at room temperature. A solution of 10% SDS was added to adjust the mixture to a final concentration of 0.1%. The samples were electrophoresed in a linear 7.5% to 15% gradient SDS slab gel using conditions described by Laemmli (16). Following electrophoresis, the slabs were subjected to radioautography to visualize radioactive bands and stained with Coomassie Brilliant Blue R.

Other Assays. Protein content of brush border membrane preparations and purified ST preparations was determined by the method of Lowry (17). Other methods for determination of ST protein (5) agreed with the Lowry method. Levels of cGMP were determined by radioimmunassay as described by Brooker, *et al.* (3).

Results

Time and Temperature. The effects of time and temperature on binding of ST to in intestinal cells were examined to establish optimal conditions prior to more detailed studies and subsequent investigation of binding kinetics. Experiments with isolated rat enterocytes incubated with ^{125}I-ST in the presence and absence of 100-fold excess native toxin showed that the most rapid rate of association, regardless of temperature, occurred during the first minute of incubation (Figure 1). Specific binding at 37°C was greater than that observed at either 20°C or 4°C. The level of intracellular cGMP reached a maximum at about 5 minutes even though the extent of binding continued to increase for 3 h (data not shown). Although not depicted in Figure 1, the level of nonspecific binding in whole cells generally ranged from 40% to 60% of the total binding. The rate of association for binding of ST to brush border membranes was essentially the same as that observed using whole cells (Figure 2). Likewise, the rate of binding correlated with the increased activity of particulate guanylate cyclase and accumulation of cGMP. In contrast to the high level of nonspecific binding observed with intact enterocytes, nonspecific binding of ^{125}I-ST to brush border membranes was consistently less than 10% of the total.

Binding of toxin as a function of the concentration of radiolabeled ST was examined using whole cells (Figure 3) and brush border membranes (Figure 4) to determine numbers of receptors and binding affinity of receptors for ST. Specific binding of ^{125}I-ST to intact cells and membranes was saturable and Scatchard analysis (21) indicated a binding capacity of 20, 475± 6125 receptors per cell and 0.8 pmol ST bound per mg brush border membrane protein (inset, Figures 3 and 4). The binding affinity (Ka of 6.3×10^{11} L/M) for whole cells was similar to that calculated for brush border membranes (Ka of 9.4×10^{11} L/M). The rate of dissociation of ST from whole cells was significantly less that the rate of association, however, dissociation was temperature dependent and specifically bound ST dissociated more rapidly at 27°C than at 4°C (Figure 5). In order to

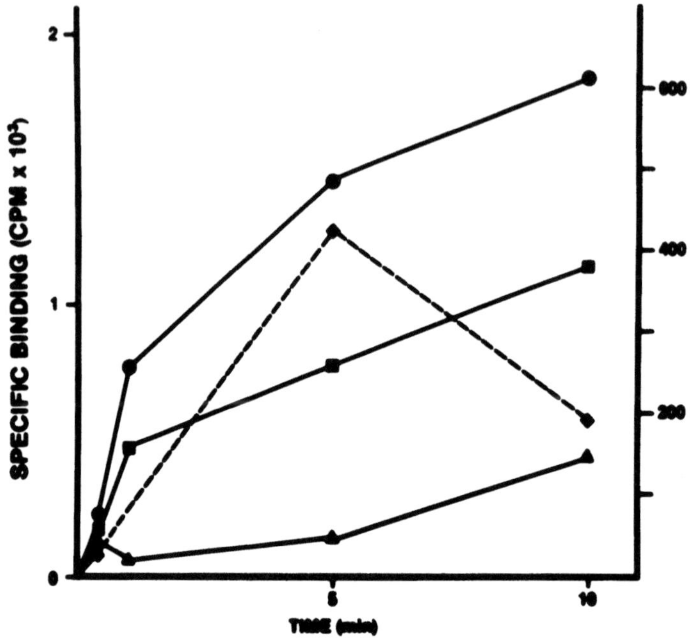

Figure 1. Time course of specific binding of ^{125}I-431 ST by rat intestinal epithelial cells. Symbols: ●—●, binding at 37°C; ■—■, binding at 20°C; ▲—▲, binding at 4°C; ■– –■, intracellular concentration of cGMP determined by RIA.

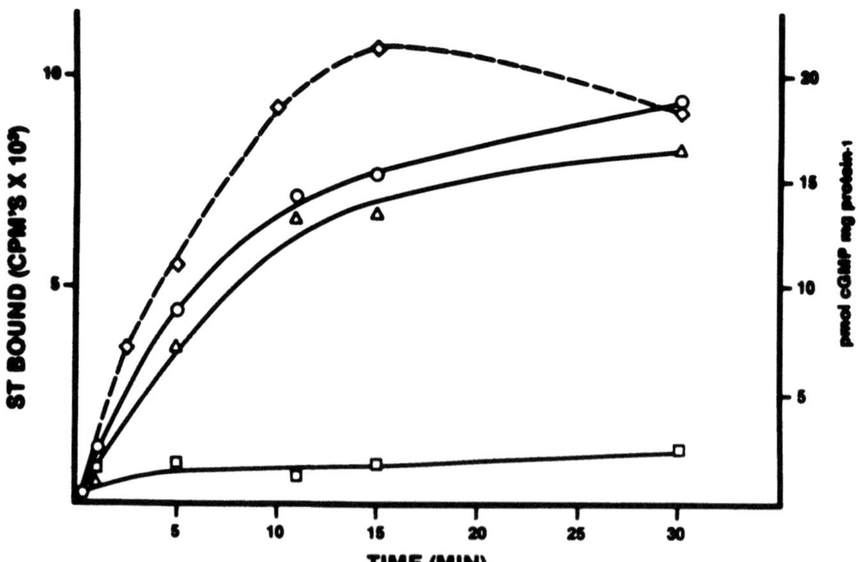

Figure 2. Time course of specific binding of ^{125}I-431 ST by rat intestinal brush border membranes. Symbols: ○—○, binding at 37°C; △—△, binding at 20°C; □—□, binding at 4°C; □– –□, amount of cGMP determined by RIA.

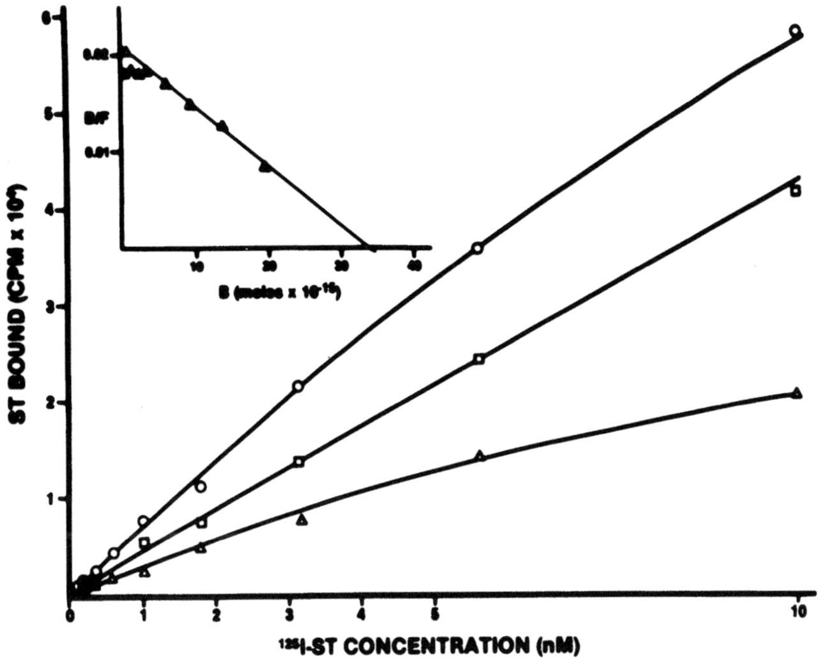

Figure 3. Effect of ^{125}I-431 ST concentration on specific binding by rat intestinal epithelial cells. Symbols: ○—○, total binding; □—□ nonspecific binding determined by addition of a 100-fold excess of native ST as described in Materials and Methods; △—△, specific binding calculated by subtracting nonspecific binding from total binding. Inset: Scatchard plot of specific binding data.

ascertain whether bound ST was internalized, intact enterocytes were lysed by ultrasonication and the sonicate subjected to ultrafiltration. All of the radioactivity remained associated with the membrane fraction which strongly suggested that specifically bound toxin remained attached to membranes and was not transferred into the interior of the cell. The dissociation of specifically bound ST from brush border membranes was similar to that observed using whole cells. Following incubation at 37°C for 10 minutes, the dissociation of ST from membranes suspended in buffer was slightly less than membranes suspended in buffer containing 2.5 uM native toxin (Figure 6).

Binding characteristics of purified STs of different host origins to rat intestinal brush border membranes were compared. The concentration of ^{125}I-431 ST was the same in each reaction mixture (10^{-9}M); whereas, the concentration of native toxins was varied between 0 and 10^{-6}M. The results showed that all purified ST_a enterotoxins exhibited similar patterns of competitive inhibition as did cold homologous 431 ST in competition with ^{125}I-431 ST (Figure 7). Scatchard analysis of these data indicated an affinity constant (Ka = 1 x 10^{12} L/M) which was virtually the same as that estimated using specific binding data.

Brush border membranes were incubated with various enzymes in order to probe the chemical nature of the receptor for ST. Most of the hydrolytic enzymes tested had no effect, while Pronase treatment had the most effect in reducing specific binding of ST to brush border membranes (Table 1). The level of inhibition observed when membranes

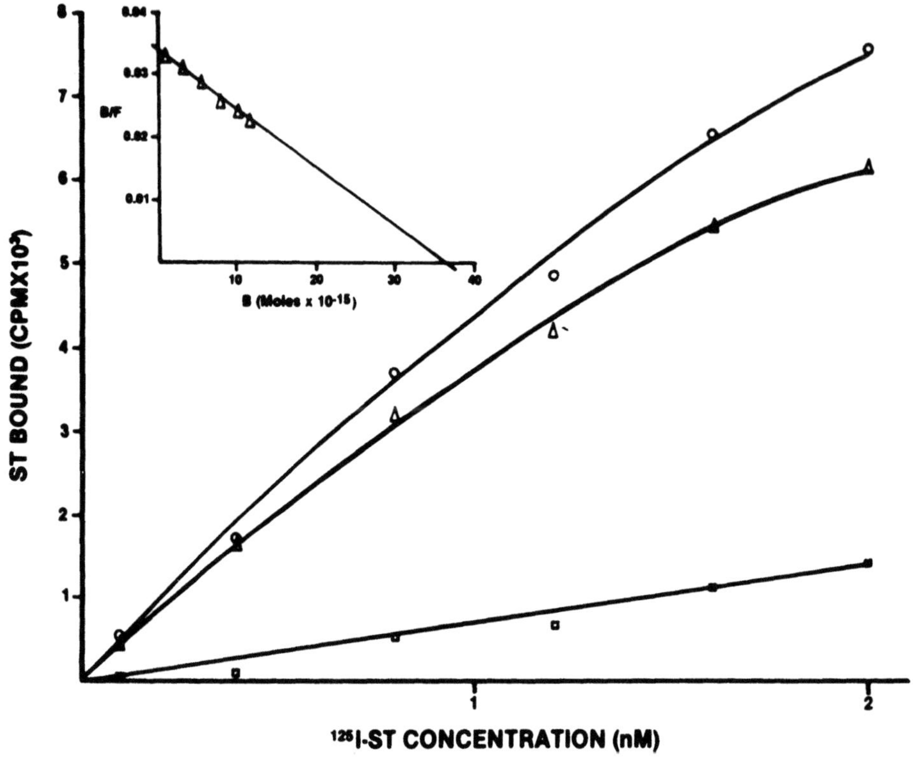

Figure 4. Effect of ^{125}I-431 binding concentration on specific binding by rat intestinal brush border membranes. Symbols: same as Figure 3. Inset: Scatchard plot of specific binding data.

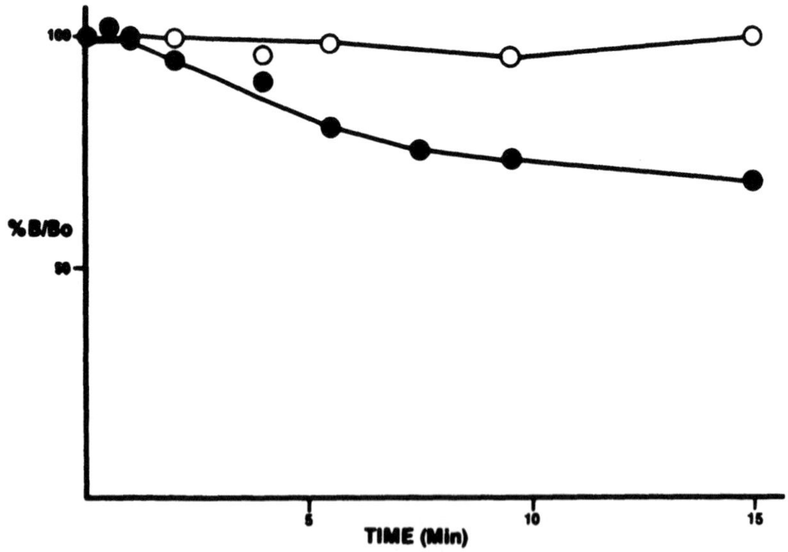

Figure 5. Dissociation of ^{125}I-431 ST from rat intestinal epithelial cells at 27°C and 4°C. Symbols: ○—○, 4°C; ●—●, 27°C.

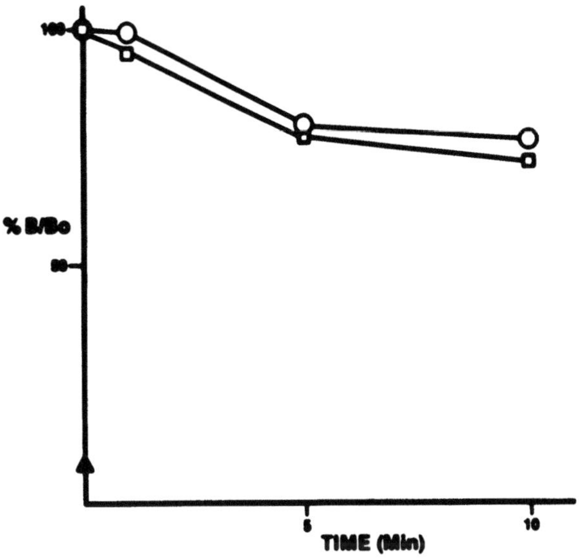

Figure 6. Dissociation of ^{125}I-431 ST from brush border membranes at 37°C. Symbols: ○—○, membranes washed and resuspended in HPBS; □—□, membranes washed and resuspended in HPBS containing a 100-fold excess of native ST.

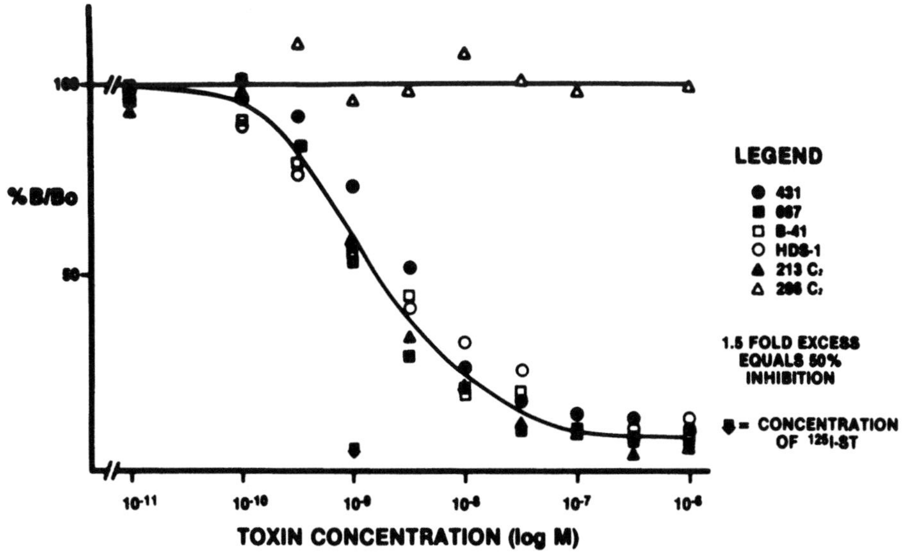

Figure 7. Competitive inhibition of binding of ^{125}I-431 ST by native 431 ST, heterologous ST_as and LT. Symbols: ●—●, 431 ST; ■—■, 667 ST; □—□, B-41 ST; ○—○, HDS-1 ST; ▲—▲, 213 C_2 ST; △—△, 286 C_2 LT.

Table 1. Enzymatic digestion of brush border membranes.

Treatment	Enzyme Concentration (ug/ml)	Residual Binding of ^{125}I-431 ST (%)
None	–	100
Phospholipase A_2	10	109
Phospholipase C	40	100
Neuraminidase	5	101
Endoglycosidase P	5	95
Papain	200	106
Trypsin	200	91
Chymotrypsin	200	90
Proteinase K	200	88
Pronase	200	67

were digested with Pronase was time dependent; however, the amount of binding did not decrease with longer incubation times.

The Ka of ST for intact enterocytes and membranes suggested that the toxin might remain bound even in the presence of detergents used to dissociate and solubilize membranes. A high molecular weight ST binding species was detected by SDS-polyacrylamide gel electrophoresis (Figure 8) of brush border membranes incubated with ^{125}I-ST and extracted with sodium deoxycholate. Migration of the putative ST receptor was distinc-

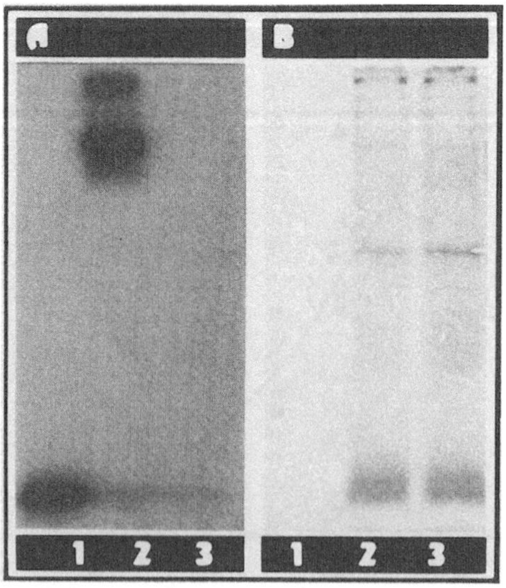

Figure 8. SDS-polyacrylamide gel electrophoresis of ST receptor extracted from brush border membranes. Panel A (radioautogram); lane 1, ^{125}I-431 ST; lane 2, soluble fraction of brush border membranes after incubation with ^{125}I-431 ST; lane 3, same as lane 2 except for addition of a 100-fold excess of native ST. Panel B, the same gel as in panel A after staining with Coomassie Brilliant Blue R.

tively different from free ST and was not evident in reaction mixtures containing a 1000-fold excess of cold native toxin. The ST binding species did not penetrate the separating gel when membranes were not extracted with sodium deoxycholate. A protein species was observed in the region of the ^{125}I-ST receptor complex which stained with both Schiff stain and Coomassie Brilliant Blue R; however, the number of bands and data in Table 1 precluded any further chemical definition of the receptor at this time.

Discussion

The association of *E. coli* ST_as was shown to be rapid, saturable, and specific as indicated by the extent of binding in the presence of 100 to 1,000-fold excess of unlabeled toxin. Further, the rate of association of ST to both whole cells and brush border membranes (Figures 1 and 2) correlated with the increase in guanylate cyclase and accumulation of cGMP.

Other workers have noted that rinsing ligated loops previously challenged with ST reduced the secretory response (7). The results reported herein are inconsistent with this observation because 1) a significant amount of specifically bound ST did not dissociate (Figures 5 and 6) and 2) high levels of native unlabeled ST did not increase the low level of toxin dissociation. Obviously, much remains to be determined as to the fate of the toxin once it interacts with its receptor and events in intestinal membranes prior to activation of particulate guanylate cyclase.

The binding affinities calculated for other bacterial toxins and selected polypeptide hormones are significantly lower than the affinity constant of ST binding to its receptor. The low number of ST specific receptors on rat enterocytes is also somewhat unusual compared with data obtained with various polypeptide hormones (2).

The results depicted in Figure 7 demonstrate that differences exist in the binding and mechanisms of action of ST and LT. G_{ml} ganglioside is the most likely receptor involved in the binding of LT to intestinal cells (18), however, high concentrations of mixed gangliosides did not alter binding of ST to intact cells or brush border membranes (data not shown). It is interesting that at a 1.5-fold excess of native toxin reduced the binding of ^{125}I-ST by 50%. In contrast to the high nonspecific binding of ST to intact enterocytes (40 to 60%), the level of nonspecific binding to brush border membranes (Figure 4) was much lower, presumably due to nonspecific attachment of ST to basal lateral membranes present in intact cells. Although comparative inhibition kinetics were not performed with basal lateral membranes, the data strongly suggested that the most likely location of the receptor for ST_as to be on microvilli. In view of the immunological similarities for human, bovine, and porcine ST previously described (9), the similar competition kinetics for ST_as of different origins shown in Figure 7 were not particularly surprising. These data strongly suggest that age-dependent host responses to different ETEC strains depend on bacterial virulence factors other than toxins (23).

The results shown in Table 1 and Figure 8 suggest that the putative ST receptor is a membrane protein probably with a close proximity to or complexed with particulate guanylate cyclase. The data also suggested that internalization of ST is not required for biological activity. Experiments are in progress to determine the relationship between ST and its receptor since the ST-binding protein was probably extracted in aggregate form.

In summary, the binding characteristics of radiolabeled porcine 431 ST and unlabeled ST_as of porcine, bovine, and human origins have been studied. The results show that 1) binding of ST_as is mediated by a single class of high affinity receptor, 2) ST_as of different host origins bind to the same rat intestinal receptor, 3) the ST receptor is very likely a protein and not related to G_{ml} ganglioside which binds LT and cholera toxin and 4) binding of ST_as to a specific receptor occurred at a rate consistent with the activation of particulate guanylate cyclase.

This investigation was supported by grant R22 AI-12357 from the National Institute of Allergy and Infectious Diseases. J.C.F. was supported by Postdoctoral Fellowship AI--06089 from the National Institute of Allergy and Infectious Diseases. The authors wish to thank Lawrence Dreyfus for cGMP determinations.

REFERENCES

1. Alderete, J. and D. C. Robertson. 1978. Purification and chemical characterization of the heat-stable enterotoxin produced by porcine strains of enterotoxigenic *Escherichia coli.* Infect. Immun. **19**:1021-1030.
2. Binder, H. J., G. F., Lemp, and J. D. Sandner. 1980. Receptors for vasoactive intestinal peptide and secretin on small intestinal epithelial cells. Am. J. Physiol. **238**:G190-G196.
3. Brooker, G., J. F. Harper, W. L. Terasaki, and R. D. Moylan. 1979. Radioimmunoassay of cAMP and cGMP. Advances in Cyclic Nucleotide Research. **10**:1-32.
4. Burgess, M. N., R. J. Bywater, C. M. Cowley, N. A. Mullan, and P. M. Newsome. 1978. Biological evaluation of a methanol-soluble, heat-stable *Escherichia coli* enterotoxin in infant mice, pigs, rabbits, and calves. Infect, and Immun. **21**:526-531.
5. Ehresmann, B., P. Imbault, and J. H. Weil. 1973. Spectrophotometric determination of protein concentration of cell extracts containing tRNAs and rRNAs. Anal. Biochem. **54**:454-463.
6. Evans, D. J. Jr., L. C. Chen, G. T. Curlin, and D. G. Evans. 1972. Stimulation of adenyl cyclase by *Escherichia coli* enterotoxin. Nature. **236**:137-138.
7. Evans, D., D. Evans Jr., and N. Pierce. 1973. Differences in the response of rabbit small intestine to heat-labile and heat-stable enterotoxins of *Escherichia coli.* Infect. Immun. **7**:873-880.
8. Field, M., L. Graf Jr., W. Laird, and P. Smith. 1978. Heat-stable enterotoxin of *Escherichia coli*: *in vitro* effects on guanylate cyclase activity, cyclic GMP concentration, and ion transport in small intestine. Proc. Natl. Acad. Sci. U. S. A. **75**:2800-2804.
9. Frantz, J. C., and D. C. Robertson. 1981. Immunological properties of *Escherichia coli* heat-stable enterotoxins: Development of a radioimmunoassay specific for heat-stable enterotoxins with suckling mouse activity. Infect. Immun. **33**:193-198.
10. Gianella, R. A., and K. W. Drake. 1979. Effect of purified *Escherichia coli* heat-stable enterotoxin on intestinal cyclic nucleotide metabolism and fluid secretion. Infect. Immun. **24**:19-23.
11. Gill, D. M., D. J. Evans, Jr., and D. G. Evans. 1976. Mechanism of action of adenylate cyclase *in vitro* by polymyxin B-released heat-labile enterotoxin of *Escherichia coli.* J. Infect. Dis. **139**: S103-S107.
12. Gill, D. M., and S. H. Richardson. 1980. Adenosine diphosphate-ribosylation of adenylate cyclase catalyzed by heat-labile enterotoxin of *Escherichia coli*: Comparison with cholera toxin. J. Infect. Dis. **141**:64-70.
13. Guerrant, R. L., J. M. Hughes, B. Chang, D. C. Robertson, and F. Murad. 1980. Activation of intestinal guanylate cyclase by heat-stable enterotoxin of *Escherichia coli*: studies of tissue specificity, potential receptors, and intermediates. J. Infect. Dis. **142**:220-228.
14. Hauser, H., K. Howell, R. M. C. Dawson, and D. E. Bowyer. 1980. Rabbit small intestinal brush border membrane preparation and lipid composition. Biochem. Biophys. Acta. **602**:567-577.
15. Kunkel, S. L. and D. C. Robertson. 1979. Purification and chemical characterization of the

heat-labile enterotoxin produced by enterotoxigenic *Escherichia coli.* Infect. Immun. **25**:586-596.

16. Laemmli, U. K. 1970. Cleavage of structural proteins during the assembly of the head of bacteriophage T4. Nature (London). **227**:680-685.
17. Lowry, O. H., N. J. Rosebrough, H. L. Farr, and R. J. Randall. 1951. Protein measurement with the Folin phenol reagent. J. Biol. Chem. **193**:265-275.
18. Moss, J., J. C. Osborne, Jr., P. H. Fishman, S. Nakaya, D. C. Robertson. 1981. *Escherichia coli* heat-labile enterotoxin, ganglioside specificity and ADP-ribosyltransferase activity. J. Biol. Chem. **256**:12861-12865.
19. Rao, M. C., S. Guandalini, P. L. Smith, and M. Field. 1980. Mode of action of heat-stable *Escherichia coli* enterotoxin. Tissue and subcellular specificities and role of cyclic GMP. Biochem. Biophys. Acta. **632**:35-46.
20. Sack, R. R. 1976. Human diarrheal disease caused by enterotoxigenic *Escherichia coli.* Ann. Rev. Microbiol. **22**:333-353.
21. Scatchard, G. 1949. The attractions of proteins for small molecules and ions. Ann. N. Y. Acad. Sci. **51**:660-672.
22. Weiger, M. M. 1973. Intestinal epithelial cell surface membrane glycoprotein synthesis. An indicator of cellular differentiation. J. Biol. Chem. **248**:2536-2541.
23. Whipp. S. C., H. W. Moon, and R. A. Argenzio. 1981. Comparison of enterotoxic activity of heat-stable enterotoxins from class 1 and class 2 *Escherichia coli* of swine origin. Infect. and Immun. **31**:245-251.

Advances in Research on Cholera and Related Diarrheas, eds., S. Kuwahara, N. F. Pierce, 259–268.

CHARACTERISTICS OF THE BINDING OF PURE HUMAN *E. COLI* HEAT-STABLE ENTEROTOXIN TO RAT INTESTINE

Ralph A. Giannella, M.D. and Marcia Luttrell

Division of Digestive Diseases, University of Cincinnati College of Medicine
Cincinnati, Ohio

Enterotoxigenic strains of *E. coli* cause diarrhea by elaborating either a large molecular weight heat-labile enterotoxin or one or more small molecular weight heat-stable enterotoxins (1). A great deal is known about the molecular actions of LT (2) but relatively little is known about the mechanism of action of ST. ST probably causes intestinal secretion by the mediation of the guanylate cyclase-cyclic GMP system (1,3-5).

We have purified STa, a suckling mouse active ST, from a human strain of *E. coli* and characterized the molecule (6,7). Figure 1 illustrates the amino acid sequence of our human ST and also lists some chracteristics of the molecule.

This ST is a peptide containing a total of 18 amino acids and is devoid of any carbohydrate or lipid. Molecular weight determined by amino acid analysis is 1972. It is a small, compact, folded molecule containing at least one disulfide bridge which is required for biologic activity. This toxin is unusual in that it contains 6 cysteine residues. It also contains two tyrosine residues, at positions 4 and 11 which are available for radioiodination.

In contrast to human ST, ST's produced by porcine strains of *E. coli* appear to be larger molecules (8-10). These various toxins are probably related in that the larger ST's probably contain the 18 amino acid peptide that we purified or the active site contained within it (7).

E. COLI ST

-AN 18 AA PEPTIDE, MW 1972
-NO CARBOHYDRATE OR LIPID
-A SMALL, COMPACT, FOLDED MOLECULE
-DISULFIDE BRIDGES REQUIRED FOR
BIOLOGIC ACTIVITY

AA SEQUENCE

```
       1   2   3   4   5   6   7   8   9
NH2 -ASN-THR-PHE-TYR-CYS-CYS-GLU-LEU-CYS-

      18  17  16  15  14  13  12  11  10
COOH-ASN-CYS-GLY-ALA-CYS-ALA-PRO-TYR-CYS
```

Figure 1. Amino acid sequence of human ST and some chemical characteristics of the molecule.

The present studies were done to determine whether a specific receptor for ST exists on intestinal cells and to characterize the ST binding process. The studies were done by studying the binding of ST to isolated rat jejunal, ileal, and colonic epithelial cells. Small intestinal cells were prepared by the method of Weiser (11) and viability was documented by trypan blue exclusion and by the preservation of active sugar transport. Isolated colonic cells were prepared by a similar method.

Figure 2 illustrates the ability of ST to stimulate cyclic GMP production in isolated jejunal villus cells.

The bottom curve are cells not exposed to ST and the level of cyclic GMP is relatively stable. In contrast, addition of ST results in the prompt and three to four fold increase in cyclic GMP concentration which persists for the duration of the experiment.

Binding studies were performed using ^{125}labeled ST. Pure ST was iodinated with ^{125}sodium iodide by the lactoperoxidase method and the iodinated ST was purified by anion exchange chromatography. These procedures resulted in a radioiodinated ST of high specific activity and the retention of biological activity as assessed by the suckling mouse assay (12).

Binding studies were carried out in one ml of an isotonic Krebs-Ringer solution containing 0.5% bovine serum albumin. Approximately 20,000 cpm of iodinated ST was added to each tube. This is approximately 0.02 pmoles of ST per tube. The binding reaction was terminated by and unbound ST separated from cell bound-ST by pressure filtration through a Whatman GFB glass fiber filter. After copious washing, the filter with adherent cell bound-ST was counted in a gamma counter. Binding is expressed at per cent of ^{125}-ST bound per milligram of protein.

Figure 3 shows the relationship between protein concentration and binding of ST to isolated jejunal villus cells.

Binding was linear with protein concentration and in all subsequent experiments, each tube contained approximately 200-500 micrograms of cell protein.

Figure 4 illustrates the time course of ST binding to jejunal villus cells.

Three binding curves are shown labeled, total, non-specific, and specific binding.

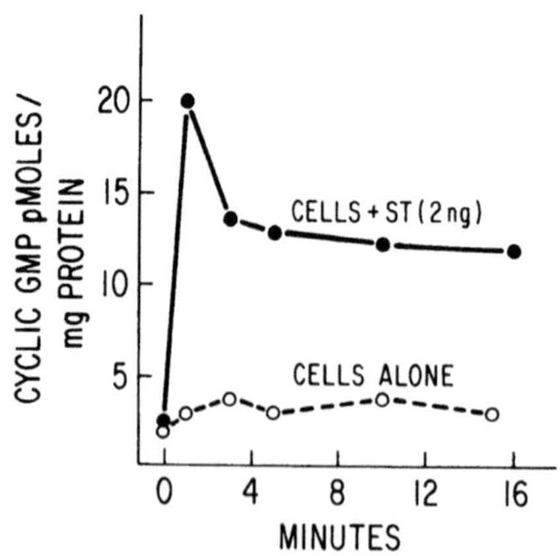

Figure 2. Effect of ST on cyclic GMP concentration in isolated jejunal villus cells.

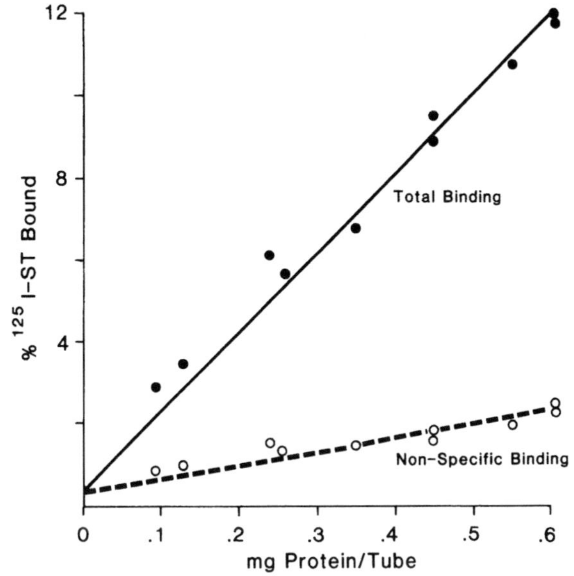

Figure 3. Relationship of protein concentration to ST binding to isolated jejunal villus cells.

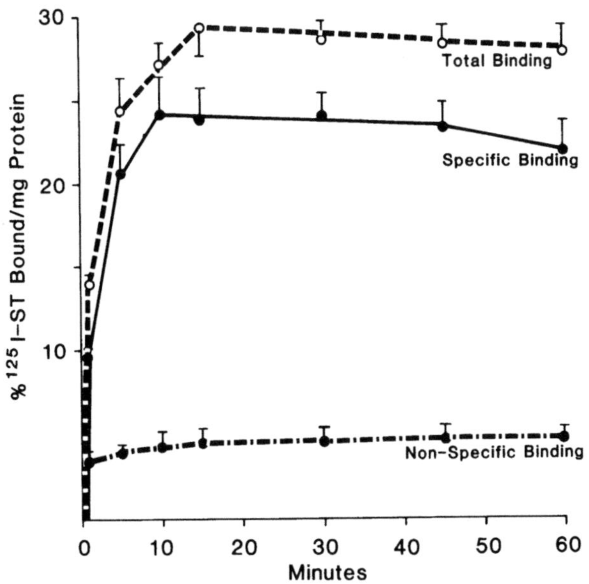

Figure 4. Time course of ST binding to jejunal villus cells.

Total binding is the amount of radioactivity bound to the cells when incubated with iodinated ST alone and represents both ST bound to receptors and ST bound in a non-specific fashion to the cell. Non-specific binding was determined by including a parallel series of tubes containing excess unlabeled ST. Under these conditions, the receptors are completely occupied and whatever binding occurs is non-receptor binding or non-specific binding. Subtracting non-specific from total binding gives a value for specific or receptor-mediated binding. All subsequent data are presented as specific binding.

Binding occurs rapidly, is largely complete by 5 minutes and plateaus by 10 to 15 minutes.

Figure 5 illustrates the effect of temperature on binding of ST to jejunal villus cells.

As shown by the top most curve--binding occurred most rapidly and reached the greatest level when done at 25°C. Binding was poorest at 37° and binding at 4° occupied an intermediate position.

Figure 6 illustrates the reversibility of the ST binding process to jejunal villus cells.

When a large quantity of unlabeled ST was added 30 minutes after binding of ^{125}I-ST had begun, ^{125}ST was dissociated from the cells by the unlabeled ST. Under the conditions of these experiments approximately 60% of bound ^{125}I-ST was dissociated by cold ST.

Figure 7 shows the results of competitive inhibition experiments, that is the ability of increasing concentrations of unlabeled ST to compete with iodinated ST for binding to jejunal and ileal villus cells.

With increasing concentration of unlabeled ST, progressively smaller amounts of ^{125}ST are bound to the villus cell resulting in a typical inhibition curve. Note that the curves for jejunal and ileal villus cells are superimposable. When association constants (Ka), a measure of affinity of the receptor for ST, were calculated by the 50% inhibition method, very similar values were obtained for jejunal and ileal cells, 4.4×10^8 versus 4.8×10^8 L/M, respectively.

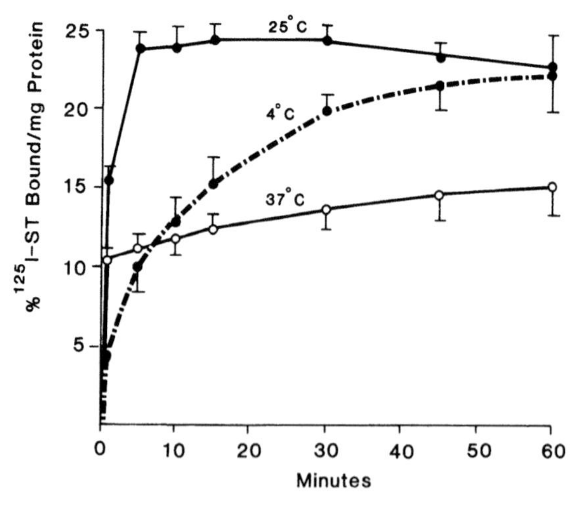

Figure 5. Effect of temperature on binding of ST to jejunal villus cells.

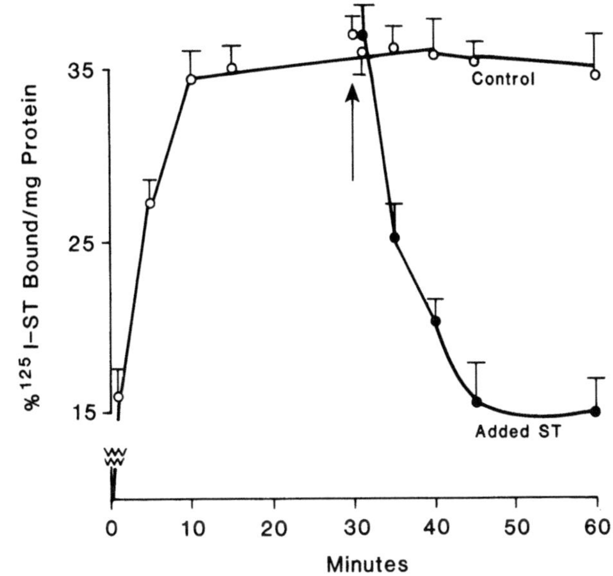

Figure 6. Reversibility of ST binding to jejunal villus cells.

When these data were subjected to analysis by the scatchard plot method, a curvilinear plot was obtained. This type of plot is consistent with either the existence of two species of receptors or with the pehnomenon of negative cooperativity. Assuming two species of receptors, one is a high affinity, low capacity receptor and the other is a low affinity but high capacity receptor.

When competitive inhibition studies were done with isolated colonic epithelial cells, a similar sigmoid shaped displacement curve was also obtained. When these colonic

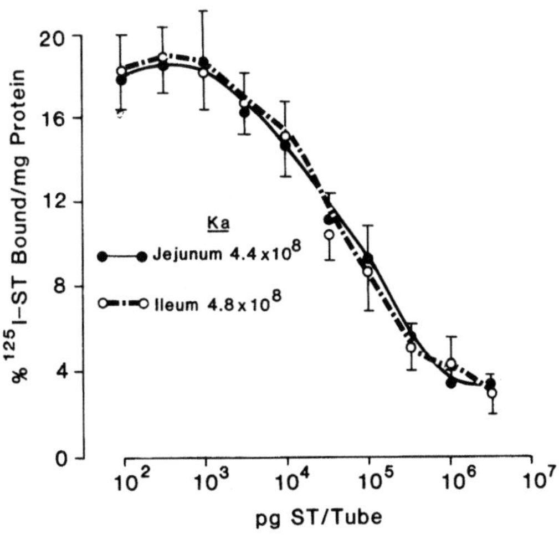

Figure 7. Competitive inhibition of ^{125}I-ST from jejunal and ileal villus cells by increasing concentrations of unlabeled ST.

Table 1. Kinetic parameters of ST binding to jejunal, ileal and colonic epithelial cells.

	Kd(molar)		Bmax (pmoles/ mg/protein)	
	A	B	A	B
Jejunal (14)	1.43×10^{-8}	1.91×10^{-7}	4.23	26.70
Ileal (3)	1.17×10^{-8}	1.77×10^{-7}	3.85	27.46
Colonic (3)	3.55×10^{-9}*	6.59×10^{-7}*	1.85*	109.45*

*p = <0.05 compared to either jejunal or ileal cells.

data were subjected to scatchard plot analysis, a curvilinear plot was also obtained indicating two species of receptor sites.

The kinetic parameters of ST binding to jejunal, ileal, and colonic cells calculated by the scatchard plot method are listed in Table 1.

The columns marked A and B refer to the high and low affinity binding sites, respectively. There are no significant differences between jejunal and ileal villus cells in either dissociation constants or in maximal binding capacity. However, the colonic high affinity binding site has a significantly higher affinity for ST and a significantly lower maximal binding capacity than either jejunal or ileal villus cells. Also note that the colonic low affinity binding site has a significantly lower affinity and a much greater binding capacity for ST than either jejunal or ileal villus cells.

Figure 8 presents data regarding the specificity of the ST binding process by illustrating the ability of other bacterial enterotoxins to interact with the ST receptor.

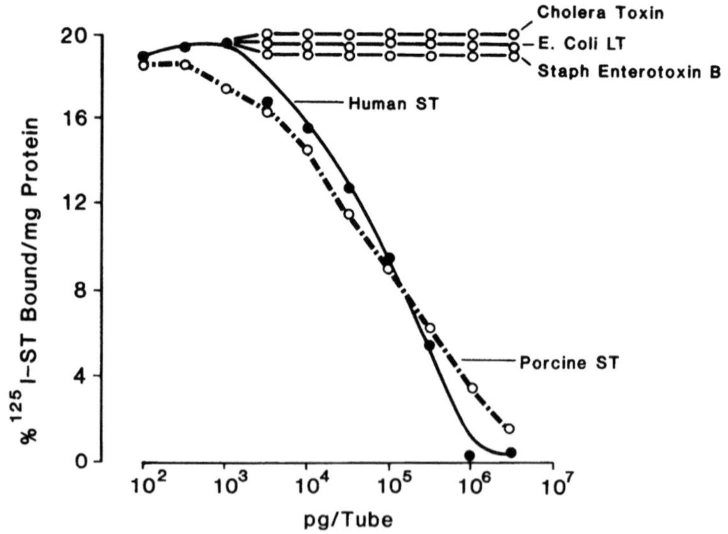

Figure 8. Competitive inhibition of ^{125}I-ST from jejunal villus cell by various purified bacterial enterotoxins.

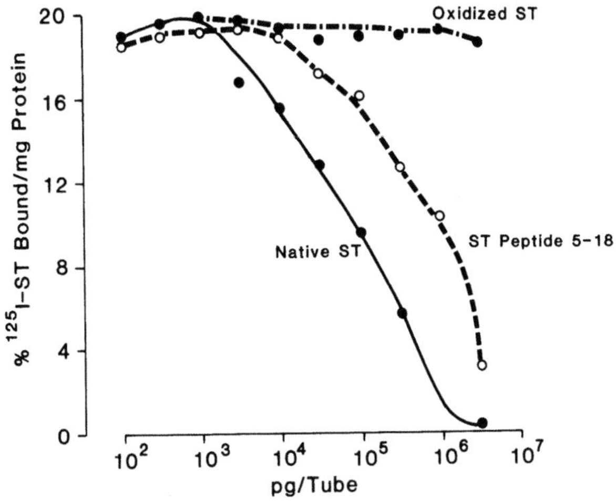

Figure 9. Effect of chemical alterations of the ST molecule on the ability to bind to jejunal villus cells.

The inhibition curve for human ST is shown by the solid line. When purified porcine ST, a larger ST molecule kindly provided by Dr. D. C. Robertson, was examined, it resulted in an identical inhibition curve, the dashed line. In contrast, pure cholera toxin, *E. coli* heat-labile toxin, or Staph enterotoxin B do not interact with the ST receptor. They cause no inhibition.

The effect of alterations of the toxin molecule on the ability to bind to these receptors is shown in Figure 9.

The typical ST inhibition curve is again shown by the solid line. As shown by the top most curve, performic acid oxidation of ST, a procedure that cleaves disulfide-bridges, results in an ST molecule that no longer can bind to the epithelial cell. In contrast, when the amino terminal 4 amino acids are removed by amino peptidase, the remaining peptide, ST 5-18, retains its ability to bind to the jejunal cell receptor.

To answer the question of whether receptors to ST exist on tissues other than the intestinal tract, we prepared crude membrane fractions from various organs and examined their ability to bind ST (Figure 10).

The typical binding curve for intact jejunal villus cells is shown by the middle dashed curve. When these cells are homogenized and the 13,000 xg membrane pellet examined, the binding specific activity is significantly increased. This suggests that the ST receptors are located on the cell membrane. In contrast, when membranes were similarly prepared from lung, liver, pancreas, they demonstrated little if any ability to bind ST. These observations are consistent with the data of Rao *et al.* (13) and of Guerrant *et al.* (14) who demonstrated that ST was unable to stimulate guanylate cyclase in any of these non-intestinal tissues. Presumably only the small intestine and colon have receptors for ST.

To determine the location of the ST receptors on the epithelial cell, we examined the ability of jejunal brush borders to bind ST. Jejunal brush borders were prepared by the method of Forstner *et al.* (15) and the purification and enrichment of the brush

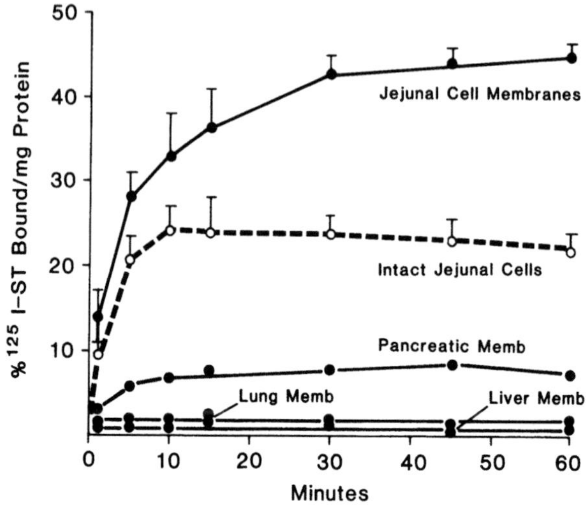

Figure 10. Binding of ^{125}I-ST to jejunal villus cells and to various membranes.

borders was monitored by measuring sucrase activity and by electron mictoscopy. The results are shown in Figure 11.

At virtually each time point, the specific activity of binding was twofold or greater in the brush borders compared to the whole cells. These data suggest that the ST receptor resides on the brush border.

We also examined the effect of goat anti-ST antisera on ST binding to jejunal villus cells. (Data not shown). Briefly, pre-incubation of goat anti-ST for one hour completely

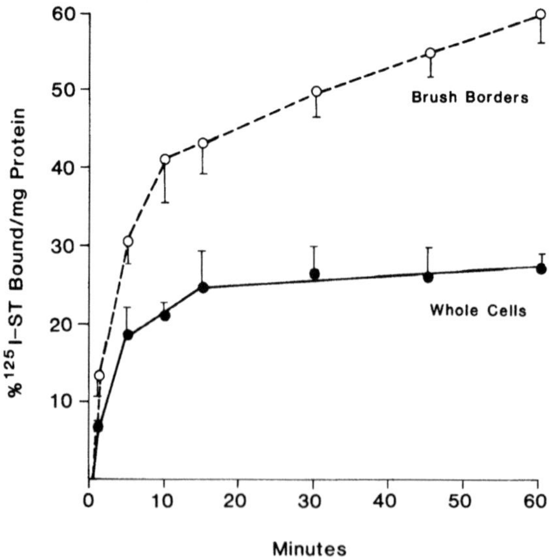

Figure 11. Binding of ^{125}I-ST to jejunal brush border membranes vs. intact jejunal villus cells.

abolished the ability of ST to bind to jejunal cells. In addition, goat anti-ST could remove ST already bound to jejunal cells.

From these data, various conclusions can be drawn. There appear to be receptors for ST on jejunal, ileal, and colonic epithelial cells. Binding of ST to these receptors is a reversible and time and temperature dependent process. The affinity of the colonic receptors for ST is significantly greater than either jejunal or ileal cells. These receptors appear to be specific for ST, are located on the cell membrane, probably on the brush border. These receptors are confined to the small and large intestine and are not present in liver, pancreas, or lung. There appear to be either two species of receptors or one receptor demonstrating negative cooperativity. Binding of ST to its receptor requires that disulfide bridges in the ST molecule be intact, but the amino terminal 4 amino acids are not required for binding. Binding of ST to goat anti-ST abolishes binding and goat anti-ST can remove ST bound to the cell.

Binding of ST to these receptors probably mediates the secretory action of ST on the intestine.

REFERENCES

1. Giannella, R. A. Pathogenesis of acute bacterial diarrheal disorders. Ann. Rev. Med. **32**:341-357, 1981.
2. Moss, J., Vaughan, M. Mechanism of activation of adenylate cyclase by choleragen and *E. coli* heat-labile enterotoxin. In Field, M., Fordtran, J. S., Schultz, S. D. (Eds.), 1980. SECRETORY DIARRHEA. Bethesda, MD: Am. Physiol. Soc. pp. 107-126.
3. Hughes, J. M., Murad, F., Chang, B., Guerrant, R. L. Role of cyclic GMP in the action of heat-stable enterotoxin of *E. coli*. Nature **271**:755-756, 1978.
4. Field, M., Graf, L. H., Laird, W. J., Smith, P. L. Heat-stable enterotoxin of *E. coli*: in vitro effects on guanylate cyclase activity, cyclic GMP concentration, and ion transport in the small intestine. Proc. Natl. Acad. Sci. (USA). **75**:2800-2804, 1978.
5. Giannella, R. A., Drake, K. W. Effect of purified *E. coli* heat-stable enterotoxin on intestinal cyclic nucleotide metabolism and fluid secretion. Infec. Immun. **24**:19-23, 1979.
6. Staples, S. J., Asher, S. E., Giannella, R. A. Purification and characterization of heat-stable enterotoxin produced by a strain of *E. coli* pathogenic for man. J. Biol. Chem. **255**:4716-4721, 1980.
7. Chan, S. K., Giannella, R. A. Amino acid sequence of heat-stable enterotoxin produced by *E. coli.* pathogenic for man. J. Biol. Chem. **256**:7744-7746, 1981.
8. Alderete, J. F., Robertson, D. C. Purification and chemical characterization of the heat-stable enterotoxin produced by porcine strains of enterotoxigenic *E. coli*. Infec. Immun. **19**:1021-1030, 1978.
9. Lathe, R., Hirth, P., DeWilde, M., Harford, N., Lecocq, J. P. Cell-free synthesis of enterotoxin of *E. coli* from a cloned gene. Nature **284**:473-474, 1980.
10. So, M., McCarthy, B. J. Nucleotide sequence of the bacterial transposon Tn 1681 encoding a heat-stable (ST) toxin and its identification in enterotoxigenic *E. coli* strains. Proc. Natl. Acad. Sic. (USA). **77**:4011-4015, 1980.
11. Weiser, M. M. Intestinal epithelial cell surface membrane glycoprotein synthesis. 1. An indicator of cellular differentiation. J. Biol. Chem. **248**:2536-2541, 1973.
12. Giannella, R. A., Drake, K. W., Luttrell, M. Development of a radioimmunoassay for *E. coli* heat-stable enterotoxin: Comparison with the suckling mouse bioassay. Infec. Immun. **33**:186-192, 1981.
13. Rao, M. C., Guandalini, S., Smith, P. L., Field, M. Mode of action of heat-stable *E. coli* enterotoxin. Tissue and subcellular specificities and role of cyclic GMP. Biochim. Biophys. Acta **632**: 35-46, 1980.
14. Guerrant, R. L., Hughes, J. M., Chang, B., Robertson, D. C., Murad, F. Activation of intestinal

guanylate cyclase by heat-stable enterotoxin of *E. coli.*: Studies of tissue specificity, potential receptors, and intermediates. J. Infec. Dis. **142**:220-228, 1980.

15. Forstner, G. G., Sabesin, S. M., Isselbacher, K. J. Rat intestinal microvillus membranes. Purification and biochemical characterization. Biochem. J. **106**:381-390, 1968.

Advances in Research on Cholera and Related Diarrheas, eds., S. Kuwahara, N. F. Pierce, 269–278.

STUDIES ON THE MECHANISM OF ACTION OF THE *ESCHERICHIA COLI* HEAT-STABLE ENTEROTOXIN (ST_a)

Lawrence A. Dreyfus and Donald C. Robertson

University of Kansas, Lawrence, KS 66045

Rat intestinal cells and brush border membranes have been shown to contain a particulate guanylate cyclase which can be stimulated by *E. coli* heat-stable enterotoxin (ST). The sequence of events prior to activation of guanylate cyclase are unknown, however, anti-inflammatory agents have been able to block secretory activity of ST (Greenberg, *et al.*, Infect. Immun. *29*:908-913, 1980) which suggested that activation of guanylate cyclase occurs via metabolism of arachidonic acid with formation of prostaglandins or other oxidized intermediates. Treatment of either intact rat enterocytes or brush border membranes with ST caused a dose dependent accumulation of cGMP. Evidence for the release and conversion of arachidonic acid to an intermediate of prostaglandin synthesis or hydroxy-derivative was not obtained by: 1) following the rate and amounts of [^{3}H]-arachidonate released from prelabeled cells incubated in the presence and absence of ST; 2) use of specific inhibitors of the cyclooxygenase and lipooxygenase pathways and 3) the fact that 0_2 was not required for activation of guanylate cyclase by ST.

Solubilization of rat intestinal brush border membranes in 3[(3-cholamidopropyl) dimethylammonio]-1-propane sulfonate (CHAPS) followed by centrifugation at 150,000 x g yielded a supernatant fraction containing both guanylate cyclase activity and a high molecular weight component which bound ^{125}I-ST. Binding of ^{125}I-ST to the solubilized component was negligible in the presence of 100-fold "cold" ST. Basal activity of guanylate cyclase did not change upon detergent solubilization, however, the solubilized enzyme could be activated by addition of ST.

The specific receptor which binds ST may initiate a transmembrane signal with rapid activation of guanylate cyclase or the putative receptor for ST may be part of a complex involved in regulation of particulate guanylate cyclase.

INTRODUCTION

The pathogenesis of enterotoxigenic *E. coli* (ETEC) is closely linked to the production of at least two kinds of enterotoxins (21). The heat-labile enterotoxin (LT) is remarkably similar in many respects to cholera toxin. Cholera toxin and *E. coli* LT 1) have an AB subunit structure (6), 2) possess shared and unique antigenic determinants (3,8,-

10), 3) bind to Gm_1 ganglioside (17), and 4) mediate intestinal secretion through activation of adenylate cyclase (21). In contrast to LT, *E. coli* heat-stable enterotoxin (ST) causes intestinal secretion by activation of guanylate cyclase, but little is known of the events which occur in the secretory response prior to and following increases in intracellular cGMP.

The binding of ST to isolated intestinal cells and membranes was studied since interaction of ST with a surface receptor is likely the first event in the mechanism of action of ST (see J.C. Frantz and D.C. Robertson, these proceedings). ST bound rapidly to intestinal cells and membranes and did not readily dissociate, and further, internalization of the toxin did not appear to be required for activation of guanylate cyclase. These data suggested that a hormone-like transmembrane signal and specific chemical mediators of the hormone-like action were involved in activation of guanylate cyclase by ST. Anti-inflammatory agents have been shown to inhibit the action of ST (7,13,16).

The objective of this investigation was to study the mechanism of activation of guanylate cyclase by ST using isolated enterocytes and intestinal brush border membrane preparations. The effects of anti-inflammatory agents on the activation of guanylate cyclase by ST were examined and a potential receptor for ST has been detected in the soluble fraction of intestinal membranes treated with detergents.

MATERIALS AND METHODS

Heat-stable enterotoxin (ST) produced by porcine ETEC strain 431 was purified as described previously (5). Purified 431 ST had an effective dose of 0.4 ng (1). Radioiodination of ST was performed by a lactoperoxidase technique as described elsewhere (5). The specific activity of the ^{125}I-ST preparations was 700-1000 Ci/mmole.

Rat intestinal epithelial cells were isolated from 120-180 gm female Sprague Dawley rats by the procedure of Weiser (27). Viability of the isolated enterocytes was determined by trypan blue exclusion and was greater than 80% in all experiments. Isolated enterocytes were labeled with [^{3}H]-arachidonic acid by incubating enterocytes (2 x 10^6/ml) in Hanks balanced salt solution (HBSS) without Ca^{++} containing 10% fetal calf serum and 1-5 μCi [^{3}H]arachidonic acid in a total volume of 50 ml. After 30 min incubation at 37 C with gentle shaking, the [^{3}H]-labeled enterocytes were centrifuged at 120 x g and washed 3X in 50 ml cold HBSS plus 10% fetal calf serum. Extraction of cell lipids and fractionation by thin layer chromatography revealed that greater than 95% of the [^{3}H]-arachidonic acid was present in triglyceride fractions.

The accumulation of cGMP in isolated enterocytes was measured in an incubation mixture containing enterocytes (5 x 10^6/ml) in HBSS containing 10% fetal calf serum, ST (100 ng/ml) and theophylline (10 mM). Following incubation for timed intervals at 37C, samples of 0.5 ml were pipetted into tubes containing 1.0 ml of absolute ethanol at 0C. After centrifugation, the supernatant fractions were dried under an air stream, resuspended in 0.5 ml acetate buffer, (pH 6.2) and assayed for cyclic GMP by a RIA procedure (2).

Metabolism of [^{3}H]-arachidonate by prelabeled enterocytes treated with ST was assayed in reaction mixtures as described above. Lipid extractions were performed at various times and extracts fractionated on silica gel G plates using the upper phase of ethyl acetate:2,2,4-trimethylpentane:acetic acid:water, 90:50:20:100 (15).

Brush border membrane vesicles were prepared from isolated intestinal epithelial cells as described by Hauser, *et al.* (9). Guanylate cyclase activity in isolated brush border membranes was assayed as described by Kimura and Murad (12). Briefly, the reaction mixtures contained brush border membranes (BBM), the soluble or particulate fraction of BBM treated with detergent (50-100 μg); Tris-Cl (pH 7.6), 5 μmole; theophylline, 1 μmole; creatine phosphate, 0.75 μmole; and ST, 10-1,000 suckling mouse units, the total volume was 0.1 ml. The reaction was started by addition of GTP-$MgCl_2$ and stopped after 10 min incubation at 37 C with 0.1 ml of 0.5 M sodium acetate (pH 4.0). The cGMP was determined using the RIA procedure as for whole cells (2). Drugs for inhibition studies were dissolved in dimethylsulfoxide (DMSO) prior to addition to reaction mixtures. The final concentration of 2-5% DMSO had no effect on basal guanylate cyclase activity or stimulation by ST.

Solubilization of intestinal brush border membranes was carried out in 5 mM 3-[(3-cholamidopropyl)dimethylammonio] 1-1-propane sulfonate (CHAPS), 154 mM NaCl, 10 mM Tris HCl, 1 mM phenylmethylsulfonylfluoride, pH 7.4, at 4 C by homogenization with 5 strokes using a Potter-Elvehjem homogenizer. The extract was centrifuged at 150,000 x g for 1 hr in a Beckman 50 Ti rotor. The supernatant fraction was assayed for ST receptor activity by incubating 50-100 μg soluble brush border membrane protein with 100,000 cpm ^{125}I-ST (0.3 ng) for 15 minutes at 37 C. The reaction mixture was then applied to a Bio-Gel P-6DG column (0.75 x 10 cm) and eluted with membrane homogenization buffer. Fractions were collected and counted in a gamma scintillation spectrometer. Sodium dodecylsulfate polyacrylamide gel electrophoresis (SDS-PAGE) used a 5-15% acrylamide gradient slab gel and a discontinuous (tris-glycine) buffer system (14).

Carrier-free Na ^{125}I and [^{3}H]-arachidonic acid were purchased from Amersham Searle. Guanosine 3′, 5′-cyclic phosphoric acid 2′-0-succinyl 3-[^{125}I] iodotyrosine methyl ester were from Collaborative Research Co., Inc., Waltham, MD. CHAPS was a product of Calbiochem, Behring Corp., San Diego, CA. All other common reagents were obtained from Sigma Chemical Co., St. Louis, MO. Anti-cGMP antiserum was prepared in goats as described by Brooker, *et al.* (2). 5,8,11,14-Eicosatetraynoic (ETYA) acid was supplied by Dr. W.E. Scott of Hoffman-LaRoche Inc., Nutley, NJ.

RESULTS

Stimulation of rat enterocyte guanylate cyclase by ST. Rat intestinal epithelial cells incubated with ST responded with a rapid dose-dependent accumulation of intracellular cGMP (Figure 1). Maximal activation of enterocyte guanylate cyclase (5 min) correlated with the binding kinetics of ST to isolated cells (J.C. Frantz and D.C. Robertson, these proceedings). The high levels of cGMP observed in enterocytes following ST treatment rapidly decreased, possibly due to phosphodiesterase activity.

Anti-inflammatory agents were incubated with isolated enterocytes since they have been shown to inhibit accumulation of cGMP and subsequent intestinal secretion mediated by ST (7,13,16). Moderate inhibition (20-40%) of ST-mediated accumulation of cGMP was observed with 0.1 mM quinacrine, a specific inhibitor of phospholipase A2. In the presence of 1.0 mM quinacrine, the level of cGMP was reduced 80-90% compared with ST-treated enterocytes not treated with the drug. Significant inhibition of cyclic GMP accumulation (85-95%) in ST-treated enterocytes was also observed with ETYA, a

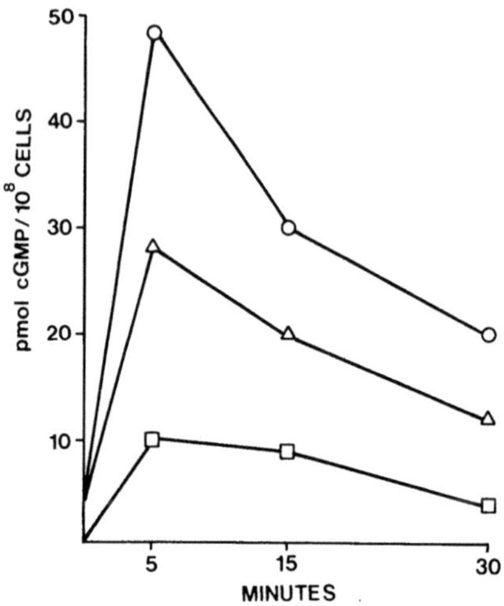

Figure 1. Activation of rat intestinal epithelial cell guanylate cyclase by ST. Symbols: □–□, 10ng/ml; △–△, 33 ng/ml; ○–○, 100 ng/ml.

structural analogue of arachidonic acid, (data not shown). These data suggested that the action of ST on rat intestinal epithelial cells may involve the release and metabolism of arachidonic acid based on the assumption that the anti-inflammatory drugs inhibited metabolism of arachidonic acid and did not directly inhibit particulate guanylate cyclase.

Metabolism of ^{3}H-arachidonic acid by ST-treated enterocytes. The rate of [^{3}H]-arachidonate release from prelabeled enterocytes treated with ST was identical to that of control cells (Figure 2). Likewise, the turnover of the [^{3}H]-label in phospholipid and diglyceride pools was not affected by treatment with ST. Treatment with as much as 1,000 suckling mouse units per 10^6 pre-labeled enterocytes, which maximally stimulated guanylate cyclase, failed to increase the release or metabolism of arachidonic acid compared with controls not treated with ST.

Guanylate cyclase activation in rat intestinal brush border membranes treated with ST. Rat enterocyte brush border membranes were isolated since the particulate guanylate cyclase of intestinal epithelial cells is known to be localized in this region of intestinal cells (26). Incubation of the brush border membranes with ST resulted in the rapid dose dependent accumulation of cGMP. The increase in cGMP was linear for 10 min and reached a maximum value by 15 min. This increase represented a 4-6 fold stimulation over the basal level of the enzyme when assayed in the presence of 1000 units $^o/_{oo}$ of ST (data not shown).

Incubation of brush border membranes with ST and anti-inflammatory agents. Indomethacin, chlorpromazine, and ETYA, anti-inflammatory agents which inhibit cyclooxygenase mediated conversion of arachidonic acid to cyclic endoperoxides, inhibited the accumulation of cGMP in brush border membrane suspensions treated with ST (Table 1). However, it should be noted that the basal level of guanylate cyclase measured in the presence of either Mg^{++} or Mn^{++} was inhibited by the anti-inflammatory agent (Table 1). These data suggested that the anti-inflammatory agents directly inhibited guanylate cyclase which prevented activation in the presence of ST.

Levels of prostaglandins in rat enterocytes and brush border membrane preparations treated with ST. Significant changes in the levels of prostaglandins PGE2, PGF2α

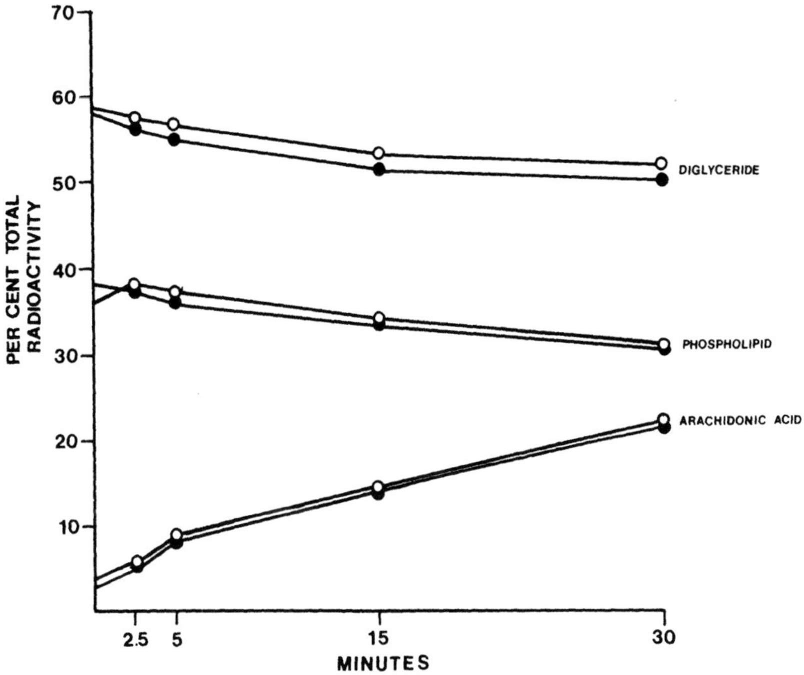

Figure 2. Release of [^{3}H]-arachidonic acid from pre-labeled rat enterocytes. Symbols: ○–○, –ST; ●–●, +ST.

Table 1. Effect of anti-inflammatory agents on activation of guanylate cyclase.

	Guanylate cyclase activity (pmol cGMP min⁻) / mg protein		
Inhibitor	Mg^{++}	Mn^{++}	Mg^{++} + ST[a]
None	6.0	31.0	15.6
Indomethacin (1.0 mM)	2.7(55.0)[b]	15.6 (49.7)[b]	2.7 (82.7)[b]
Chlorpromazine (1.0 mm)	0.2 (96.7)	1.9 (98.1)	0.3 (93.9)
5,8,11,14-Eicosatetraynoic acid (2.5 mM)	1.7 (72.7)	23.8 (23.2)	4.9 (68.6)

[a]100 suckling mouse units added to each reaction mixture.

[b]Percent inhibition

and thromboxane B2 were not observed either in isolated enterocytes or rat brush border membranes incubated with ST (Table 2). Even though an increase in prostaglandin levels could not be detected, there was a dose dependent accumulation of cGMP. If the activation of guanylate cyclase by ST involves a free radical or oxidized intermediate 0_2 should be required, however, the level of guanylate cyclase activity in brush border membranes treated with ST was not decreased by anoxygenic conditions (data not shown).

Detergent solubilization of rat intestinal brush border membranes. In order to determine if ST binds to a specific receptor and initiates a transmembrane signal, or interacts more directly with guanylate cyclase, rat intestinal brush border membranes were solubilized in CHAPS, a non-denaturing zwiterionic detergent. The soluble fraction was incubated with ^{125}I-ST and fractionated on Bio-Gel P-6. The soluble fraction of brush border membranes treated with CHAPS contained a component which bound ^{125}I-ST (Figure 3). The void volume fraction represented approximately 25% of the total radioactivity in the reaction mixture (Figure 3). The inclusion volume peak contained free ^{125}I-ST. Specificity of binding was demonstrated by incubating ^{125}I-ST and the putative receptor in the presence of 10- and 100-fold "cold" ST. The association of ^{125}I-ST with the receptor was reduced by 83% in the presence of 10-fold "cold" ST and was negligeable in the presence of 100-fold "cold" ST. Reduced and carboxymethylated ST did not compete with the labeled native toxin (data not shown).

Characterization of the Bio-Gel P-6 void volume material by SDS-PAGE followed by radioautography revealed a single band of radioactivity (other than free ^{125}I-ST) with an apparent molecular weight of 100,000 (Figure 4, lane A). Boiling the ^{125}I-ST-receptor complex in SDS before electrophoresis released ^{125}I-ST from its receptor (Figure 4, lane B).

The CHAPS solubilized membrane fraction also contained guanylate cyclase activity. Incubation of the solubilized membrane fraction with ST resulted in a 4-fold activa-

Table 2. Prostaglandin levels in rat enterocytes and brush border membranes treated with ST.

	PGE_2[a]		$PGF_{2\alpha}$[a]		TxB_2[a]	
	-ST	+ST[b]	-ST	+ST[b]	-ST	+ST[b]
Intact erythrocytes (5 x 10^6)						
0 min	1.0	0.9	0.09	0.10	0.01	0.01
0.25	1.23	1.14	0.08	0.11	0.01	0.01
0.5	1.18	0.93	0.10	0.10	0.01	0.01
2.5	0.84	0.98	0.09	0.09	0.01	0.01
Membranes (500 ng)						
10 min	0.11	0.09	0.04	0.04	0.01	0.01

[a]nanograms per milliliter

[b]500 ng/ml

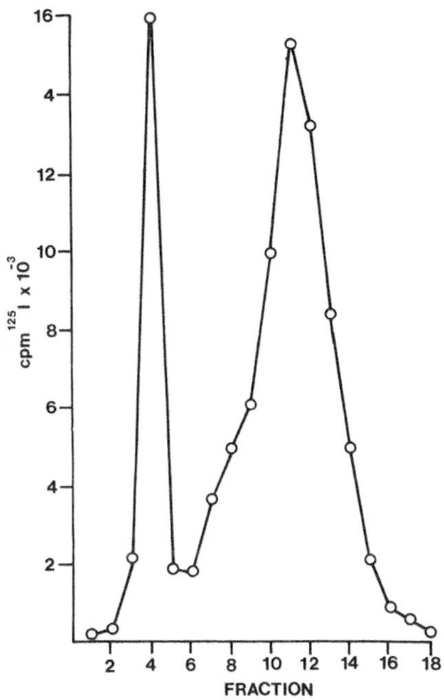

Figure 3. Fractionation of rat intestinal brush border membranes with CHAPS detergent.

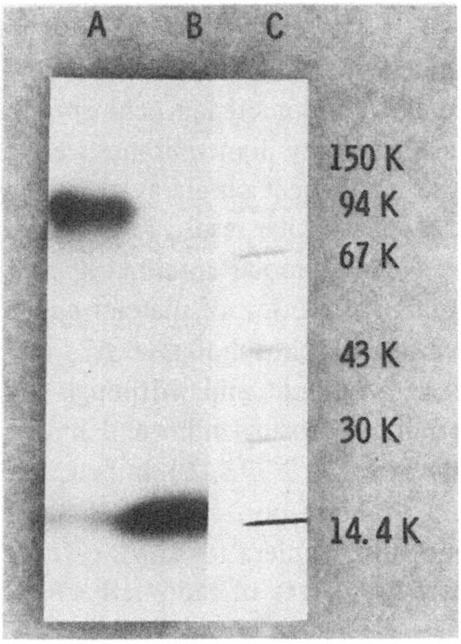

Figure 4. Sodium dodecylsulfate-polyacrylamide gel electrophoresis of CHAPS soluble fraction of rat brush border membranes incubated with ^{125}I-431 ST.

Table 3. Effect of detergent solubilization on rat enterocyte brush border membrane guanylate cyclase activity.

Fraction	Addition	pmol cGMP min^{-1} mg $Protein^{-1}$	Fold Stimulation
Membranes	None	1.00	–
	ST[a]	3.81	3.81
150,000 x g Supernatant	None	0.45	–
	ST[a]	1.83	4.07
150,000 x g Pellet	None	3.88	–
	ST[a]	10.20	2.63

[a]1000 u ST/ml

tion of guanylate cyclase which was comparable to a level of activation seen in intact membrane vesicles (Table 3).

A CHAPS extract of liver plasma membrane was prepared and tested for guanylate cyclase activity and binding of ^{125}I-ST. Although the preparation contained guanylate cyclase activity, it could not be activated by ST and lacked an ST-binding component as found in extracts of intestinal brush border membranes.

The rapid dose-dependent accumulation of cGMP in enterocytes and membranes treated with ST was decreased by indomethacin, chlorpromazine, and ETYA. However, basal levels of guanylate cyclase activity in membranes were also decreased which suggested that the agents exerted a direct effect on guanylate cyclase and may have nothing to do with secretion mediated by ST. Similar results have been observed when platelets were treated with ascorbic acid (20). Micromolar amounts of aspirin, indomethacin, or ETYA inhibited the ascorbate-mediated activation of platelet guanylate cyclase, but the activation was not due to activation of phospholipase A2, or the formation of cyclic endoperoxides or hydroperoxyarachidonic acid. Although indomethacin, chlorpromazine and ETYA are known to inhibit prostaglandin and hydroperoxyeicosatetraenoic acid formation, other activities do exist (19,22,23,25). In fact, Smith, *et al.* (23) demonstrated that indomethacin inhibited ion transport changes in the rabbit ileum treated with a number of secretagogues, including cholera toxin, *E. coli* LT and ST (23). These authors concluded that the anti-secretory effect of indomethacin was not due to inhibition of prostaglandin synthesis.

Activation of intestinal guanylate cyclase by ST may occur either by a direct interaction with a specific receptor or due to a soluble secondary messenger. Our data indicated that the soluble fraction of intestinal brush border membranes homogenized with CHAPS contained a component which specifically bound ST. Native ST, but not reduced and carboxymethylated ST, competed with ^{125}I-labeled native ST which suggested that disulfide bonds are required for the interaction of ST with its receptor. Once bound, ST remained avidly associated with its receptor as shown by the inability of electrophoresis in SDS to dissociate the complex. In fact, heat treatment at 100 C was required to dissociate ^{125}I-ST from the soluble receptor. It is not known whether guanylate cyclase activity is associated with the solubilized ST receptor.

If the component solubilized from rat intestinal brush border membranes is indeed the biological receptor for ST, binding must occur prior to activation of guanylate cyclase. Guanylate cyclase activity was present in the soluble fraction of rat intestinal brush border membranes which could be stimulated by ST. Apparently, the ST receptor was still active even in the presence of detergent. Liver membranes did not contain an ST-specific receptor, thus it seems likely that non-intestinal tissues do not respond to ST because they lack the specific receptor present in the small intestine and colon.

In summary, recent work in our laboratory suggests that ST exerts its biological effect at the surface of rat enterocytes. This study demonstrated that the trans-membrane signal does not appear to be mediated by the release and metabolism of arachidonic acid. A biologically active receptor for ST has been identified and partially characterized after solubilization from rat intestinal brush border membranes. Previous data showed that treatment of ST with reducing agents abolished biological activity of the toxin which suggested that disulfide bonds were necessary for biological activity in suckling mice (L.A. Dreyfus and D.C. Robertson, unpublished observations). Intact disulfide bonds are also required for binding of ST to its receptor. Activation of guanylate cyclase by ST appears to involve a receptor mediated trans-membrane signal. The nature of the ST receptor and its association with particulate intestinal guanylate cyclase are now under investigation.

REFERENCES

1. Alderete, J. F. and D. C. Robertson. 1978. Purification and chemical characterization of the heat-stable enterotoxin produced by porcine strains of enterotoxigenic *Escherichia coli*. Infect. Immun. **19**:1021-1030.
2. Brooker, G., J. F. Harper, W. L. Terasaki, and R. D. Moylan. 1979. Radioimmunoassay of cAMP and cGMP. Advances in Cyclic Nucleotide Research. **10**:1-32.
3. Clements, J. C. and R. A. Finkelstein. 1978. Immunological cross-reactivity between a heat-labile enterotoxin(s) of *Escherichia coli* and subunits of *Vibrio cholera* enterotoxin. Infect. Immun. **21**: 1036-1039.
4. Field, M., L. H. Graf, Jr., W. L. Laird, and P. L. Smith. 1978. Heat-stable enterotoxin of *Escherichia coli*: In vitro effects on guanylate cyclase activity, cGMP concentration, and ion transport in small intestine. Proc. Natl. Acad. Sci. USA **75**:2800-2804.
5. Frantz, J. C. and D. C. Robertson. 1981. Immunological properties of *Escherichia coli* heat-stable enterotoxins: Development of a radioimmunoassay specific for heat-stable enterotoxins with subkline mouse activity. Infect. Immun. **33**:193-198.
6. Gill, D. M., J. D. Clements, D. C. Robertson, and R. A. Finkelstein. 1981. Subunit number and arrangement in *Escherichia coli* heat-labile enterotoxin. Infect. Immun. **33**:677-682.
7. Greenberg, R. N., F. Murad, B. Chang, D. C. Robertson, and R. L. Guerrant. 1980. Inhibition of *Escherichia coli* heat-stable enterotoxin by indomethacin and chlorpromazine. Infect. Immun. **29**:908-913.

8. Gyles, C. L. 1974. Immunological study of the heat-labile enterotoxins of *Escherichia coli* and *Vibrio cholerae*. Infect. Immun. **9**:564-570.
9. Hauser, H., K. Howell, R. M. C. Dawson, and D. E. Bowyer. 1980. Rabbit small intestinal brush border membrane preparation and lipid composition. Biochim. Biochphys. Acta. **602**:567-577.
10. Honda, T., Y. Takeda, and T. Miwatani. 1981. Isolation of special antibodies which react only with homologous enterotoxins from *Vibrio cholerae* and enterotoxigenic *Escherichia coli* heat-labile enterotoxin. Infect. Immun. **33**:677-682.
11. Hughes, J. M., F. Murad, B. Chang and R. L. Guerrant. 1978. Role of cGMP in the action of heat-stable enterotoxin of *Escherichia coli*. Nature (Lond.) **271**:755-756.
12. Kimura, H. and F. Murad. 1974. Evidence for two different forms of guanylate cyclase in rat heart. J. Biol. Chem. **249**:6910-6919.
13. Knoop, F. C. and D. M. Abbey. 1981. Effect of chemical and pharmacological agents on the secretory activity induced by *Escherichia coli* heat-stable enterotoxin. Can. J. Microbiol. **27**:754-758.
14. Laemmli, U. K. 1970. Cleavage of structural proteins during the assembly of the head of bacteriophage T4. Nature (London) **227**:680-685.
15. Lapetina, E. G., C. J. Schmitges, K. Chandrabose and P. Cuatrecasas. 1977. Cyclic adenosine 3′, 5′-monophosphate and prostacyclin inhibit membrane phospholipase activity in platelets. Biochem. Biophys. Res. Comm. **76**:828-835.
16. Madsen, G. L. and F. C. Knoop. 1978. Inhibition of the secretory activity of *Escherichia coli* heat-stable enterotoxin by indomethacin. Infect. Immun. **22**:143-147.
17. Moss, J., J. C. Osborne, Jr., P. H. Fishman, S. Nakaya, and D. C. Robertson. 1981. *Escherichia coli* heat-labile enterotoxin: Ganglioside specificity and ADP-ribosyltransferase activity. J. Biol. Chem. (in Press).
18. Newsome, P. M., M. N. Burgess, and N. A. Mullan. 1978. Effects of *Escherichia coli* heat-stable enterotoxin on cGMP levels in mouse intestine. Infect. Immun. **22**:290-291.
19. Nickander, R., F. G. McMahon, and A. S. Ridolfo. 1979. Non-steroidal anti-inflammatory agents. Ann. Rev. Pharmacol. Toxicol. **19**:469-490.
20. Pickett, W. C., K. F. Austen, and E. J. Goetzl. 1979. Inhibition by non-steroidal anti-inflammatory agents on the ascorbate-induced elevations of platelet cGMP levels.
21. Sack, R. B. 1975. Human diarrheal disease caused by enterotoxigenic *Escherichia coli*. Ann. Rev. Microbiol. **29**:333-353.
22. Smith, P. L. and M. Field. 1980. In vitro antisecretory effects of trifuoperazine and other neuroleptics in rabbit and human small intestine. Gastroenterology **78**:1545-1553.
23. Smith, P. L., J. B. Blumberg, J. S. Stoff and M. Field. 1981. Antisecretory effects of indomethacin on rabbit ileal mucosa in vitro. Gastroenterology **80**:356-365.
24. Staples, S. J., S. E. Asher, and R. A. Gianella. 1980. Purification and characterization of heat-stable enterotoxin produced by a strain of *E. coli* pathogenic for man. J. Biol. Chem. **255**:4716-4721.
25. Tobias, L. D. and J. G. Hamilton. 1978. The effects of 5, 8, 11, 14-eicosatetraynoic acid on lipid metabolism. Lipids **14**:181-193.
26. Walling, M. W., A. K. Mircheff, C. H. Van Os, E. M. Wright. 1978. Subcellular distribution of nucleotide cyclases in rat intestinal epithelium. Am. J. Physiol. **235**:E539-E545.
27. Weiser, M. M. 1973. Intestinal epithelial cell surface membrane glycoprotein synthesis. I. An indicator of cellular differentiation. J. Biol. Chem. **248**:2536-2541.

Advances in Research on Cholera and Related Diarrheas, eds., S. Kuwahara, N. F. Pierce, 279–284.

DEVELOPMENT OF A SIMPLE TEST (BIKEN TEST) FOR DETECTION OF LT-PRODUCING *ESCHERICHIA COLI* AND APPLICATION OF THIS TEST

Takeshi Honda, Sekiko Taga, Michiko Arita, Yoshifumi Takeda and Toshio Miwatani

Department of Bacteriology and Serology, Research Institute for Microbial Diseases, Osaka University, 3-1, Yamada-oka, Suita, Osaka 565, Japan

It has been established that enterotoxigenic *Escherichia coli* is one of the most important causative bacteria of diarrhea in developing countries and of traveller's diarrhea (18, 20). Although we need further informations on epidemiology of enterotoxigenic *E. coli,* they are limited because of difficulties of performing the identification of the organisms.

For detection of the LT of enterotoxigenic *E. coli*, various assay methods have been developed, including the ileal loop test (15), vascular permeability test (6), Chinese hamster ovary (CHO) cell assay (8), Y-1 adrenal cell assay (3, 19), passive immune hemolysis (5, 21, 25), reversed passive hemagglutination (14) staphylococcal coagglutination method (1), solid-phase radioimmunoassay (7), ganglioside G_{M1} enzyme-linked immunosorbent assay (22), and DNA probe assay (16). However, many of these assay methods are unsuitable for routine clinical purposes because they need special material or techniques or both, such as a large number of animals, stocks of special tissue culture cells, and radioisotopes. In this paper, we report a simple, reproducible and inexpensive method, the Biken test (9, 11) for detection of enterotoxigenic *Escherichia coli* producing heat-labile enterotoxin (LT). This method is based on the principles of the Elek test (4) and Ouchterlony double gel diffusion test (17) and was used in a field study in Bangladesh with good results (9). We also developed a method for obtaining heat-stable enterotoxin (ST) from the culture agar used for the Biken test and demonstrated usefulness of this ST-sampling method.

MATERIALS AND METHODS

Strains

All the *E. coli* strains used in this study were isolated at Osaka Airport Quarantine Station between May 1979 and April 1981 from persons with traveller's diarrhea who had just come back from cholera-infected areas of Sourth-East Aria. Cultures were kept on Dorset agar slants before use.

LT and anti-LT antiserum

LT was isolated and purified from an LT-producing strain of *E. coli*, 536-5, essentially as described by Clements and Finkelstein (2). The purification procedure was as described in detail previously (23). Antiserum against purified LT was prepared essentially as described previously (12). The antiserum obtained was purified by immunoaffinity column chromatography as described previously (12). The purified anti-LT immunoglobulin was diluted with 0.2M borate buffer (pH 8.0) to give a titer of 1 : 1.5, which means that a maximal dilution of the antiserum giving a precipitin line against 2 μg of purified LT in an Ouchterlony gel diffusion test was 1.5-fold. The gel diffusion test was performed as described previously (13) with 0.9% Noble agar (Difco) plate in phosphate buffered saline (pH 7.0) containing 0.2% sodium azide as a preservative.

Chemicals

Polymyxin B (Taito Pfizer Co., Tokyo), lincomycin (Japan Upjohn Co., Tokyo) and other chemicals for preparing Biken agar No. 2 were described previously (9, 11).

Chinese hamster ovary (CHO) cell assay

CHO cell assay was carried out as described previously (10). Eagle's minimal essential medium was used in place of the F12 medium originally described by Guerrant *et al.* (8), since this modification decreased the extent of elongation of CHO cells in the absence of LT.

Biken agar No. 2

The composition of the Biken agar No. 2 for the Biken test is as follows: casamino acids (Difco), 2%; yeast extract (Difco), 1%; NaCl, 0.25%; K_2HPO_4, 1.5%; glucose, 0.5%; trace salts solution (5% $MgSO_4$, 2% $CoCl_2 \cdot 6H_2O$ and 0.5% $FeCl_3$), 0.05%; Noble agar (Difco), 1.5%; lincomycin, 90 μg/ml; pH 7.5.

Biken test

The Biken test was carried out essentially as described previously (9, 11) but anti-LT antiserum was used instead of the anti-cholera enterotoxin (CT) antiserum used previously (11). Four isolates of *E. coli* to be tested were plated onto a single plate of Biken agar No. 2 (11). A typical example of the inoculation is shown in Fig. 1. The plate was incubated at 37°C for 48 hours, and then paper discs (Whatmann AA) containing polymyxin B (about 500 IU) were placed on each colony and the plate was incubated for an additional 5 hours. Then anti-LT antiserum was put into a well (6-7 mm in diameter) cut near each colony (about 5 mm distant, see Fig. 1) and the plate was further incubated at 37°C for 24 hours. Precipitin lines between anti-LT antiserum and bacterial colonies were examined by naked eye, preferably with an immunodiffusion view box. Results were confirmed after incubation for additional 24 hours.

Sampling for ST assay from the agar plate

After polymyxin B treatment and just before the anti-LT antiserum was placed in the center well during the Biken test, either 2 pieces of agar (7 mm in diameter) or 3 pieces (5.5 mm in diameter) were punched out from just outside the periphery of each colony (see Fig. 1). These pieces of agar were put into 0.4 ml of phosphate buffered saline (0.01 M, pH 7.0) and allowed to stand overnight at 4°C to extract ST. Then the phosphate buffered saline solution was used for ST assay.

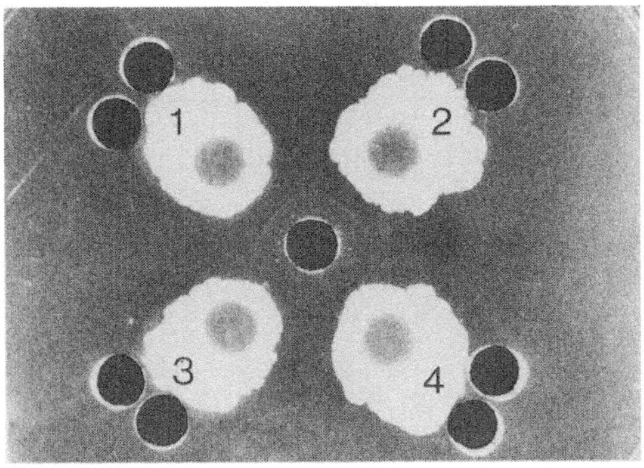

Fig. 1. A typical example of the Biken test on Biken agar No. 2. Four strains were spread around the center well for anti-LT antiserum. Round circles on colonies are paper discs containing polymyxin B. Precipitin lines were observed between the center well and strains 1 and 2. Two circular portions of agar (7 mm in diameter) were punched out from near the periphery of each colony for ST assay.

Liquid culture for ST sampling

E. coli cells were grown in tryptic soy broth (2 ml in 12 mm x 100 mm test tubes) with rotary shaking (40 rpm) at 37°C for 22 hours. The culture was centrifuged at 10,000 rpm for 15 minutes and the supernatant was used for ST assay.

Suckling mouse assay

ST activity of samples was assayed in suckling mice as described previously (24). The fluid accumulation (FA) ratio was calculated as the ratio of the weight of the entire intestine to that of the rest of the body.

RESULTS

A total of 2,229 strains of *E. coli* isolated from patients with traveller's diarrhea were tested for LT production by both the Biken test and CHO cell assay. As summarized in Table 1, the results of the two assays correlated very well: 578 strains gave positive results in both tests and 1,629 strains gave negative results in both. Only 22 strains gave discrepant results: 12 were positive by the Biken test only and 10 were positive by CHO

Table 1. Comparison of the results of the Biken test and CHO assay for detection of LT-producibility in 2,229 strains of *E. coli.*

Assay method		No. of strains
Biken test	CHO cells	
+	+	578
–	–	1,629
+	–	12
–	+	10

Table 2. Comparison of results on ST activity of samples from Biken plates and standard liquid cultures of 2,229 strains of *E. coli*.

Samples from: Biken plate	standard culture	No. of strains
+[1]	+	1,140
–[2]	–	1,081
+	–	3
–	+	5

[1]FA ratio, more than 0.080.
[2]FA ratio, less than 0.079.

cell assay only. The coincidence rate calculated from these results was 99.0%. Further analysis showed that the discrepancies were partly due to mixed culture of strains of LT-producing and -nonproducing cells (data not shown).

Pieces of agar plate (7 mm in diameter) were punched out from just outside the periphery of colonies (see Fig. 1) and tested for ST as described in the Materials and Methods. Samples from 2,229 strains were tested for ST activity in suckling mice and results were compared with those obtained from liquid cultures. As shown in Table 2, the results obtained with the two series of samples correlated very well: only 8 strains (0.4%) gave discrepant results.

DISCUSSION

The usefulness of the Biken test for detection of LT-producing *E. coli* was demonstrated in a large scale field study. In this study, we used anti-LT antiserum instead of the anti-CT antiserum used previously (11), and found that it gave a sharper and clearer precipitin line than anti-CT antiserum. This was probably because, in addition to an antigenic determinant(s) common to both LT and CT, LT and CT both have a specific antigenic determinant (12). Recently, we reported that LT from human enterotoxigenic *E. coli* (LT_h) is immunologically not identical with LT from porcine enterotoxigenic *E. coli* (LT_p) (13), and thus anti-LT_h antiserum gave better results than anti-LT_p antiserum with isolates from humans. Although not examined in detail, it seems likely that anti-LT_p antiserum should be used for detecting LT-producing *E. coli* of porcine origin.

From our experience, the following points are important in the Biken test. 1) The volume of the medium, Biken agar No. 2, in the petri dish: If the agar is too thick the precipitin line is faint, and if the agar is too thin bacterial growth is poor and thus the precipitin line is also faint. The best results were obtained with 12 - 15 ml of agar/petri dish of 90 mm diameter. 2) The strains tested should not be inoculated as a pin-point, but spread out as shown in Fig. 1. 3) The bacteria should be incubated for at least 48 hours. Addition of antiserum at too early a time decreses the sensitivity of this test. 4) The titer of the anti-LT antiserum is important. If the titer of the antiserum is too high, hypotoxigenic strains do not produce a precipitin line. An appropriate titer of the antiserum was found to be 1 : 1.5, which means that the maximal dilution of the antiserum to give a precipitin line against 2 μg of purified LT in the Ouchterlony gel diffusion test is 1.5-fold.

Vigorous shaking of cultures was reported to be necessary for obtaining samples for ST assay (24). In this study, we found that pieces of agar from Biken agar No. 2 obtained during the course of LT production were good sources of ST. Almost identical results were obtained with samples from Biken agar and from standard liquid culture. Sampling from the Biken agar simplifies the test for ST-producing *E. coli*, since no separate liquid culture with shaking is necessary, and strains on a single agar plate, Biken agar No. 2, can be tested for both LT and ST production.

This work was supported by a Grant-in-Aid for Scientific Research from the Ministry of Education, Science and Culture of Japan.

REFERENCES

1. Brill, B. M., B. L. Wasilauskas, and S. H. Richardson. 1979. Adaptation of the staphylococcal coagglutination technique for detection of heat-labile enterotoxin of *Escherichia coli*. J. Clin. Microbiol. **9**: 49-55.
2. Clements, J. D., and R. A. Finkelstein. 1979. Isolation and characterization of homogeneous heat-labile enterotoxins with high specific activity from *Escherichia coli* cultures. Infect. Immun. **24**: 760-769.
3. Donta, S. T., H. W. Moon, and S. C. Whipp. 1974. Detection of heat-labile *Escherichia coli* enterotoxin with the use of adrenal cells in tissue culture. Science **183**: 334-336.
4. Elek, S. 1948. The recognition of toxinogenic bacterial strains in vitro. Br. Med. J. **1**: 493-496.
5. Evans, D. J., Jr., and D. G. Evans. 1977. Direct serological assay for the heat-labile enterotoxin of *Escherichia coli* using passive immune hemolysis. Infect. Immun. **16**: 604-609.
6. Evans, D. J., Jr., D. G. Evans, and S. L. Gorbach. 1973. Production of vascular permeability factor by enterotoxigenic *Escherichia coli* isolated from man. Infect. Immun. **8**: 725-730.
7. Greenberg, H. B., D. A. Sack, W. Rodriguez, R. B. Sack, R. G. Wyatt, A. R. Kalica, R. S. Horswood, R. M. Chanock, and A. Z. Kapikian. 1977. Microtiter solid-phase radioimmunoassay for detection of *Escherichia coli* heat-labile enterotoxin. Infect. Immun. **17**: 541-545.
8. Guerrant, R. L., L. L. Brunton, T. C. Schnaitman, L. I. Rebhun, and A. G. Gilman. 1974. Cyclic adenosine monophosphate and alteration of Chinese hamster ovary cell morphology: a rapid, sensitive in vitro assay for the enterotoxin of *Vibrio cholerae* and *Escherichia coli*. Infect. Immun. **10**: 320-327.
9. Honda, T., Q. Akhtar, R. I. Glass, and A. K. M. G. Kibriya. 1981. A simple assay to detect *Escherichia coli* producing heat-labile enterotoxin: results of a field study of the Biken test in Bangladesh. Lancet, ii, 609-610.
10. Honda, T., M. Shimizu, Y. Takeda and T. Miwatani. 1976. Isolation of a factor causing morphological changes of Chinese hamster ovary cells from culture filtrate of *Vibrio parahaemolyticus*. Infect. Immun. **14**: 1028-1033.
11. Honda, T., S. Taga, Y. Takeda, and T. Miwatani. 1981. Modified Elek test for detection of heat-labile enterotoxin of enterotoxigenic *Escherichia coli*. J. Clin. Microbiol. **13**: 1-5.
12. Honda, T., Y. Takeda and T. Miwatani. 1981. Isolation of special antibodies which react only with homologous enterotoxins from *Vibrio cholerae* and enterotoxigenic *Escherichia coli*. Infect. Immun. **34**: 333-336.
13. Honda, T., T. Tsuji, Y. Takeda, and T. Miwatani. 1981. Immunological nonidentity of heat-labile enterotoxins from human and porcine enterotoxigenic *Escherichia coli*. Infect. Immun. **34**: 337-340.
14. Kudoh, Y., S. Yamada, S. Matsushita, K. Ohta, M. Tsuno, T. Muraoka, N. Ohtomo, and M. Ohashi. 1979. Detection of heat-labile enterotoxin of *Escherichia coli* by reversed passive hemagglutination test with specific immunoglobulin against cholera toxin, p. 266-273. *In* K.

Takeya and Y. Zinnaka (eds.), Proceedings of the 14th Joint Conference of the US-Japan Cooperative Medical Science Program, Cholera Panel, Toho University, Tokyo.

15. Moon, H. W., S. C. Whipp, G. W. Engstrom, and A. L. Baetz. 1970. Response of the rabbit ileal loop to cell-free products from *Escherichia coli* enteropathogenic for swine. J. Infect. Dis. **121**: 182-187.

16. Moseley, S. L., I. Huq, A. R. M. A. Alim, M. So, M. Samadpour-Motalebi, and S. Falkow. 1980. Detection of enterotoxigenic *Escherichia coli* by DNA colony hybridization. J. Infect. Dis. **142**: 892-898.

17. Ouchterlony, Ö. 1949. Antigen-antibody reactions in gels. Acta Pathol. Microbiol. Scand. **26**: 507-515.

18. Ouchterlony, Ö., and J. Holmgren. (eds.) 1980. Cholera and related diarrheas. 43rd Nobel Symposium, Stockholm. 1978, S. Karger, Basel.

19. Sack, D. A., and R. B. Sack. 1975. Test for enterotoxigenic *Escherichia coli* using Y1 adrenal cells in miniculture. Infect. Immun. **11**: 334-336.

20. Sack, R. B. 1975. Human diarrheal disease caused by enterotoxigenic *Escherichia coli*. Ann. Rev. Microbiol. **29**: 233-353.

21. Serafim, M. B., A. F. Pestana de Castro, L. R. Reis, and L. R. Travulsi. 1979. Passive immune hemolysis for detection of heat-labile enterotoxin produced by *Escherichia coli* isolated from different sources. Infect. Immun. **24**: 606-610.

22. Svennerholm, A. -M., and J. Holmgren. 1978. Identification of *Escherichia coli* heat-labile enterotoxin by means of a ganglioside immunosorbent assay (G_{M1}-ELISA) procedure. Curr. Microbiol. **1**: 19-23.

23. Takeda, Y., T. Honda, S. Taga, and T. Miwatani. 1981. In vitro formation of hybrid toxins between subunits of *Escherichia coli* heat-labile enterotoxin and those of cholera enterotoxin. Infect. Immun. **34**: 341-346.

24. Takeda, Y., T. Takeda, T. Yano, K. Yamamoto, and T. Miwatani. 1979. Purification and partial characterization of heat-stable enterotoxin of enterotoxigenic *Escherichia coli*. Infect. Immun. **25**: 978-985.

25. Tsukamoto, T., Y. Kinoshita, S. Taga, Y. Takeda, and T. Miwatani. 1980. Value of passive immune hemolysis for detection of heat-labile enterotoxin produced by enterotoxigenic *Escherichia coli* J. Clin. Microbiol. **12**: 768-771.

Advances in Research on Cholera and Related Diarrheas, eds., S. Kuwahara, N. F. Pierce, 285–292.

IMMUNOLOGICAL AND MOLECULAR HETEROGENEITY OF HEAT-LABILE ENTEROTOXINS FROM HUMAN AND PORCINE ENTEROTOXIGENIC *ESCHERICHIA COLI*

Takao Tsuji, Takeshi Honda, Yoshifumi Takeda and Toshio Miwatani

Department of Bacteriology and Serology, Research Institute for Microbial Diseases, Osaka University, Yamada-oka, Suita, Osaka 565, Japan

The molecular structure of heat-labile enterotoxin (LT) of enterotoxigenic *Escherichia coli* is similar to that of cholera enterotoxin (CT). Dallas and Falkow (5) showed that LT synthesized by minicells containing Ent plasmid DNA was composed of two distinct proteins with molecular weights of 25,000 and 11,500 daltons, values similar to those of the A and B subunits of CT. Clements and Finkelstein (3) demonstrated more directly that the subunit structure of purified LT was very similar to that of CT; that is, LT consisted of two subunits, A and B, with molecular weights of 28,000 and 11,500, respectively. Moreover, similarities in the amino acid sequences of the A and B subunits of CT and LT were reported by Spicer et al. (17) and Dallas and Falkow (6), respectively.

The immunological similarity of LT to CT is also well established. Gyles and Barnum (11) first reported the immunological kinship of CT and LT, by showing cross neutralization of the ability of cell lysates to cause fluid accumulation in rabbit ileal loops. Gyles (10) confirmed the partial identity of CT and LT by the Ouchterlony double gel diffusion test. Subsequently, Clements and Finkelstein (1, 2) demonstrated the immunological cross-reactivity of LT with the A and B subunits of CT.

All the above experiments were carried out with LT produced by a strain of porcine enterotoxigenic *E. coli*. Kunkel and Robertson (13) have suggested, however, that there are molecular and immunological differences between LT's from human and porcine enterotoxigenic *E. coli*. In this work, we demonstrate immunological and molecular heterogeneity of LT's from human strain (LT_h) and porcine strains (LT_p) of enterotoxigenic *E. coli*.

MATERIALS AND METHODS

Bacterial strains

LT-producing human strains of *E. coli* were isolated from diarrheal patients and porcine strains were provided by Dr. A. F. Pestana de Castro, University of Campinas, Brazil.

Preparation of purified LT_h and LT_p

LT_h and LT_p were isolated and purified from whole-cell lysates of a human strain (*E. coli* 536-5) and a porcine strain (either *E. coli* 0-149-26 or G7-17), respectively. The procedures for purification were essentially as described by Clements and Finkelstein (3).

Details of the culture of cells, isolation of LT from the cells and purification by successive column chromatographies on Bio-Gel A5m and Sephacryl S-200 were described previously (18). For separation of spontaneous aggregates of B subunits of LT_h and LT_p, Sephacryl S-200 eluates were further chromatographed on a Sephadex G-75 column (superfine, 1.5 x 150 cm) in 0.05 M Tris-HCl buffer (pH 7.4) containing 1 mM EDTA, 3 mM sodium azide and 0.2 M NaCl (TEAN buffer) (9). Fractions containing biological activities, such as activities to induce morphological change of Chinese hamster ovary cells (12) and rabbit skin vascular permeability (4), were collected, concentrated by Amicon PM-10 membrane filtration and used as purified LT_h and LT_p.

Purified CT

CT from the culture filtrate of *Vibrio cholerae* 569B, purified by the method of Ohtomo et al. (15), was purchased from Sanko Junyaku Co., Tokyo.

Treatment of LT_h and LT_p with trypsin

Purified LT_h and LT_p were treated with trypsin as described by Rappaport et al. (16), since these preparations were isolated and purified from whole-cell lysates. About 10 μg of purified preparation in 0.2 ml of 50 mM ammonium bicarbonate was incubated with about 0.5 μg of trypsin (Sigma Chemical Co., St. Louis, Mo.; Type Xl; diphenyl carbamyl chloride treated bovine pancrease trypsin) at 37°C for 60 minutes.

Double gel diffusion test

The Ouchterlony double gel diffusion test was carried out with 1.2% Noble agar (Difco) in TEAN buffer. After the samples were applied, the plates were placed in a humidified incubator at room temperature for about 16 to 24 hours. The plates were washed extensively against a solution containing 0.4% NaCl and 0.4% $Na_2B_4O_7$. Then they were dried, stained with 0.5% Coomassie brilliant blue in a solution containing 50% methanol and 10% acetic acid, and destained in a solution containing 50% methanol and 10% acetic acid.

Isoelectric focusing of purified toxin

Electrofocusing of the purified toxin on ampholine carrier ampholytes was carried out in an LKB electrofocusing system 8100-10, using a pH gradient of 3 to 10. A sample of about 2 mg of purified toxin was applied and electrophoresis was performed at a constant voltage of 300 v for 72 hours. Then fractions were collected and their absorbance at 280 nm and ability to cause morphological changes of Chinese hamster ovary cells were measured.

Polyacrylamide gel electrophoresis

Polyacrylamide gel disc electrophoresis was carried out as described by Davis (7) on 7% acrylamide gel. Electrophoresis was performed at a constant current of 2 mA per tube for 3 hours at 4°C.

Electrophoresis on an SDS-polyacrylamide gel slab (0.2 x 13.5 x 12.0 cm) in 0.1% SDS was carried out as described by Laemmli (14) with 12% acrylamide gel. Electrophoresis was performed at a constant current of 25 mA for 4.5 hours.

Gels were stained with Coomassie brilliant blue and then destained as described previously (8).

Amino acid analysis

The amino acid compositions of purified toxins were determined in a Hitachi type 835 analyzer using samples hydrolyzed in 4 M methanesulfonic acid at 110°C for 24 hours in evacuated sealed tubes.

RESULTS

Immunological heterogeneity of LT_h and LT_p

The double gel diffusion test against anti-LT_h antiserum showed that LT_h and LT_p were antigenically related but not identical. As shown in Fig. 1A, the precipitin line between purified LT_h and anti-LT_p antiserum and that between LT_p and anti-LT_h antiserum formed a spur. This showed that LT_h possessed an antigenic determinant(s) that was not found in LT_p. Similarly, the precipitin line between purified LT_h and anti-LT_p antiserum and that between LT_p and anti-LT_p antiserum formed a spur (Fig. 1B), which indicated that LT_p possessed an antigenic determinant(s) that was not found in LT_h.

To determine whether strains of human *E. coli* and porcine *E. coli*, respectively, produce immunologically identical LT's, we prepared crude LT's from several human and porcine *E. coli* and examined them by the double gel diffusion test. As shown in Fig. 2A, the LT's from all the human *E. coli* strains tested, which were randomly selected, gave pricipitin lines that fused (Fig. 2A), indicating that they were identical. All the porcine *E. coli* strains were also found to produce immunologically identical LT's as shown in Fig. 2B.

Differences in the physicochemical properties of LT_h and LT_p

Since we demonstrated the immunological heterogeneity of LT_h and LT_p, we concluded that their physicochemical properties must also be different. We examined the ionic charges of LT_h and LT_p, by polyacrylamide gel disc electrophoresis without SDS.

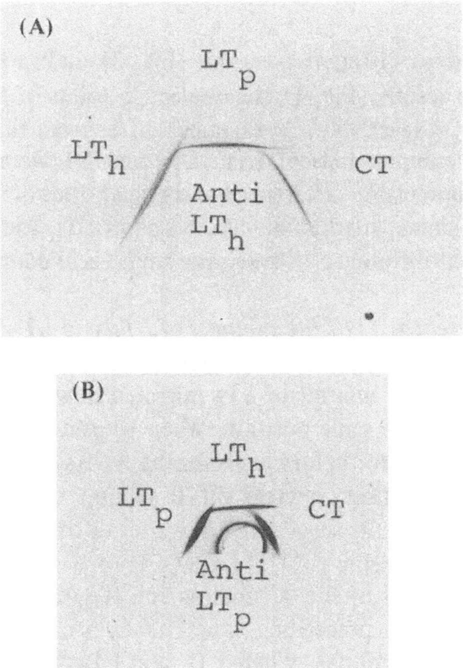

Fig. 1. Double gel diffusion test of LT_h, LT_p and CT with anti-LT_h (A) anti-LT_p (B).

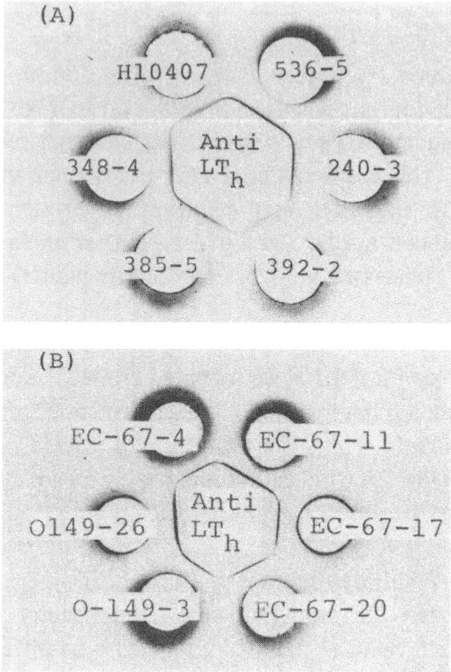

Fig. 2. Double gel diffusion test of crude LT preparations of various strains of human *E. coli* (A) and porcine *E. coli* (B).

LT_h and LT_p migrated to different positions (Fig. 3), indicating that they differed in ionic charge. From the results (Fig. 4), the isoelectric points of LT_h and LT_p were calculated as 7.50 and 8.10, respectively; both values differ from that of CT, which is 6.80.

The amino acid compositions of LT_h, LT_p and CT were compared, as shown in Table 1. There were appreciable differences in the quantities of several amino acids, such as threonine, serine, alanine, methionine and lysine in LT_h and LT_p. It was also found that there was a marked difference between the amino acid compositions of LT_h and CT and of LT_p and CT.

Demonstration of different sizes of the subunits of LT_h and LT_p

SDS-polyacrylamide slab gel electrophoresis showed that LT_h and LT_p differed in size. As seen in Fig. 5, the B subunit of LT_h migrated slower than those of LT_p and CT, which migrated to almost the same position. When trypsin-treated LT_h and LT_p and CT were treated with dithiothreitol before analysis, the A_1 fragments of these toxins migrated to almost the same position, whereas the B subunit of LT_h migrated slower than that of LT_p or CT. These results suggest that the sizes of the B subunits of LT_h, LT_p and CT have the following relationship: $LT_h > LT_p = CT$.

Although the mobilities of the A subunits and A_1 fragments of LT_h, LT_p and CT were indistinguishable in the preceeding experiments, a careful examination showed a slight difference in their mobilities. When LT_h and LT_p were treated with trypsin and subjected to electrophoresis after dithiothreitol treatment, the A subunit gave two bands attributable to A_1 and A_2 fragments. As shown in Fig. 6, the mobility of fragment A_1 of

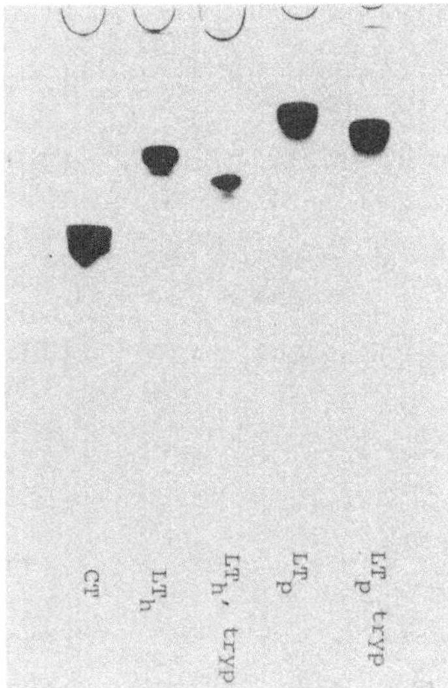

Fig. 3. Polyacrylamide disc gel electrophoresis of CT, LT_h and LT_p. Samples of 5 – 10 μg with or without trypsin treatment were subjected to electrophoresis.

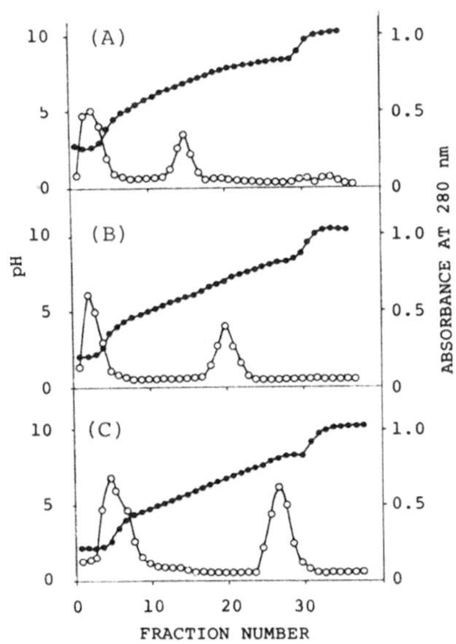

Fig. 4. Isoelectric focusing of CT, LT_h and LT_p. ●, pH; ○, absorbance at 280nm. (A) CT; (B) LT_h; (C) LT_p.

Table 1. Amino acid composition of LT_h, LT_p and CT

Amino acid	Concentration (%) LT_h	LT_p	CT
Aspartic acid/asparagine	11.11	11.12	11.62
Threonine	8.36	9.24	7.70
Serine	8.09	7.54	5.72
Glutamic acid/glutamine	12.45	12.61	11.73
Proline	3.76	3.76	4.32
Glycine	5.16	5.04	5.55
Alanine	5.78	5.23	9.36
Cystine	1.55	1.52	1.57
Valine	3.65	3.63	4.02
Methionine	2.77	3.02	2.30
Isoleucine	9.14	9.10	7.21
Leucine	5.40	5.41	6.07
Tyrosine	5.64	5.42	4.36
Phenylalanine	2.17	2.23	2.57
Histidine	1.71	1.47	3.78
Lysine	6.61	7.08	6.75
Arginine	5.47	5.53	4.20
Tryptophan	1.17	1.05	1.17

LT_p was slightly less than that of LT_h or CT, the latter two migrating to almost the same position. As shown in Fig. 7, the bands of fragments A_2's, the fastest band, also had different mobilities. Fragment A_2 of LT_p migrated slightly faster than that of LT_h or CT, which migrated to almost the same position. From these results it is concluded that the sizes of the A_1 fragments are in the order $LT_p > LT_h = CT$ and those of the A_2 fragment are in the order $LT_h = CT > LT_p$.

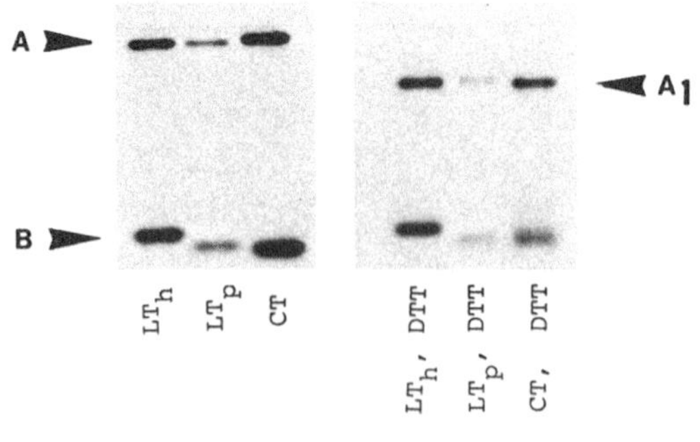

Fig. 5. SDS-polyacrylamide slab gel electrophoresis of LT_h, LT_p and CT. Samples (about 2 μg) were heated at 100°C for 2 minutes in the absence or presence of 10 mM dithiothreitol and subjected to electrophoresis.

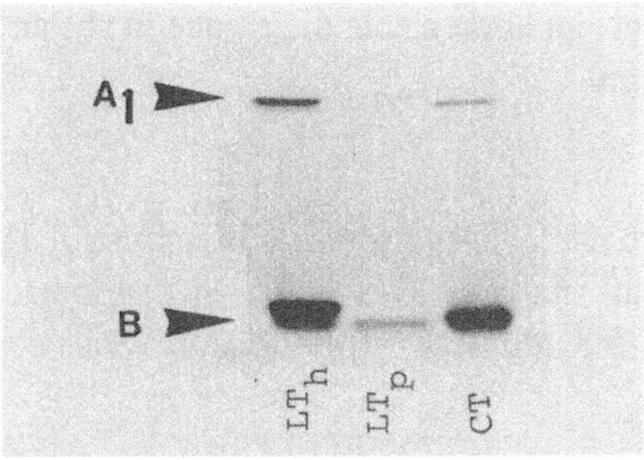

Fig. 6. Different mobilities of the A_1 fragments of LT_h, LT_p and CT on SDS-polyacrylamide slab gel electrophoresis. Samples (about 2 – 5 μg) were treated with dithiothreitol as described in the legend of Fig. 5 and subjected to electrophoresis.

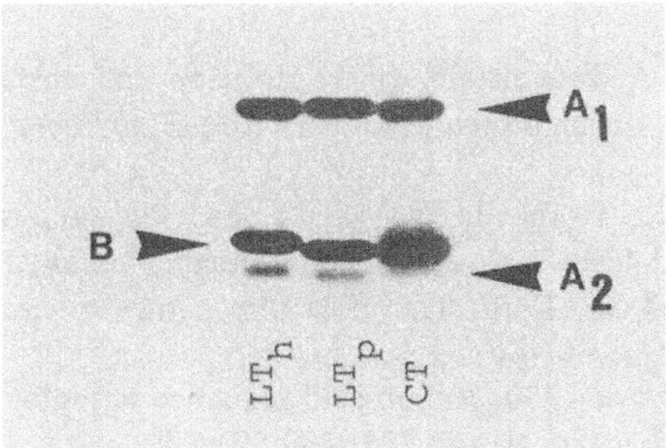

Fig. 7. Different mobilities of the A_2 fragments of LT_h, LT_p and CT on SDS-polyacrylamide slab gel electrophoresis. Samples of about 8 μg were used. Other experimental conditions were as for Fig. 6.

DISCUSSION

The present study demonstrated that LT_h and LT_p are antigenically related, but not identical. These LT's share a common antigen determinant(s). In addition, LT_h has an antigen determinant(s) that is not present in LT_p, and LT_p has an antigen determinant(s) that is not present in LT_h. It was also shown that LT_h and LT_p had a common antigen determinant(s) that was not found in CT. These results suggest that LT_h, LT_p, and CT share a common antigen determinant(s) and, in addition, that each enterotoxin possesses its own antigen determinant(s). There is also an antigen determinant(s) common to LT_h and LT_p.

Similarity in the molecular structure of LT_p and CT has been reported by several workers. Dallas and Falkow (5) showed that LT synthesized in minicells containing porcine Ent plasmid was composed of two distinct proteins with molecular weights of 25,500 and 11,500 daltons. Clements and Finkelstein (3) obtained purified LT_p and demonstrated that it consists of A and B subunits, with molecular weights of 28,000 and 11,500, respectively. Similarities in the amino acid sequences of the A and B subunits of LT_p and CT were reported by Spicer et al. (17) and Dallas and Falkow (6), respectively. However, Kunkel and Robertson (13) examined the physicochemical properties of purified LT_h and found that its amino acid composition was quite different from that of CT. In this paper, we present evidence that the ionic charges of the toxin molecule of LT_h, and LT_p and CT are different and that the sizes of the B and A subunits of LT_h and

LT_p are different. Moreover, an appreciable difference in the amino acid compositions of LT_h and LT_p is demonstrated.

We thank Dr. Saburo Hara, Department of Chemistry, Faculty of Science, Osaka University for amino acid analysis. This work was supported by a Grant-in-Aid for Scientific Research from the Ministry of Education, Science and Culture of Japan.

REFERENCES

1. Clements, J. D., and R. A. Finkelstein. 1978. Immunological cross-reactivity between a heat-labile enterotoxin(s) of *Escherichia coli* and subunits of *Vibrio cholerae* enterotoxin. Infect. Immun. **21**: 1036-1039.
2. Clements, J. D., and R. A. Finkelstein. 1978. Demonstration of shared and unique immunological determinants in enterotoxins from *Vibrio cholerae* and *Escherichia coli*. Infect. Immun. **22**: 709-713.
3. Clements, J. D., and R. A. Finkelstein. 1979. Isolation and characterization of homogeneous heat-labile enterotoxins with high specific activity from *Escherichia coli* cultures. Infect. Immun. **24**: 760-769.
4. Craig, J. P., K. Yamamoto, T. Takeda, Y. Takeda, and T. Miwatani. 1981. Vascular permeability activity of *Escherichia coli* heat-stable enterotoxin. Infect. Immun. **33**: 473-476.
5. Dallas, W. S., and S. Falkow. 1979. The molecular nature of heat-labile enterotoxin (LT) of *Escherichia coli*. Nature **277**: 406-407.
6. Dallas, W. S., and S. Falkow. 1980. Amino acid sequence homology between cholera toxin and *Escherichia coli* heat-labile toxin. Nature **288**: 499-501.
7. Davis, B. J. 1964. Disc electrophoresis. II. Method and application to human serum protein. Ann. N. Y. Acad. Sci. **121**: 404-427.
8. Fairbanks, G., T. L. Steck, and D. F. H. Wallach. 1971. Electrophoretic analysis of the major polypeptide of the human erythrocyte membrane. Biochemistry, **10**: 2606-2617.
9. Finkelstein, R. A., and J. J. LoSpalluto. 1969. Pathogenesis of experimental cholera. Preparation and isolation of choleragen and choleragenoid. J. Exp. Med. **130**: 185-202.
10. Gyles, C. L. 1974. Immunological study of the heat-labile enterotoxins of *Escherichia coli* and *Vibrio cholerae*. Infect. Immun. **9**: 564-570.
11. Gyles, C. L., and D. A. Barnum. 1969. A heat-labile enterotoxin from strains of *Escherichia coli* enteropathogenic for pigs. J. Infect. Dis., **120**: 419-426.
12. Honda, T., M. Shimizu, Y. Takeda, and T. Miwatani. 1976. Isolation of a factor causing morphological changes of Chinese hamster ovary cells. Infect. Immun. **14**: 1028-1033.
13. Kunkel, S. L., and D. C. Robertson. 1979. Purification and chemical characterization of the heat-labile enterotoxin produced by enterotoxigenic *Escherichia coli*. Infect. Immun. **25**: 586-596.
14. Laemmli, U. K. 1970. Cleavage of structural proteins during the assembly of the head of bacteriophage T4. Nature **227**: 680-685.
15. Ohtomo, N., T. Muraoka, H. Inoue, H. Sasaoka, and H. Takahashi. 1974. Preparation of cholera toxin and immunization studies with cholera toxoid, p. 132-142. *In* Proceedings of the 9th Joint Conference of the US-Japan Cooperative Medical Science Program, Cholera Panel. National Institutes of Health, Bethesda, Md.
16. Rappaport, R. S., J. F. Sagin. W. A. Pierzchala, G. Bonde, B. A. Rubin, and H. Tint. 1976. Activation of heat-labile *Escherichia coli* enterotoxin by trypsin. J. Infect. Dis. **133**: s41-s54.
17. Spicer, E. K., W. M. Kavanaug. W. S. Dallas, S. Falkow, W. H. Konigobe, and D. E. Schafer. 1981. Sequence homologies between A subunits of *Escherichia coli* and *Vibrio cholerae* enterotoxins. Proc. Natl. Acad. Sci. U.S.A. **78**: 50-54.
18. Takeda, Y., T. Honda, S. Taga, and T. Miwatani. 1981. In vitro formation of hybrid toxins between subunits of *Escherichia coli* heat-labile enterotoxin and those of cholera enterotoxin. Infect. Immun. **34**: 341-346.

Advances in Research on Cholera and Related Diarrheas, eds., S. Kuwahara, N. F. Pierce, 293–300.

ANTIGENIC HETEROGENEITY AMONG HEAT-LABILE ENTEROTOXINS FROM *ESCHERICHIA COLI*

Randall K. Holmes, Edda M. Twiddy, and Michael G. Bramucci[1)]

Department of Microbiology, Uniformed Services University of the Health Sciences, Bethesda, Maryland

We have previously described a solid phase radioimmunoassay for quantitative measurements of cholera enterotoxin (CT) and other antigenically related enterotoxins (1). The heat-labile enterotoxin (LT) of *Escherichia coli* cross-reacts with CT and can be measured in this assay system. The solid phase radioimmunoassay is performed in polyvinyl microtiter plates and involves four sequential steps: immobilization of purified equine anti-choleragenoid antibody; binding of enterotoxin antigen; binding of rabbit anti-enterotoxin; and binding of radioiodinated goat anti-rabbit IgG (γ) (hereafter designated $[^{125}I]$GARG).

We modified this solid phase radioimmunoassay and used it for preliminary studies concerning the immunochemistry of CT and LT. The rationale for these experiments can be summarized in the following manner. If each of the specific reagents is used at a saturating concentration, the amount of $[^{125}I]$GARG bound should reach a maximum that will be determined both by the amount of bound enterotoxin antigen and by its antibody binding capacity. Because CT and LT are partially cross-reacting antigens, we expected the maximum amount of bound $[^{125}I]$GARG to be greater with CT than with LT in assays using anti-CT antibodies. Figure 1 illustrates the results obtained when purified CT (choleragen) was compared with LT antigens in concentrated culture supernatants from several enterotoxigenic *E. coli* strains of independent origin. As expected, the maximum amount of bound $[^{125}I]$GARG was greater with CT than with any of the LT antigens. However, the maximum amounts of $[^{125}I]$GARG bound were also found to differ significantly and in a reproducible manner with the LT antigens from different enterotoxigenic *E. coli* strains. These observations led us to test the hypothesis that the LTs produced by enterotoxic strains of *E. coli* of independent origin might be cross-reacting but not identical variants of LT.

We selected *E. coli* strains HE12, a hypertoxinogenic mutant of KL320(pCG86) isolated in our laboratory (1), and Throop D for further study. HE12 is an *E. coli* K12 derivative harboring plasmid pCG86, an LT^+, ST^+, multiply antibiotic resistant plasmid from a porcine enteropathogenic *E. coli* strain (5). Throop D was isolated from a human

1) Present address : Department of Microbiology and Immunology, Hahneman Medical College and Hospital, Philadelphia, PA 19102

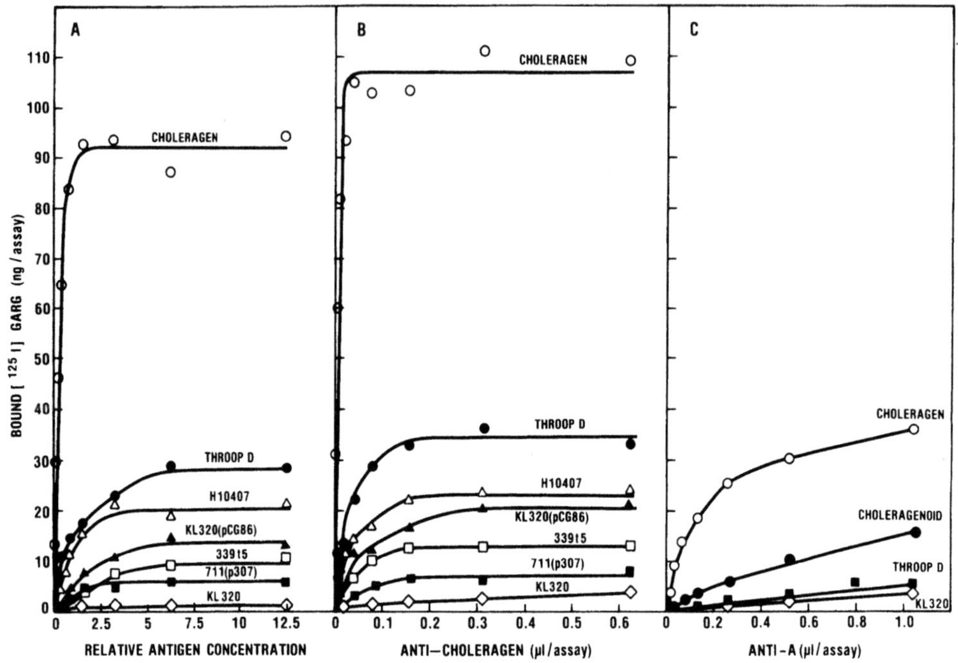

Fig. 1 Comparison of binding of anti-CT antibodies to purified CT (choleragen) and to LT antigens in concentrated culture supernatants from several enterotoxigenic strains of *E. coli*. KL320 is a nonenterotoxigenic *E. coli* K12 strain. The solid phase radioimmunoassay method was modified from reference 1. Titration of each reagent was performed under conditions where all other reagents were used at saturating concentrations. A) Titrations of CT and LT antigens. The highest concentration of CT was 0.25 µg/ml. B) Titrations of rabbit anti-CT (serum A23). C) Titration of anti-A serum prepared by absorbing anti-CT serum with the purified B subunit of CT. The anti-A serum reacted with CT but did not give detectable reactions with the LTs from *E. coli* Throop D or from other enterotoxigenic *E. coli* strains under the standardized conditions for this assay.

patient with cholera-like secretory diarrhea (4). For convenience we have designated the LTs from HE12 and Throop D as porcine LT (pLT) and human LT (hLT), respectively. CT was purified from Syncase broth cultures of *V. cholerae* 569B Inaba by published methods (10). For purification of pLT or hLT, bacteria from glucose-Syncase broth cultures were disrupted by sonication, and cell-associated LT was purified by affinity chromatography on agarose (2) followed by ion-exchange chromatography on phosphocellulose (6). Specific hyperimmune antisera were prepared in rabbits against the purified pLT, hLT, and CT.

The polypeptide subunits of purified pLT, hLT, and CT were compared by polyacrylamide gel electrophoresis in the presence of sodium dodecylsulfate (Figure 2). The electrophoretic mobilities of the monomeric A and B subunits and of the A_1 fragment of pLT were very similar to the mobilities of the corresponding polypeptides of CT (6). In contrast, the electrophoretic mobilities of the A_1 and B polypeptides of the

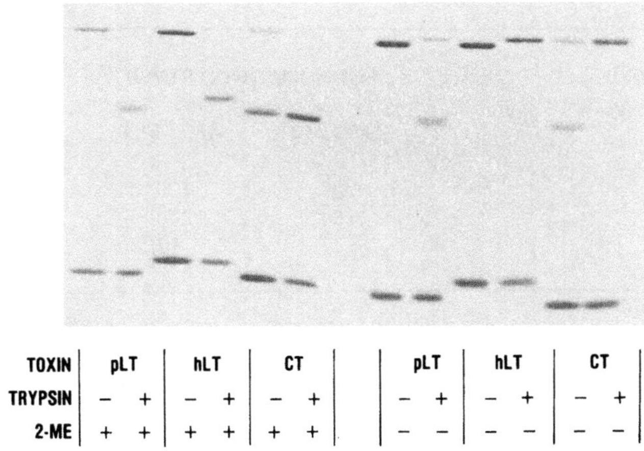

Fig. 2 Samples of pLT, hLT, and CT were boiled in sample treatment mix and subjected to electrophoresis in 13% polyacrylamide gel containing sodium dodecylsulfate in a discontinuous buffer system (8). Samples were analyzed before or after trypsin treatment and in the presence or absence of 2-mercaptoethanol, as indicated. Polypeptides were stained with Coomassie brilliant blue. The small A_2 polypeptides stained poorly. The A_1 and B polypeptides of hLT had significantly slower mobilities than the A_1 and B polypeptides of pLT and CT.

hLT were significantly slower than those for the corresponding polypeptides of pLT and CT.

The cytotoxicities of the purified CT, pLT, and hLT were tested using a modification of the Y1 adrenal cell assay (9). The minimal toxic dose for each of the three toxins was approximately 25 pg per assay. Pretreatment of pLT and hLT with trypsin under conditions that resulted in complete conversion of the intact A polypeptides to the nicked form (see Figure 2) did not result in enhanced toxicity of these enterotoxins for Y1 adrenal cells. In contrast, treatment of pLT and hLT with trypsin and with dithiothreitol did activate the adenosine diphosphate ribosyl transferase activity (11) associated with the A subunits of these toxins (data not shown). Neutralization tests were performed with 100 pg test doses of each toxin and with serial two-fold dilutions of each antitoxin (Table 1). The neutralizing titer of each antitoxin was highest for the homologous enterotoxin. For each antitoxin only slight differences in titer (twofold or less) were observed with pLT and with hLT as the test antigens, whereas larger differences in titer (8-fold to 16-fold) were seen when either pLT or hLT was compared with CT as the test antigen.

The immunologic cross-reactions between pLT, hLT, and CT were analyzed further by Ouchterlony-type immunodiffusion tests with hyperimmune anti-pLT, anti-hLT, and anti-CT (Figure 3). Each of these antitoxins reacted best with its homologous enterotoxin antigen. Reactions of partial identity were demonstrated using each possible pair of enterotoxins with each of the three specific antitoxins. Thus, in spite of the striking similarities between purified pLT and hLT with respect to potency, mode of action, and

Table 1. Neutralization of purified heat-labile enterotoxins by homologous and heterologous anti-enterotoxic sera.

Enterotoxin	Neutralizing titer (units/ul)[a]		
	ANTI-pLT	ANTI-hLT	ANTI-CT
pLT	200	100	12.5
hLT	100	200	12.5
CT	25	12.5	200

a) Antisera were tested in twofold serial dilutions. The unit of neutralizing antitoxin was defined as the smallest volume of antiserum required to decrease the cytotoxic response from 4+ to 1+ or less.

cross-neutralization, there are also significant differences between these two enterotoxins in terms of their unique antigenic determinants and the electrophoretic mobilities of their Al and B polypeptides in SDS-polyacrylamide gels.

Additional studies were performed to analyze the immunochemistry of the A and B subunits of pLT and hLT. Each purified enterotoxin was radioiodinated with ^{125}I by the chloramine T method (7), and the ^{125}I-labeled A and B subunits were isolated by gel filtration chromatography under dissociating conditions. The results of a representative purification of radiolabeled pLT subunits are presented in Figure 4. The purified A and B subunits of pLT and hLT were designated pLT-A, pLT-B, hLT-A, and hLT-B.

Next, we titrated the anti-pLT, anti-hLT, and anti-CT sera for binding to the purified, radiolabeled polypeptides [^{125}I]pLT-A, [^{125}I]pLT-B, [^{125}I]hLT-A, and [^{125}I]hLT-B (Figure 5). Each of the radiolabeled polypeptides was immunoprecipitated by all three antitoxins. Thus, shared antigenic determinants exist both on the A poly-

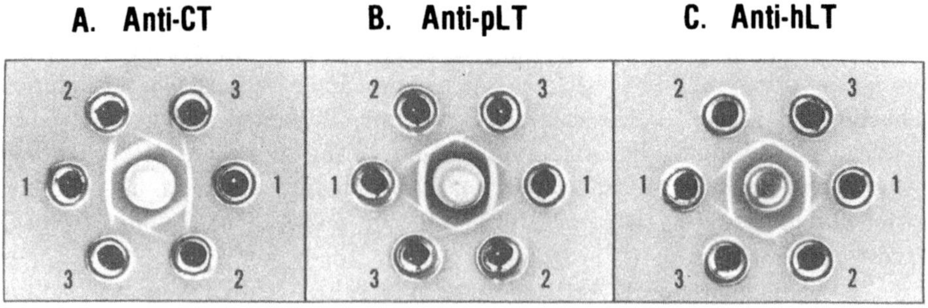

Fig. 3 Comparison of antigenic determinants of pLT, hLT, and CT by Ouchterlony type immunodiffusion tests. Rabbit antitoxins were added to the center wells as follows: A) Anti-CT (serum A23, 1:2 dilution), B) Anti-pLT (serum A45, undiluted), and C) Anti-hLT (serum B59, undiluted). Samples of purified enterotoxin at 200 μg/ml were added to the outer wells of each plate and were numbered as follows: 1) CT, 2) pLT, and 3) hLT.

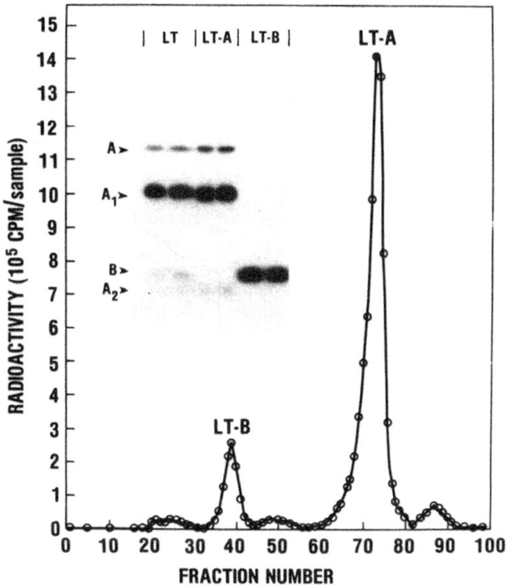

Fig.4 Purification of subunits of [^{125}I]pLT. A 100 μg sample of purified pLT was radioiodinated by the chloramine T method (7). After dialysis to remove unreacted Na^{125}I, the [^{125}I]pLT was subjected to gel filtration chromatography on Biogel P60 in 0.1 M glycine buffer at pH 3.2 in the presence of 1.0 M urea and 100 μg of bovine serum albumin/ml. Samples were removed from each fraction for measurement of radioactivity, and the fractions containing [^{125}I]pLT-A or [^{125}I]pLT-B were pooled. Samples of the radioiodinated pLT, pLT-A, and pLT-B were analyzed by electrophoresis in SDS-polyacrylamide gels in the presence of 2-mercaptoethanol as described in the legend for Figure 2, followed by autoradiography (see insert).

peptides and on the B polypeptides of pLT, hLT, and CT.

Finally, specific competitive-binding radioimmunoassays were developed for pLT-A, pLT-B, hLT-A, and hLT-B (Figure 6). Each assay mixture contained one of the specific radiolabeled enterotoxin subunits, a sufficient volume of the homologous antitoxin to precipitate 50-70% of the radiolabeled polypeptide in the absence of competing antigen, and a variable amount of non-radioactive pLT, hLT, or CT as the competing antigen. In the specific assays for pLT-B and hLT-B (Figures 6B and 6D), complete competition was observed only with the homologous enterotoxins. Partial crossreactions were observed with the heterologous LT enterotoxins and, to a lesser extent, with CT. The results obtained in the specific competitive-binding radioimmunoassays for the antigenic determinants of pLT-A and hLT-A were different (Figures 6A and 6C). Complete competition was observed in both assays when either pLT or hLT was used as the non-radioactive competing antigen, although differences in the dose response curves were noted. Partial cross-reactions between CT and hLT-A or pLT-A were observed, but the extent of competition by CT was greater with hLT-A than with pLT-A.

In summary, we have developed a modification of our solid phase radioimmunoassay for heat-labile enterotoxins that is useful as a rapid screening test to identify variants of LT that differ in the extent of their cross-reactions with one another

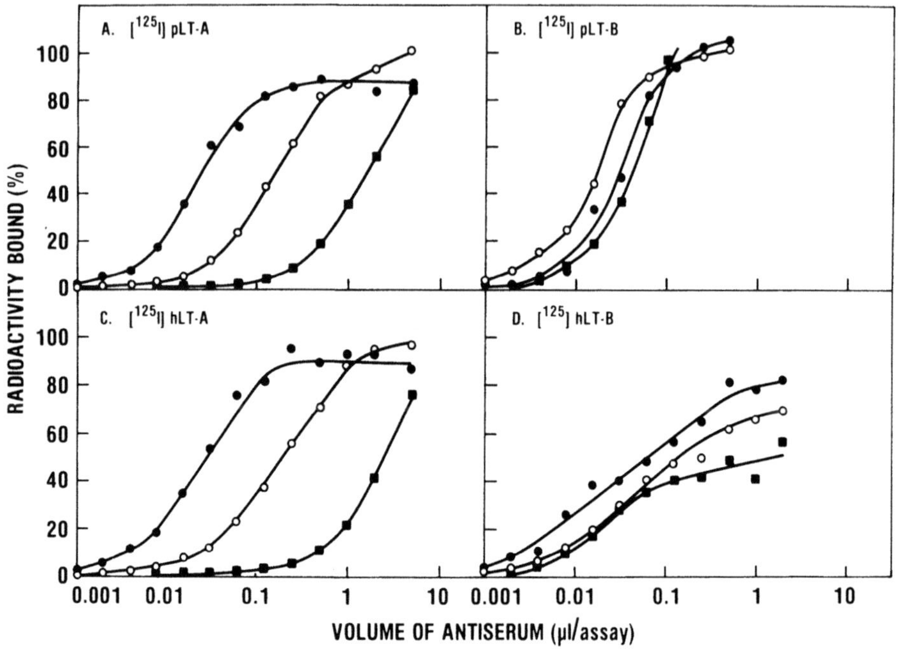

Fig. 5 Binding of purified [^{125}I] pLT-A, [^{125}I] pLT-B, [^{125}I] hLT-A, and [^{125}I] hLT-B by anti-pLT (○; serum A45), anti-hLT (●; serum B59), and anti-CT (■; serum A23). Each reaction mixture contained either 20,000 CPM of radiolabeled pLT-A or hLT-A or 10,000 CPM of radiolabeled pLT-B or hLT-B. Samples of anti-pLT, anti-hLT or anti-CT were added to the reaction mixtures in the volumes noted. After incubation, radioactivity in immune complexes bound to *Staphylococcus aureus* bearing protein A was measured. Assay procedures were based on methods described in reference 3.

or with CT. We have purified two partially cross-reacting LTs (pLT and hLT) coded by plasmids from human and porcine enterotoxigenic *E. coli* strains, and we have compared their polypeptide subunits, their biologic activities, and their immunochemical properties. Although these two enterotoxins are closely related to each other and to CT, their B polypeptide subunits and A_1 polypeptide fragments are not identical in size. The B subunits of pLT and hLT have unique antigenic determinants in addition to shared antigenic determinants, but the immunodominant determinants of the A polypeptides of these two LTs are very similar. The A and B subunits of both LTs crossreact partially with CT. Our data support the concept that the structural genes for LTs on Ent plasmids in *E. coli* strains from various sources are homologous genes among which significant evolutionary divergence has occurred.

This study was supported in part by Public Health Service research grant 5 R22 AI14107 from the National Institute of Allergy and Infectious Diseases and in part by the Uniformed Services University of the Health Sciences. The opinions expressed are the private views of the authors and should not be construed as official or as necessarily reflecting the views of the Department of Defense. We thank the following investigators

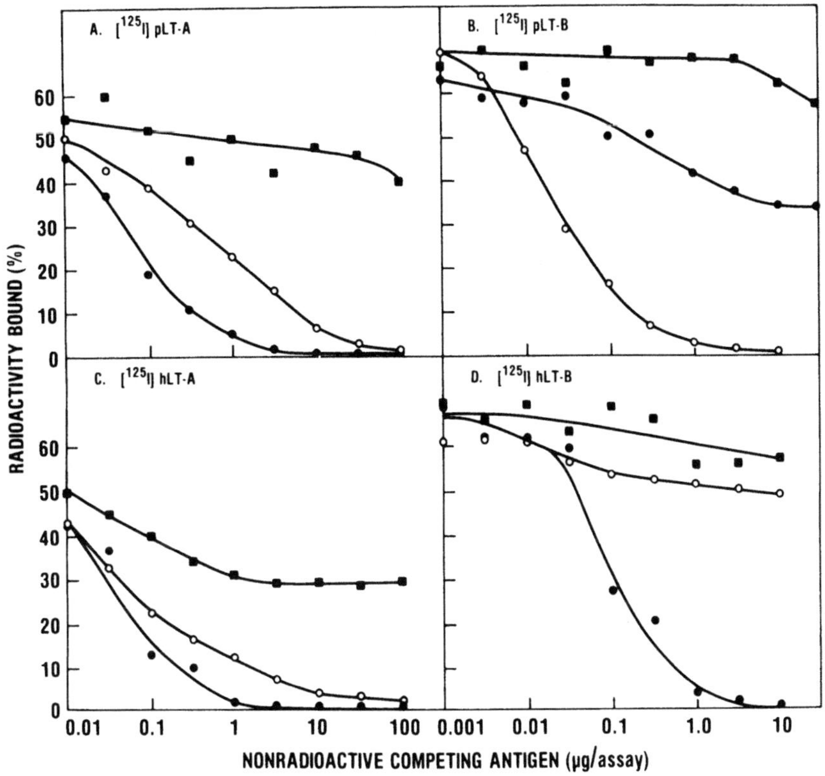

Fig. 6 Competitive-binding radioimmunoassays for pLT-A (panel A), pLT-B (panel B), hLT-A (panel C), and hLT-B (panel D). Assay procedures were based on methods described in reference 3. Each reaction mixture contained the specific radioiodinated ligand indicated (either 20,000 CPM of pLT-A or hLT-A or 10,000 CPM of pLT-B or hLT-B), an appropriate volume of the homologous antitoxin (anti-pLT for panels A and B; anti-hLT for panels C and D), and the amount of nonradioactive competing ligand indicated (○, pLT; ●, hLT; ■, CT).

for providing the bacterial strains indicated: R. Finkelstein (*E. coli* Throop D, H10407, and 339t5), S. Falkow (*E. coli* 711(p307)), and W. Maas (*E. coli* KL320 and KL320(pCG86)).

REFERENCES

1. Bramucci, M. G., E. M. Twiddy, W. B. Baine, and R. K. Holmes. 1981. Isolation and characterization of hypertoxinogenic (htx) mutants of *Escherichia coli* KL320(pCG86). Infect. Immun. **32**: 1034-1044.
2. Clements, J. D., and R. A. Finkelstein. 1979. Isolation and characterization of homogeneous heat-labile enterotoxin with high specific activity from *Escherichia coli* cultures. Infect. Immun. **24**:760-769.
3. Cryz, S. J., Jr., S. L. Welkos, and R. K. Holmes. 1980. Immunochemical studies of diphtherial toxin and related nontoxic mutant proteins. Infect. Immun. **30**:835-846.
4. Finkelstein, R. A., M. L. Vasil, J. R. Jones, R. A. Anderson, and T. Barnard. 1976. Clinical

cholera caused by enterotoxigenic *Escherichia coli*. J. Clin. Microbiol. **3**:382-384.

5. Gyles, C. L., S. Palchaudhuri, and W. K. Maas. 1977. Naturally occurring plasmid carrying genes for enterotoxin production and drug resistance. Science **198**:198-199.
6. Holmes, R. K., M. G. Bramucci, and E. M. Twiddy. 1980. Genetic and biochemical studies of heat-labile enterotoxin of *Escherichia coli*, p. 189-201. *In* Proceedings of the 15th Joint Conference on Cholera. NIH Publication 80-2003. National Institutes of Health, Bethesda, MD.
7. Hunter, W. M., and F. C. Greenwood. 1962. Preparation of iodine-131 labelled human growth hormone of high specific activity. Nature **194**:495-496.
8. Maizel, J. V. 1971. Polyacrylamide gel electrophoresis of viral proteins. *In* Methods in Virology. K. Maramorosch and H. Kaprowski, editors. Academic Press, Inc., New York. **5**:179-246.
9. Maneval, D. R., Jr., R. R. Colwell, S. W. Joseph, R. Grays, and S. T. Donta. 1980. A tissue culture method for the detection of bacterial enterotoxins. J. Tissue Culture Methods **6**:85-90.
10. Mekalanos, J. J., R. J. Collier, and W. R. Romig. 1978. Purification of cholera toxin and its subunits: new methods of preparation and use of hypertoxinogenic mutants. Infect. Immun. **20**: 552-558.
11. Mekalanos, J. J., R. J. Collier, and W. R. Romig. 1979. Enzymatic activity of cholera toxin. I. New methods of assay and the mechanism of ADP-ribosyl transfer. J. Biol. Chem. **254**:5849-5854.

Author Index

Subject Index

GPSR Compliance

The European Union's (EU) General Product Safety Regulation (GPSR) is a set of rules that requires consumer products to be safe and our obligations to ensure this.

If you have any concerns about our products, you can contact us on ProductSafety@springernature.com

In case Publisher is established outside the EU, the EU authorized representative is:

Springer Nature Customer Service Center GmbH
Europaplatz 3
69115 Heidelberg, Germany

Batch number: 10607320

Printed by Printforce, the Netherlands